FIRST AID™ CASES FOR THE USMLE STEP 1

TAO LE, MD, MHS
Assistant Clinical Professor of Pediatrics and Medicine
Division of Allergy and Clinical Immunology
Department of Pediatrics
University of Louisville

KENDALL KRAUSE
Yale University School of Medicine
Class of 2007

JOSHUA KLEIN, MD, PhD
Resident in Neurology
Massachusetts General Hospital
Brigham and Women's Hospital

ANIL SHIVARAM, MD
Resident in Ophthalmology
Boston University

McGraw-Hill
MEDICAL PUBLISHING DIVISION

New York / Chicago / San Francisco / Lisbon / London / Madrid / Mexico City
Milan / New Delhi / San Juan / Seoul / Singapore / Sydney / Toronto

The **McGraw·Hill** *Companies*

First Aid™ Cases for the USMLE Step 1

2 3 4 5 6 7 8 9 0 QPD/QPD 0 9 8 7 6

ISBN 0-07-146410-7
ISSN 1559-5757

NOTICE

Medicine is an ever-changing science. As new research and clinical experience broaden our knowledge, changes in treatment and drug therapy are required. The authors and the publisher of this work have checked with sources believed to be reliable in their efforts to provide information that is complete and generally in accord with the standards accepted at the time of publication. However, in view of the possibility of human error or changes in medical sciences, neither the authors nor the publisher nor any other party who has been involved in the preparation or publication of this work warrants that the information contained herein is in every respect accurate or complete, and they disclaim all responsibility for any errors or omissions or for the results obtained from use of the information contained in this work. Readers are encouraged to confirm the information contained herein with other sources. For example and in particular, readers are advised to check the product information sheet included in the package of each drug they plan to administer to be certain that the information contained in this work is accurate and that changes have not been made in the recommended dose or in the contraindications for administration. This recommendation is of particular importance in connection with new or infrequently used drugs.

This book was set in Electra LH by Rainbow Graphics.
The editor was Catherine A. Johnson.
The production supervisor was Phil Galea.
Project management was provided by Rainbow Graphics.
Quebecor Dubuque was printer and binder.

This book is printed on acid-free paper.

DEDICATION

To the contributors to this and future editions, who took time to share their knowledge, insight, and humor for the benefit of all those who yearn to pass their boards.

and

To our families, friends, and loved ones, who encouraged and assisted us in the task of assembling this guide.

CONTENTS

CONTRIBUTING AUTHORS

Mary Allison Arwady
Yale University School of Medicine
Class of 2007

Arianne Boylan
Yale University School of Medicine
Class of 2007

Joanna Chin
Yale University School of Medicine
MD/PhD program
Class of 2009

Maria Mazzeo
Yale University School of Medicine
Class of 2007

Andrew Nerlinger, MD
Resident in Emergency Medicine
University of California at Los Angeles

Craig Platt
Yale University School of Medicine
MD/PhD program
Class of 2009

Akash Shah, MD
Resident in Radiology
Cornell University

Lindsey Sukay, MD
Resident in Pediatrics
The Children's Hospital Denver
University of Colorado School of Medicine

Sadhna Vora, MD
Resident in Internal Medicine
Massachusetts General Hospital

J. Dawn Waters, MD
Resident in Neurosurgery
Department of Surgery
University of California, San Diego Medical Center

SENIOR REVIEWERS

Andrew J. Armstrong, MD
Fellow, Division of Hematology & Oncology
Johns Hopkins School of Medicine
Sidney Kimmel Comprehensive Cancer Center
Hematology and Oncology

Robert D. Auerbach, MD, FACOG
Associate Clinical Professor
Obstetrics, Gynecology & Reproductive Sciences
Yale University School of Medicine
Reproductive System

Susan J. Baserga, MD, PhD
Associate Professor
Departments of Molecular Biophysics & Biochemistry, Genetics, and Therapeutic Radiology
Yale University School of Medicine
Biochemistry

Peter Chin-Hong, MD
Assistant Professor, Division of Infectious Diseases
Department of Medicine
University of California, San Francisco
Microbiology and Immunology

Tracey Cho, MD
Resident, Department of Neurology
Massachusetts General Hospital and Brigham and Women's Hospital
Harvard Medical School
Neurology and Psychiatry

Rachel Chong, MD
Fellow, Division of Endocrinology
Department of Medicine
Johns Hopkins School of Medicine
Endocrine System

Niccolò D. Della Penna, MD
Director, General Hospital Psychiatry Consultation Service
Department of Psychiatry
The University of Chicago Hospitals
Behavioral Science

JoAnne Micale Foody, MD, FACC, FAHA
Assistant Professor
Section of Cardiovascular Medicine, Department of Internal Medicine
Yale University School of Medicine
Cardiovascular System

Karen Jacobson, MD
Staff Attending
Beth Israel Deaconess Medical Center
Microbiology and Immunology

Shanta E. Kapadia, MBBS, MSurg
Anatomy Lecturer
Section of Anatomy and Experimental Surgery
Yale University School of Medicine
Anatomy

Nayer Khazeni, MD
Fellow, Pulmonary and Critical Care Medicine
Department of Internal Medicine
Yale University School of Medicine
Respiratory System

Geoffrey Nguyen, MD
Fellow, Division of Gastroenterology
Johns Hopkins School of Medicine
Gastrointestinal System

Alan Pao, MD
Fellow, Division of Nephrology
Department of Medicine
University of California, San Francisco
Renal System

Marcus M. Reidenberg, MD, FACP
Professor of Pharmacology, Medicine, and Public Health
Head, Division of Clinical Pharmacology
Weill Medical College of Cornell University
Attending Physician, New York Presbyterian Hospital
Editor Emeritus, Clinical Pharmacology and Therapeutics
Pharmacology

PREFACE

With *First Aid Cases for the USMLE Step 1*, we continue our commitment to providing students with the most useful and up-to-date preparation guides for the USMLE Step 1. This new addition to the *First Aid* series represents an outstanding effort by a talented group of authors and includes the following:

- Commonly asked question stems on the USMLE Step 1 integrated into a single USMLE-style case
- Concise yet complete explanations
- Two-column format for easy self-quizzing
- High-yield images, diagrams, and tables to complement the questions and answers
- Organized as a perfect supplement to *First Aid for the USMLE Step 1*

We invite you to share your thoughts and ideas to help us improve *First Aid Cases for the USMLE Step 1*. See How to Contribute, p. xxi.

Louisville Tao Le
New Haven Kendall Krause
Boston Joshua Klein
Boston Anil Shivaram

ACKNOWLEDGMENTS

This has been a collaborative project from the start. We gratefully acknowledge the thoughtful comments and advice of the residents, international medical graduates, and faculty who have supported the authors in the development of *First Aid Cases for the USMLE Step 1.*

For support and encouragement throughout the process, we are grateful to Thao Pham and Selina Bush. Thanks to our publisher, McGraw-Hill, for the valuable assistance of their staff. For enthusiasm, support, and commitment to this challenging project, thanks to our editor, Catherine A. Johnson. For outstanding editorial work, we thank Emma D. Underdown. A special thanks to Rainbow Graphics for remarkable production work.

Louisville Tao Le
New Haven Kendall Krause
Boston Joshua Klein
Boston Anil Shivaram

HOW TO CONTRIBUTE

To continue to produce a high-yield review source for the USMLE Step 1 exam, we invite you to submit any suggestions or corrections. We also offer **paid internships** in medical education and publishing ranging from three months to one year (see below for details). Please send us your suggestions for

- High-yield USMLE Step 1 cases
- New facts, mnemonics, diagrams, and illustrations
- Low-yield cases to remove

For each entry incorporated into the next edition, you will receive a $10 gift certificate, as well as personal acknowledgment in the next edition. Diagrams, tables, partial entries, updates, corrections, and study hints are also appreciated, and significant contributions will be compensated at the discretion of the authors. Also let us know about material in this edition that you feel is low yield and should be deleted.

The preferred way to submit entries, suggestions, or corrections is via electronic mail. Please include your name, address, institutional affiliation, phone number, and e-mail address (if different from the address of origin). If there are multiple entries, please consolidate into a single e-mail or file attachment. Please send submissions to:

firstaidteam@yahoo.com

Otherwise, please send entries, neatly written or typed or on disk (Microsoft Word), to:

First Aid Team
914 North Dixie Avenue, Suite 100
Elizabethtown, KY 42701
Attention: Step 1 Casebook

All entries become property of the authors and are subject to editing and reviewing. Please verify all data and spellings carefully. In the event that similar or duplicate entries are received, only the first entry received will be used. Include a reference to a standard textbook to facilitate verification of the fact. Please follow the style, punctuation, and format of this edition if possible.

INTERNSHIP OPPORTUNITIES

The author team is pleased to offer part-time and full-time paid internships in medical education and publishing to motivated medical students and physicians. Internships may range from three months (e.g., a summer) up to a full year. Participants will have an opportunity to author, edit, and earn publication credit on a wide variety of projects, including the popular *First Aid* series. Writing/editing experience, familiarity with Microsoft Word, Internet access, and a passion for education are desired. For more information, e-mail a résumé or a short description of your experience along with a cover letter to **firstaidteam@yahoo.com.**

SECTION I

General Principles

- Behavioral Science
- Biochemistry
- Microbiology & Immunology
- Pharmacology

Behavioral Science

▶ Case 1

A 58-year-old man is brought to the emergency department by his supervisor after he was found stumbling and confused at work. On physical examination, the patient appears slightly sedated and admits to recent heavy drinking, but says his last drink was 1–2 days earlier. He also says he vomited three times earlier that morning. He denies chest and abdominal pain. He is afebrile but tremulous. CT scan of the head is negative for mass lesions or bleeding. Relevant laboratory findings are as follows:

Aspartate aminotransferase: 57 U/L
Alanine aminotransferase: 18 U/L
Lactate dehydrogenase: 398 U/L

- **What is the most likely diagnosis?**

Alcohol withdrawal.

- **What is the pathophysiology of this condition?**

Alcohol is a central nervous system depressant that causes neuronal changes, including downregulation of γ-aminobutyric acid receptors, when chronically abused. The withdrawal of alcohol can lead to hyperactivity of the neurons, thereby decreasing cortical inhibition. Additionally, increased serum norepinephrine and altered serotonin levels have been implicated in both alcohol craving and tolerance.

- **What are the symptoms of this condition?**

Minor symptoms (occurring 6–36 hours after the last drink) include:

- Diaphoresis
- Gastrointestinal upset
- Headache
- Nausea and vomiting
- Palpitations
- Tremulousness

Seizures can occur within 6–48 hours of the last drink. Visual (or less commonly, tactile or auditory) hallucinations can occur within 12–48 hours of the last drink, and delirium tremens may occur within 48–96 hours.

- **What is delirium tremens?**

About 5% of patients with alcohol withdrawal symptoms develop **delirium tremens,** which is a collection of symptoms that includes delirium, tachycardia, hypertension, agitation, low-grade fever, and diaphoresis. Untreated, the mortality rate of patients who develop delirium tremens is around 20%; major causes of death are arrhythmias and infection.

- **What treatment is appropriate for this condition?**

Benzodiazepines, particularly lorazepam and diazepam, are the treatment of choice for all types of alcohol withdrawal symptoms, including withdrawal seizures and delirium tremens. Barbiturates and propofol are used if the patient is refractory to benzodiazepines.

▶ Case 2

A 17-year-old girl presents to her physician with right foot pain. She states she has been exercising quite frequently recently. She has not had menses for several months now. Upon further questioning, she reluctantly states she is afraid of gaining weight and is on a new strict diet consisting exclusively of cereal and vegetables. Her weight is currently 44.1 kg (97 lb) with an associated body mass index of 17 kg/m^2. An x-ray of her foot is taken (see Figure 1-1 below). Relevant laboratory findings are as follows:

Hemoglobin: 10.8 g/dL
Hematocrit: 33.5%
Mean corpuscular volume (MCV): 78.5 fl

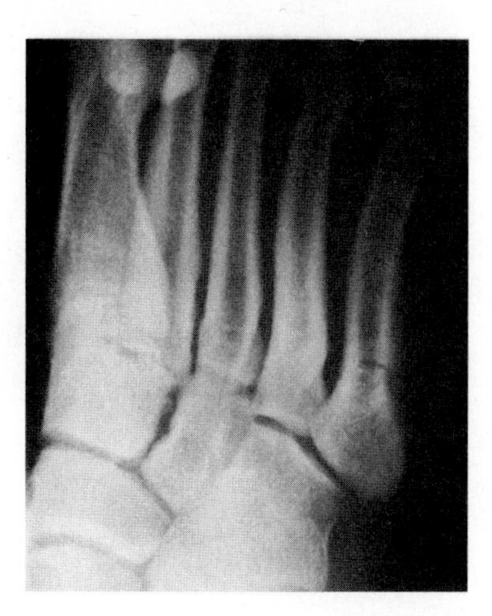

FIGURE 1-1. (Reproduced, with permission, from Knoop KJ, Stack LB, Storrow AB. *Atlas of Emergency Medicine*, 2nd ed. New York: McGraw-Hill, 2002: 343.)

What is the most likely diagnosis?	Anorexia nervosa.
What other symptoms of this condition are common at presentation?	Patients typically present with severe weight loss and clinical manifestations of multiple nutritional deficiencies. Dental caries and erosions (see Figure 1-2 on the following page) may be present if patients are also vomiting. Additional purging via laxative abuse may cause palpitations, lightheadedness, or chest pain because of electrolyte abnormalities.
What diagnosis would be of concern if this patient were of normal weight?	**Bulimia nervosa** can present with similar findings, with its fundamental feature being uncontrollable binge eating, often with subsequent purging. These patients are usually of normal weight and have irregular menses. Nutritional deficiencies, however, are uncommon.
What kind of anemia does this patient likely have?	Low hematocrit and low MCV suggest a **microcytic anemia,** most likely due to iron deficiency, which is common in these patients. Vitamin B_{12} and folate deficiency because of inadequate nutritional intake usually causes a **macrocytic anemia.** Some patients may have an overall **normocytic anemia** because of a mixed picture of both microcytic and macrocytic anemias from these various deficiencies.
What nutritional deficiency may contribute to the radiographic findings in Figure 1-1?	Fractures of the fifth metatarsal bone in these patients are often related in part to osteopenia or osteoporosis secondary to vitamin D and calcium deficiency.

- **What region of the brain regulates appetite and is thought to play a role in eating disorders?**

The **hypothalamus.** The "feeding center" is located in the lateral nucleus. When stimulated, it promotes eating/appetite. The "satiety center" is located in the ventromedial nucleus. When stimulated, it signals the body to stop eating. Lesions to this area cause hyperphagia and obesity.

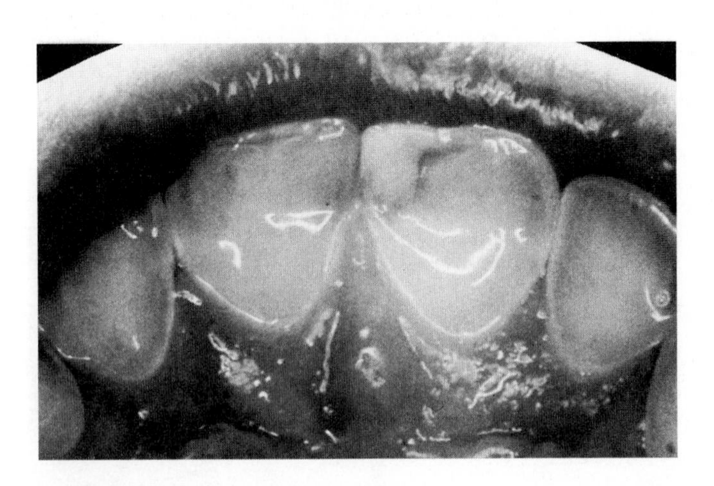

FIGURE 1-2. Dental erosions in patients with vomiting. (Courtesy of David P. Kretzschmar, DDS, MS.)

► Case 3

A 24-year-old woman is brought to the emergency department with confusion, blurred vision, dizziness, and somnolence. She recently lost her job as a finance consultant. Her friend states the woman is generally healthy, but is taking medication for occasional episodes of intense fear, sweating, nausea, and abdominal and chest pain. Physical examination reveals a respiratory rate of 8 breaths per minute.

■ **What is the most likely diagnosis?**	Benzodiazepine toxicity, as characterized by respiratory depression, confusion, and other symptoms of central nervous system depression.
■ **What class of drugs might be responsible for this patient's symptoms?**	Her friend's description is consistent with a diagnosis of panic disorder. Benzodiazepines (such as clonazepam, lorazepam, and alprazolam) are commonly used in the short-term treatment of panic disorder.
■ **What treatment was likely administered to this patient in the emergency department?**	Flumazenil, a competitive antagonist at the γ-aminobutyric acid (GABA) receptor, is effective in reversing symptoms of benzodiazepine overdose.
■ **How does the mechanism of action of benzodiazepines differ from that of barbiturates?**	Normally, $GABA_A$ receptors respond to GABA binding by opening chloride channels, which leads to hyperpolarization. Binding of benzodiazepines to γ subunits or to an area of the α unit influenced by the γ unit facilitates channel opening, but does not directly initiate chloride current. Both benzodiazepines and barbiturates enhance the affinity of GABA for $GABA_A$ receptors. Benzodiazepines act by increasing the **frequency** of opening of chloride channels. In contrast, barbiturates act by increasing the **duration** of opening of chloride channels.
■ **What are the advantages of using benzodiazepines vs. using barbiturates?**	Benzodiazepines have a lower risk of dependence, P450 system involvement, respiratory depression, coma, and loss of rapid eye movement sleep. They are considered much safer than barbiturates in cases of overdose.
■ **What drugs, when taken with benzodiazepines, increase the likelihood of developing toxicity?**	■ Acetaminophen ■ Alcohol ■ Cimetidine ■ Disulfiram ■ Isoniazid ■ Valproic acid

GENERAL PRINCIPLES

BEHAVIORAL SCIENCE

▶ **Case 4**

A 65-year-old man with diabetes is admitted to the hospital for repair of a hip fracture. On postoperative day 4, his wife reports he seems very confused and he could not remember her name. Evaluation reveals the patient is inattentive and generally confused. However, his nurse notes that he was fine both the day before and 3 hours earlier. The patient has been taking morphine, and is continuing to take his previously prescribed β-blocker and angiotensin-converting enzyme inhibitor for hypertension. He is afebrile, and his blood pressure is 105/51 mm Hg. Relevant laboratory findings are as follows:

Sodium: 133 mEq/L	Phosphate: 3.0 mg/dL
Calcium: 8.9 mg/dL	Blood urea nitrogen: 18 mg/dL
Potassium: 3.9 mEq/L	Creatinine: 1.5 mg/dL
Chloride: 99 mEq/L	Glucose: 58 mg/dL
Magnesium: 1.9 mg/dL	Urinalysis: unremarkable
Bicarbonate: 25.1 mEq/L	

- **What is the most likely diagnosis?**

Delirium. The *Diagnostic and Statistical Manual of Mental Disorders*, 4th edition, lists the key features of delirium as:

- Altered consciousness with reduced attention
- Altered cognition of perceptual disturbance not accountable for by dementia
- Development over a short time with waxing and waning
- Evidence that the change is caused by a medical condition, drug, or other substance.

- **What is the differential diagnosis of this condition?**

Delirium should be distinguished from depression, psychotic illness, and dementia. This is difficult because delirium is often superimposed on dementia, and is often mistaken for dementia in elderly persons. The acuity of presentation and the waxing and waning course are the most helpful ways to differentiate delirium from dementia. Furthermore, delirium is caused by a medical or pharmacological entity, and this cause must be excluded before a change in mental status can be labeled as something other than delirium.

- **What risk factors are associated with this condition?**

- Advanced age
- Dehydration
- Hypoglycemia
- Institutionalization
- Metabolic and electrolyte disturbances
- Particular medications
- Postoperative state

- **What are the most common drugs that cause this condition?**

Major classes of drugs that commonly cause delirium are opioids (especially morphine and meperidine), anticholinergic agents (including benztropine for Parkinson's disease), anticonvulsants (phenytoin), antidepressants (tricyclic antidepressants, selective serotonin reuptake inhibitors), β-blockers, digoxin, corticosteroids, dopamine agonists, H_2-receptor blockers, and sedative hypnotics. This list is not complete, as many more drugs can cause delirium.

- **What treatments are most appropriate for this condition?**

The key to treating delirium is to treat the underlying etiology. The most common disturbances include fluid and electrolyte imbalances, infections (especially urinary tract infections), drug or alcohol toxicity, alcohol withdrawal, psychoactive drug withdrawal, metabolic disorders, and low perfusion states. The most important first step is a thorough medication review and reversal of any metabolic abnormalities.

▶ Case 5

A 19-year-old male college student is brought to the emergency department by his roommate, who found him sitting outside their room breathing very shallowly. The patient is difficult to understand because he is intoxicated, has slurred speech, and is drowsy. Physical examination reveals pinpoint pupils. The roommate admits they were both at a party earlier in the evening, but he lost track of the patient and is not sure what he could have taken.

What drugs of abuse could be involved in this case?	▪ Alcohol ▪ Amphetamines ▪ Benzodiazepines or barbiturates ▪ Cocaine ▪ Heroin (opioids) ▪ Lysergic acid diethylamide (LSD) ▪ Phencyclidine (PCP)
What signs and symptoms are associated with alcohol intoxication and withdrawal?	▪ Intoxication: disinhibition, decreased cognition, unsteady gait ▪ Withdrawal: tremor, seizures, delirium tremens (benzodiazepines)
What signs and symptoms are associated with opioid intoxication and withdrawal?	▪ Intoxication: intense euphoria, drowsiness, slurred speech, decreased memory, pupil constriction, decreased respirations ▪ Withdrawal: nausea, vomiting, pupil dilation, insomnia
What signs and symptoms are associated with benzodiazepine or barbiturate intoxication and withdrawal?	▪ Intoxication: respiratory and cardiac depression, disinhibition, unsteady gait ▪ Withdrawal: agitation, anxiety, depression, tremor, seizures, delirium
What signs and symptoms are associated with PCP and LSD intoxication and withdrawal?	▪ PCP intoxication: intense psychosis, violence, rhabdomyolysis, hyperthermia ▪ LSD intoxication: increased sensation, colors richer, tastes heightened, visual hallucinations ▪ There are no withdrawal symptoms from PCP and LSD

▶ Case 6

A mother of 15-month-old fraternal male twins consults her pediatrician because she is concerned about the development of one twin. Her concern lies in the fact that the older twin began to walk at approximately 12 months of age, but the younger twin still is unable to walk by himself. Physical examination reveals no significant issues.

- **Is it appropriate that the younger twin has not yet walked?**

Yes. The approximate age children achieve the motor milestone of walking is 15 months. However, the child should be able to sit alone—a milestone that should occur between 6 and 9 months of age.

- **By what age should the infant reflexes have disappeared?**

These reflexes normally disappear within the first year. They include the Moro reflex (extension of limbs when startled), the rooting reflex (nipple seeking when cheek brushed), the palmar reflex (grasps objects in palm), and the Babinski reflex (large toe dorsiflexes with plantar stimulation).

- **What cognitive/social milestones should these infants have reached?**

Social smile (3 mo), recognizes people (4–5 mo), stranger anxiety (7–9 mo), orients to voice (7–9 mo), separation anxiety (15 mo), and the ability to speak a few words (15 mo).

- **When evaluating the development of the twins, the physician was interested in the brothers' Apgar scores at birth. What are the components of the Apgar score?**

Apgar is a useful acronym for the scoring system—Appearance, Pulse, Grimace, Activity, and Respiration (see Table 1-1 below). Each category is scored from 0–2, with 10 being a perfect score. The scoring is done at 1 and 5 minutes after birth.

- **What upcoming motor and social milestones should the mother expect to see?**

Upcoming motor milestones include climbing stairs (12–24 mo), the ability to stack 6 blocks (18–24 mo), riding a tricycle (3 yrs), simple drawings (4 yrs), and hopping on one foot (4 yrs). Upcoming cognitive/social milestones include object permanence (12–24 mo), parallel play (24–48 mo), core gender identity (24–36 mo), toilet training (30–36 mo), group play (3 yrs), and cooperative play (4 yrs).

TABLE 1-1. Apgar scoring system.

CATEGORY	SCORE 0	SCORE 1	SCORE 2
Appearance (color)	Blue/pale	Trunk pink	All pink
Pulse	None	<100	>100
Grimace (reflex irritability)	None	Grimace	Grimace + cough
Activity (muscle tone)	Limp	Some	Active
Respiration (effort)	None	Irregular	Regular

► Case 7

A couple is eating dinner at home with their quiet 6-year-old son. The couple gets into an argument and the father starts to yell at his son, who begins to cry. His mother gives the child candy, which temporarily relieves the crying. His mother continues to give him candy every time the child cries. The father then yells at the child and takes away the candy because children who cry should not be eating candy.

What defense mechanism is the father using?	**Displacement,** characterized by transferral of feelings from one object to another. In this case, the father's anger at the mother is displaced onto the child.
What type of reinforcement is the child using on the mother?	This is an example of **positive reinforcement,** in which the consequences of a response increase the likelihood that the response will recur. Specifically, the child cries because crying makes it more likely the mother will continue to give him candy.
How does negative reinforcement differ from punishment?	In **negative reinforcement,** behavior is encouraged or reinforced so as to remove an aversive stimulus. In **punishment,** behavior is discouraged and reduced by virtue of administration of an aversive stimulus.
Which method of conditioning is the father using by removing the reward?	The father is employing **extinction,** characterized by elimination of a behavior by nonreinforcement. The child may stop crying after discovering that there is no reward for the behavior.

► Case 8

A male newborn who was delivered at home is brought to the emergency department by his grandmother 30 minutes after his birth. The grandmother says "the baby isn't acting right." The baby weighs 2700 g (about 6 pounds) and was born at 38 weeks' gestational age. However, the baby is limp, unresponsive, and breathing infrequently, with bluish skin and pupils 2 mm in diameter. The infant is immediately resuscitated and stabilized for transfer to the Newborn Intensive Care Unit (NICU) for monitoring. By day 3 of life, his nurse reports the infant is vomiting, has diarrhea, and cries excessively. Physical examination reveals tachycardia, tachypnea, pinpoint pupils, diaphoresis, tremors, increased muscle tone, and piloerection.

What is the most likely diagnosis for the newborn's presentation in the ED?	Opioid intoxication, heralded by the triad of (1) respiratory depression, (2) central nervous system depression, and (3) pinpoint pupils. Importantly, **pinpoint pupils** due to opioid intoxication will be present despite opioid tolerance.
What pharmacologic treatment should this patient receive in the ED to specifically target the cause of his symptoms?	Naloxone, an opioid antagonist, will reverse the effects of opioid agonists in this patient by selectively binding to opioid receptors.
What is the most likely diagnosis on day 3 of life?	The newborn is demonstrating symptoms of opiate withdrawal, also known as **neonatal abstinence syndrome.** Tachycardia, dilated pupils, diaphoresis, and other opiate withdrawal symptoms are related to sympathetic hyperactivity.
What is the most appropriate long-term treatment for this patient?	An opioid agonist, such as methadone, will relieve symptoms of acute opiate withdrawal. Methadone administration can then be tapered, as the baby is weaned.
What opioid drugs are most commonly used to treat this condition?	■ Codeine ■ Fentanyl ■ Hydromorphone ■ Meperidine ■ Methadone ■ Morphine ■ Oxycodone

GENERAL PRINCIPLES

BEHAVIORAL SCIENCE

▶ Case 9

A 21-year-old man and his mother visit the clinic because his daytime sleepiness is starting to interfere with his studies. The man is slightly obese and has a history of pulmonary hypertension. His mother mentions he was prescribed a medication "for sleep," but he does not use it. On questioning, the man says he has a prescription for amphetamines and is taking sertraline. His mother also mentions that while they were sitting in the waiting room for their appointment, the young man said he heard "bells ringing," which no one else heard. Shortly thereafter, the young man fell asleep during their conversation.

▪ **Why does the patient have a prescription for amphetamines?**	The hallucinations, sudden onset of sleep, and amphetamine treatment is consistent with a diagnosis of **narcolepsy.** This condition has a strong genetic component.
▪ **What kind of hallucinations is the patient having?**	Hallucinations prior to falling asleep are termed **hypnagogic hallucinations** ("gogic"—"go" to sleep). **Hypnopompic hallucinations,** which occur during waking, are also associated with narcolepsy.
▪ **What stage of sleep is this patient likely to experience immediately upon falling asleep?**	Narcolepsy is associated with rapid eye movement (REM) sleep within 10 minutes after falling asleep.
▪ **What other electroencephalographic (EEG) abnormalities might be expected in this patient?**	Sertraline, a selective serotonin reuptake inhibitor, suggests the possibility of depression. **Depression** is associated with decreased REM latency and decreased stage 4, slow-wave sleep. Effective treatment with antidepressants, however, usually reverses any EEG abnormalities caused by major depression.
▪ **What other common sleep abnormality might account for poor quality of sleep?**	Obesity and pulmonary hypertension are associated with **sleep apnea,** which can be very disruptive and can lead to significant daytime fatigue. Arrhythmias and loud snoring are also associated with sleep apnea.

► **Case 10**

An 8-year-old boy who has been consistently incontinent at night has been diagnosed with primary nocturnal enuresis. After several months of unsuccessful nonpharmacologic therapy, the child is brought back to the pediatrician. The boy will be going to a 3-week-long summer camp in 1 month, and his parents are concerned about the social and psychological implications of his enuresis. They are interested in pharmacologic therapy to prevent his bed-wetting while he is at summer camp.

- **In what stage of sleep is this patient's enuresis occurring?**

Enuresis occurs during stage 4 sleep, which is the deepest non–rapid eye movement (non-REM) sleep (see Table 1-2 below).

- **What pharmacologic treatment is most appropriate for this patient?**

Imipramine is a tricyclic antidepressant that has been successfully used to treat primary nocturnal enuresis in children. It works by decreasing the duration of stage 4 sleep.

- **Which neurotransmitters influence sleep?**

Serotonin (from the raphe nucleus) initiates sleep. Acetylcholine is the principal neurotransmitter promoting REM sleep. Conversely, norepinephrine reduces REM sleep.

- **What physiologic changes occur in REM sleep?**

Pulse increases in rate and variability, REMs occur, blood pressure rises and has increased variability, and penile or clitoral tumescence occurs. The percentage of sleep spent in REM sleep decreases with increasing age.

- **What class of drugs is useful for treating night terrors and sleepwalking?**

Benzodiazepines are useful for this purpose. Night terrors and sleepwalking occur during stage 4 sleep, and benzodiazepines shorten stage 4 sleep.

TABLE 1-2. Stages of Sleep

Stage (% of sleep)	Description	EEG Waveform
Awake	Active mentally, alert	Beta (highest frequency, lowest amplitude)
Awake/eyes closed		Alpha
Stage 1 (5%)	Light sleep	Theta
Stage 2 (45%)	Deeper sleep	Sleep spindles and K complexes
Stage 3–4 (25%)	Deepest non-REM sleep	Delta (lowest frequency, highest amplitude; slow-wave sleep)
REM (25%)	Dreaming, loss of motor tone, increased brain oxygen use; may represent a memory processing function	Beta

Biochemistry

▶ **Case 1**

A 45-year-old man comes to a community health clinic for his annual physical. He has no major complaints other than his chronic arthritis, which is worsening and is affecting his lower back, hips, and knees. On physical examination, the patient's sclerae are noted to be brownish-blue, and his ear cartilage is similarly discolored. An x-ray of the spine reveals disc degeneration and dense calcification that is most prominent in the lumbar region. Upon voiding for urinalysis, the man's urine is a normal color; however, after standing, the urine turns dark.

What is the most likely diagnosis?	Alkaptonuria (ochronosis).
What is the biochemical defect in this condition?	This disease is characterized by the absence of **homogentisate oxidase,** an enzyme of tyrosine metabolism that catalyzes the conversion of homogentisate to maleylacetoacetate (see Figure 2-1 below). The accumulation of homogentisate in cartilage leads to arthritis as well as to the discoloration of sclerae and other areas of the body.
From which essential amino acid is the accumulated metabolite involved in this defect derived?	Homogentisate is derived from phenylalanine. The defective enzyme is necessary for the metabolism of this amino acid, which is both glucogenic and ketogenic. Homogentisate is normally metabolized to acetoacetate (a ketone) and fumarate (part of the tricarboxylic acid cycle).
Given this patient's extent of joint disease, how might his mental functioning be affected?	Alkaptonuria has no effect on cognitive functioning. Aside from its effects on joints and discoloration of sclerae and skin, the disease is benign.
What is the most appropriate treatment for this condition?	There are no known ways to prevent the buildup of homogentisate. Dietary restriction of tyrosine and phenylalanine will reduce the production of homogentisate, but there has been no demonstrated benefit to this approach. Treating the symptoms of the patient's arthritis is the only recommended therapy in this case.

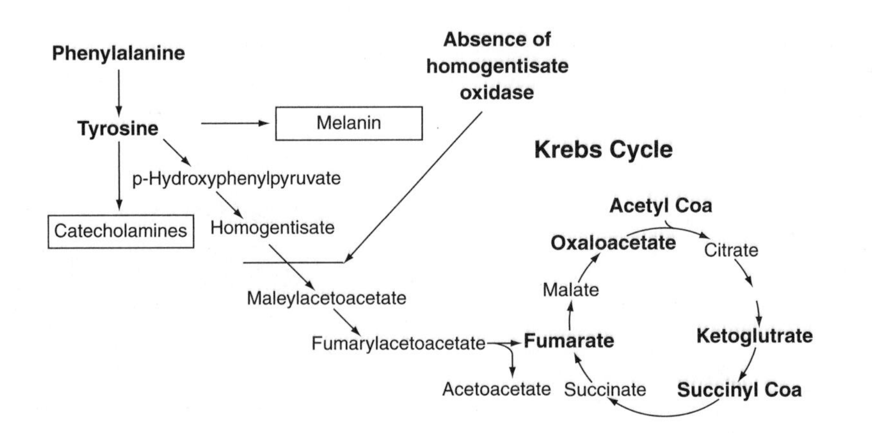

FIGURE 2-1. Flow chart showing conversion of homogentisate to maleylacetoacetate in phenylalanine metabolism.

▶ Case 2

A 37-year-old chemist with a 20-year history of bipolar disorder is rushed to the emergency department by his wife, who found him lying unconscious in the living room of their home. The man's skin is bright red, and he is breathing rapidly. Upon presentation, his breath smells like bitter almonds.

▪ **What is the most likely diagnosis?**	This man has ingested cyanide (the "bitter almond" breath is pathognomonic).
▪ **What biochemical process is disrupted in this condition?**	Cyanide is a direct inhibitor of one step in the electron transport chain (see Figure 2-2 below). Cyanide inhibits cytochrome oxidase (CoQ).
▪ **Does this patient have a greater-than-normal or lower-than-normal proton concentration in the intermembrane space of his mitochondria?**	The man will have a lower proton concentration. The electron transport chain fuels the transport of protons from the mitochondrial matrix to the intermembrane space. Because this patient has ingested cyanide and has thus inhibited this process, his proton gradient is weakened, and therefore he will have a smaller concentration of protons in the intermembrane spaces of his mitochondria.
▪ **What is the most appropriate treatment for this condition?**	Amyl nitrite. Amyl nitrate oxidizes hemoglobin to methemoglobin. This is normally undesirable because this form of hemoglobin binds oxygen less avidly. However, methemoglobin strongly binds cyanide, preventing it from further disrupting electron transport.
▪ **What other substances inhibit the electron transport chain?**	Amytal, rotenone, antimycin A, azide, and **carbon monoxide** also inhibit the electron transport chain.
▪ **What additional substances disrupt oxidative phosphorylation?**	▪ ATPase inhibitors such as oligomycin can directly inhibit the mitochondrial ATPase. Although the proton gradient forms, ATP is not produced. As a result, electron transport ceases. ▪ Uncoupling agents such as 2,4-dinitrophenol (2,4-DNP) increase the permeability of the inner mitochondrial membrane, thereby disrupting the formation of a proton gradient. In this case, electron transport is not disrupted.

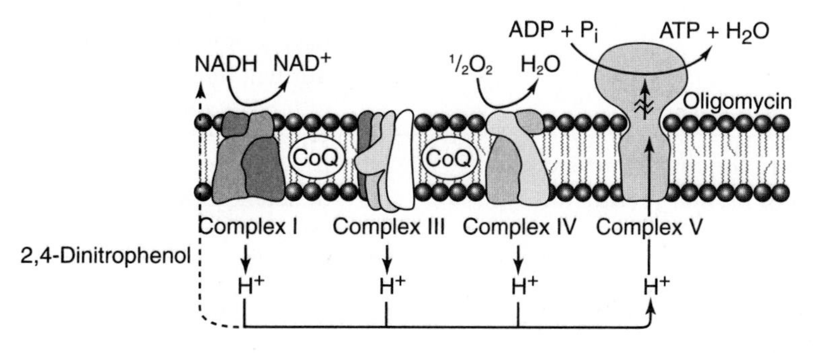

FIGURE 2-2. Cyanide inhibition of oxidative phosphorylation in the electron transport chain. (Reproduced, with permission, from Bhushan V, Le T, et al. *First Aid for the USMLE Step 1: 2006*. New York: McGraw-Hill, 2006: 91.)

▶ **Case 3**

A 6-year-old boy is followed by his pediatrician for delayed language acquisition and behavioral problems at school. His mother reports a normal pregnancy with adequate prenatal care and adds that she did not use drugs or alcohol during the pregnancy. Genetic analysis reveals a normal 46,XY karyotype but an abnormal-appearing X chromosome. Polymerase chain reaction (PCR) analysis reveals an abnormal region on the X chromosome with 200 CGG trinucleotide repeats.

- **What is the most likely diagnosis?**

This boy has fragile X syndrome, in which methylation of DNA sequences in the promoter area (where the expanded CGG triplets reside) causes silencing of the *FMR1* gene and complete loss of FMR1 protein. The FMR1 protein is involved in mRNA stabilization and transport.

- **What is PCR?**

PCR is a laboratory method used to amplify copies of genes to facilitate detection. First, the patient's DNA is denatured by heat to promote strand separation. During cooling, primers specific for the target gene (in this case the *FMR1* gene) anneal to the patient's DNA and are elongated using a specialized DNA polymerase. The number of copies of the gene is thus doubled. Cycles of heating, annealing, and elongation are then repeated using a thermocycler to produce a logarithmic increase in copies of the target gene.

- **What is the inheritance pattern of this condition?**

Fragile X syndrome is an X-linked genetic disorder. The hallmark of X-linked disorders is the absence of father-to-son disease transmission. X-linked recessive disorders are much more common in males than in females, as females would need two abnormal copies of the gene to show the disease phenotype. In X-linked dominant disorders, males and females are equally affected. Fragile X syndrome is unique in that it is not fully penetrant, and many families show a maternal transmission pattern.

- **What are other trinucleotide repeat disorders, and why are they associated with "premutations"?**

In addition to fragile X, other disorders with a triplet gene (typically CAG) mutation are Huntington's disease, several types of spinocerebellar ataxia, Friedreich's ataxia, and myotonic dystrophy. Typically, higher numbers of trinucleotide repeats result in more severe and earlier onset of the phenotypic expression of disease. Patients with an intermediate number of repeats are said to have a **premutation** because while they themselves are clinically normal, their children are at risk of further increasing the number of repeats and thus expressing clinical disease.

- **What are the major preventable causes of mental retardation?**

In utero infections, maternal drug or alcohol use, and nutritional deficiencies are preventable causes of mental retardation in the fetus.

▶ Case 4

A 5-month-old girl is brought to the pediatrician by her parents because she has been very sleepy lately and has been vomiting and sweating profusely at night. The infant's mother remarks their daughter was doing fine during the first months of her life, but began showing these changes shortly after she began weaning from breast milk. Laboratory testing reveals a serum glucose level of 30 mg/dL, and urinalysis is positive for reducing sugar but negative for glucose.

■ **What is the most likely diagnosis?**	Fructose intolerance.
■ **What intermediate is elevated within the liver cells in this condition?**	Fructose-1-phosphate.
■ **What enzyme is deficient in this condition?**	Aldolase B.
■ **How does this condition cause hypoglycemia?**	Aldolase B splits fructose-1-phosphate into glyceraldehyde and dihydroxyacetone phosphate (DAP) (see Figure 2-3 below). Its absence leads to an accumulation of fructose-1-phosphate in liver cells. The lack of available phosphate inhibits glycogenolysis and gluconeogenesis.
■ **What is the most appropriate treatment for this condition?**	The condition is treated through the removal of sucrose, fructose, and sorbitol from the diet.

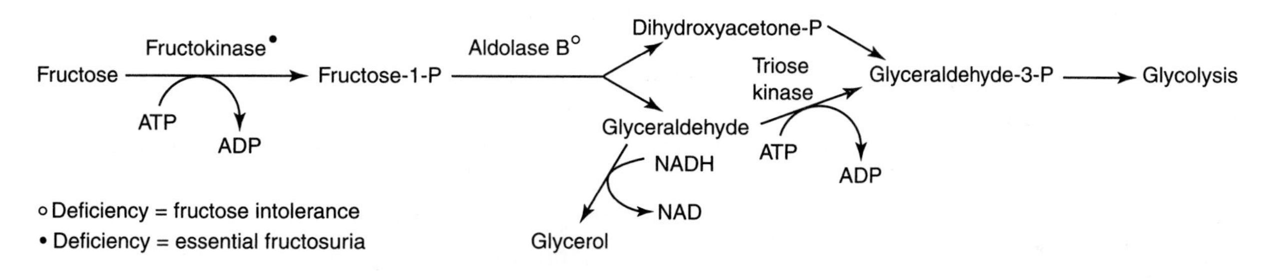

FIGURE 2-3. Aldolase B splitting fructose-1-P into glyceraldehydes and DAP. (Reproduced, with permission, from Bhushan V, Le T, et al. *First Aid for the USMLE Step 1: 2006*. New York: McGraw-Hill, 2006: 93.)

GENERAL PRINCIPLES

BIOCHEMISTRY

▶ Case 5

A 12-year-old mentally retarded boy is brought into a health clinic in Peru. His parents have noted that he seems to have difficulty with his vision. Physical examination reveals bilateral dislocated lenses and a marfanoid body habitus. Laboratory studies show increased levels of serum methionine and serum homocysteine.

▪ **What is the most likely diagnosis?**	Homocystinuria.
▪ **What is the biochemical defect in this condition?**	The most common form of inherited homocystinuria results from reduced activity of **cystathionine synthase,** an enzyme that converts homocysteine to cystathionine (see Figure 2-4 below).
▪ **What vitamin supplementation would be appropriate in this condition?**	**Vitamin B_6** is a necessary cofactor in cystathionine synthase. **Vitamin B_6** supplementation has been successful in many patients with this enzyme deficiency.
▪ **For which conditions is this patient at greatly increased risk?**	▪ **Cardiovascular disease:** Elevated plasma homocysteine leads to an increased risk of coronary artery disease, stroke, and peripheral artery disease. ▪ **Osteoporosis:** Homocysteine inhibits collagen cross-linking and over time can cause osteoporosis.
▪ **What enzyme deficiency is most likely to be found in a patient with increased serum homocysteine but decreased serum methionine?**	This could be caused by a deficiency of methionine synthase. This enzyme catalyzes the conversion of homocysteine to methionine. Like patients with cystathionine synthase deficiency, these patients often have central nervous system dysfunction and vascular disease.

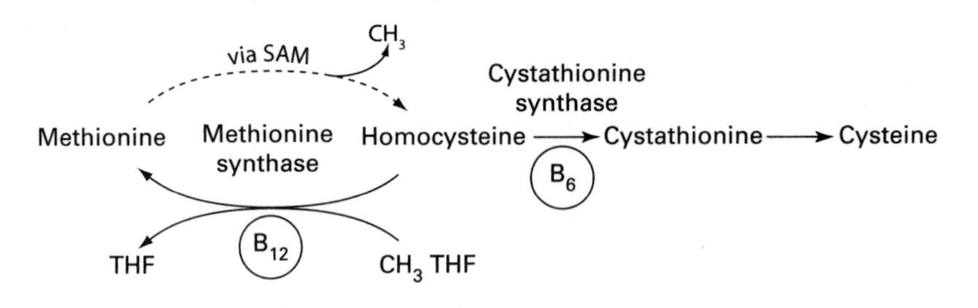

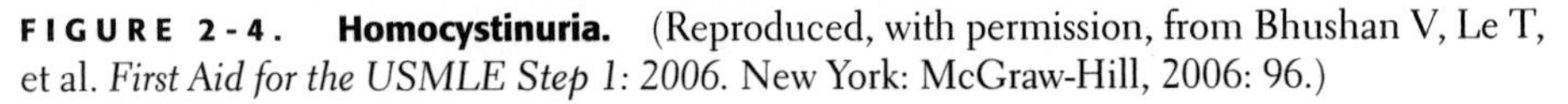

FIGURE 2-4. Homocystinuria. (Reproduced, with permission, from Bhushan V, Le T, et al. *First Aid for the USMLE Step 1: 2006.* New York: McGraw-Hill, 2006: 96.)

► Case 6

A 1-year-old boy is brought to the pediatrician because his parents have recently noted a number of abnormalities. Although the child was normal at birth, he does not interact with others as his older sister did at the same age. The parents also note that the child has an abnormally large tongue and coarse facial features. Physical examination reveals multisystem abnormalities. Funduscopic examination shows corneal clouding, and cardiac examination is significant for a 3/5 systolic ejection murmur. Additionally, the baby's liver seems to be enlarged, and his joints are stiff.

What is the most likely diagnosis?	Hurler's syndrome.
What is the pathophysiology of this condition?	This syndrome results from a defect in α-L-iduronidase, an enzyme essential to the degradation of dermatan sulfate and heparin sulfate. This disease is one of the **mucopolysaccharidoses,** a group of hereditary disorders characterized by defects in glycosaminoglycan (GAG) metabolism. In Hurler's syndrome, the GAGs are not appropriately degraded in the lysosomes and are therefore deposited in various tissues. The disease is inherited in an autosomal recessive manner.
What disease has a similar presentation, but is typically milder?	**Hunter's syndrome** is another mucopolysaccharidosis. It is due to a deficiency of iduronate sulfatase and has X-linked inheritance. Unlike Hurler's syndrome, Hunter's syndrome does not present with corneal clouding.
What are the typical findings on electron microscopy?	The lysosomal vesicles will be swollen with partially degraded polysaccharides.
A researcher who wants to use gene therapy to treat this condition successfully clones the defective gene and integrates it into an effective viral vector. After the in vitro experiments fail, the researcher discovers that the cultured cells are secreting the gene product. What went wrong?	α-L-iduronidase is a lysosomal enzyme. These enzymes must be tagged by mannose-6-phosphate in the Golgi apparatus to be targeted to the lysosomes. It is likely that the researcher's gene product is not being tagged properly and has entered the default secretory pathway.

► Case 7

A 2-year-old boy is brought to the pediatrician by his mother, who is visibly upset. The mother reports that her son has recently been biting his fingers and scratching his face incessantly. She says he was normal for the first few months of his life but has become increasingly irritable since about 3 months of age. The mother also mentions that her son often has "orange-colored sand" in his diapers. Laboratory studies reveal a serum uric acid level of 55 mg/dL. Urinalysis reveals crystalluria and microscopic hematuria.

- **What is the most likely diagnosis?**

  Lesch-Nyhan syndrome.

- **What is the biochemical defect in this condition?**

  Lesch-Nyhan syndrome is characterized by a deficiency in hypoxanthine-guanine phosphoribosyltransferase (HGPRT).

- **What is the function of the deficient enzyme?**

  HGPRT plays a key role in the purine salvage pathway (see Figure 2-5 below), recycling hypoxanthine and guanine to the purine nucleotide pool. In the absence of this enzyme, these purine bases are degraded into uric acid, resulting in the development of hyperuricemia.

- **What is the most appropriate treatment for this condition?**

  Allopurinol inhibits xanthine oxidase, which prevents the formation of uric acid from the more soluble hypoxanthine and xanthine. Doses should be titrated to normalize serum uric acid levels.

- **What other conditions can be expected if this disease is not treated?**

  Kidney stones, renal failure, gouty arthritis, and subcutaneous tophi deposits will result if the disorder is left untreated.

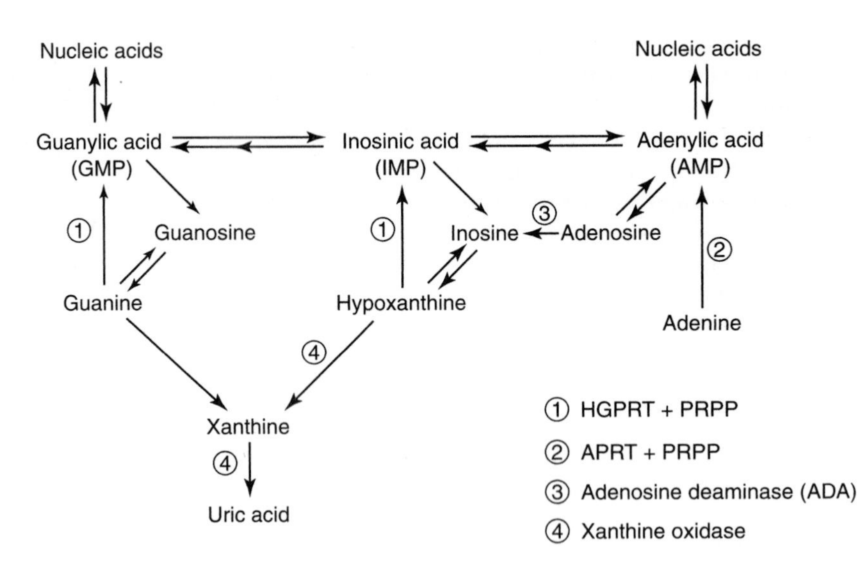

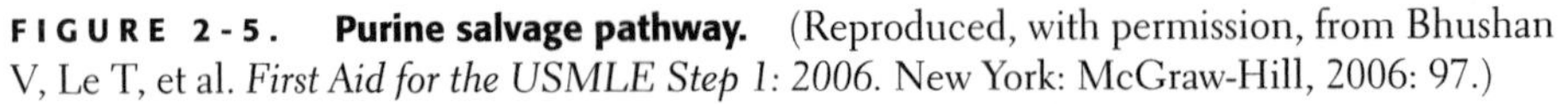
FIGURE 2-5. Purine salvage pathway. (Reproduced, with permission, from Bhushan V, Le T, et al. *First Aid for the USMLE Step 1: 2006*. New York: McGraw-Hill, 2006: 97.)

► Case 8

A 19-year-old female college student comes to the university health clinic complaining of muscle aches. She recently began an exercise program in an attempt to lose the 6–8 kg (15 lb) that that she had gained over the past year. After her first day of weight lifting, however, she became extremely sore. Several hours later, her urine was the color of "cherry soda pop." Physical examination is unremarkable. Laboratory tests reveal a serum creatine kinase level of 93,970 IU/L. Urinalysis is negative for blood and positive for myoglobin.

▪ **What is the most likely diagnosis?**	McArdle's disease (type V glycogen storage disease).
▪ **What is the biochemical defect in this condition?**	McArdle's disease is caused by a deficiency of muscle glycogen phosphorylase. Although glycogen formation is not affected, glycogen cannot be broken back down to glucose (glycogenolysis) because the α-1,4-glycosidic bonds cannot be broken in the muscle to release glucose-1-phosphate.
▪ **What are the most likely findings on biopsy of the liver and muscle?**	A liver biopsy will be normal, as the defective enzyme is present only in muscle. Muscle biopsy will show subsarcolemmal and intermyofibrillar accumulation of glycogen.
▪ **After the patient completes an exercise tolerance test, her lactic acid levels do not increase normally. Why?**	Lactic acid is a product of anaerobic glucose metabolism. Failure of lactic acid levels to elevate after exercise is an indication of a defect in the metabolism of glycogen or glucose to lactate. This response can be seen in other disorders of glycogenolysis or glycolysis as well.
▪ **What is the most appropriate treatment for this condition?**	Oral ingestion of sucrose before exercise has been demonstrated to improve exercise tolerance and reduce the risk of myoglobinuria.

▶ Case 9

A 2-year-old boy is brought to a health clinic in Peru because of poor development as well as vomiting, irritability, and a skin rash. The boy's mother also notes that his urine has a strange "mousy" odor. Physical examination reveals the child has an eczema-like rash, is hyperreflexive, and has increased muscle tone. He is surprisingly fair-skinned in comparison to the rest of his family. Laboratory studies reveal a positive Guthrie test and a serum phenylalanine level of 28 mg/dL.

▪ **What is the most likely diagnosis?**	Phenylketonuria (PKU).
▪ **What is the pathophysiology of this condition?**	PKU is caused by a defect in the metabolism of **phenylalanine** (see Figure 2-6 below). Normally, this essential amino acid is converted to tyrosine by phenylalanine hydroxylase. However, when phenylalanine hydroxylase activity is reduced or absent, phenylalanine builds up, leading to excess phenyl ketones in the blood and resulting in the symptoms seen in this patient. In patients with PKU, tyrosine cannot be derived from phenylalanine, so it becomes an essential amino acid. PKU is inherited in an autosomal recessive fashion.
▪ **What additional physical characteristics are common at presentation?**	Other physical findings include failure to thrive, mental retardation, microcephaly, large cheek and upper jaw bones, and widely spaced teeth with poorly developed enamel.
▪ **What is the cofactor for the defective enzyme in this disease that, when deficient, can also lead to increased levels of phenylalanine in the blood?**	A deficiency in tetrahydrobiopterin can also lead to increased blood levels of phenylalanine.
▪ **What is the most appropriate treatment for this condition?**	PKU should be treated with decreased dietary phenylalanine (which is contained in NutraSweet) and increased dietary tyrosine. Studies suggest continuation of dietary restrictions throughout life is necessary for optimal outcomes.

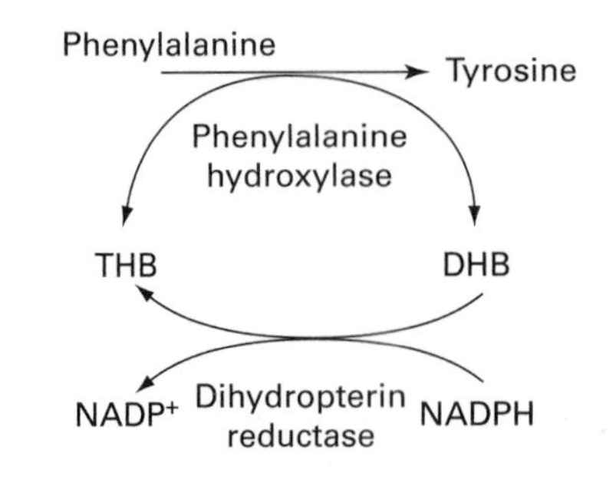

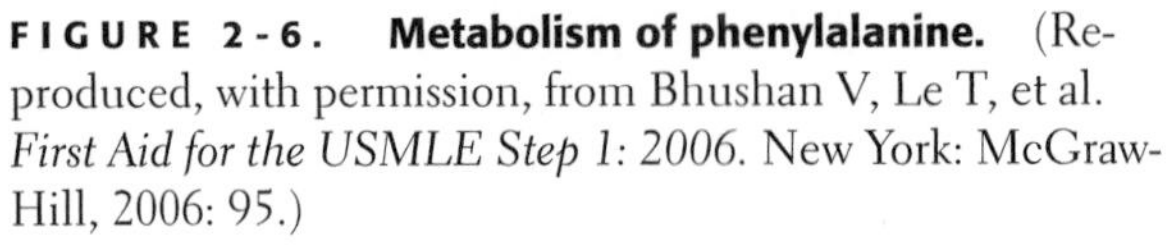

FIGURE 2-6. Metabolism of phenylalanine. (Reproduced, with permission, from Bhushan V, Le T, et al. *First Aid for the USMLE Step 1: 2006*. New York: McGraw-Hill, 2006: 95.)

► Case 10

A 6-month-old baby is brought to the pediatrician because she has been feeding poorly and has been lethargic for the past several months. The baby has also started breathing more rapidly than normal and recently had a seizure. Laboratory studies reveal a serum pH of 7.20, an anion gap of 19, elevated levels of pyruvate and alanine, and decreased levels of citrate.

■ **What is the most likely diagnosis?**	Pyruvate dehydrogenase deficiency.
■ **What is the pathophysiology of this condition?**	Pyruvate dehydrogenase converts pyruvate to acetyl-CoA (see Figure 2-7 below). Without it, glucose and amino acids cannot be shunted to the tricarboxylic acid (TCA) cycle to be used for energy. This baby has a lactic acidosis because she is relying heavily on glycolysis for energy.
■ **Why are alanine levels high and citrate levels low in this condition?**	Pyruvate levels are high because much of the excess pyruvate is converted to alanine in a reversible reaction by alanine aminotransferase. Citrate levels are low because pyruvate cannot be converted to acetyl-CoA to replenish the TCA cycle intermediates. Citrate is one such intermediate.
■ **What is the most appropriate treatment for this condition?**	Treatment involves increased intake of ketogenic nutrients (foods with high fat content). These foods will provide energy without necessitating use of the citric acid cycle. Oral citrate is also helpful in replenishing the substrates of the citric acid cycle.
■ **Which are the only purely ketogenic amino acids?**	Leucine and lysine are the only purely ketogenic amino acids.

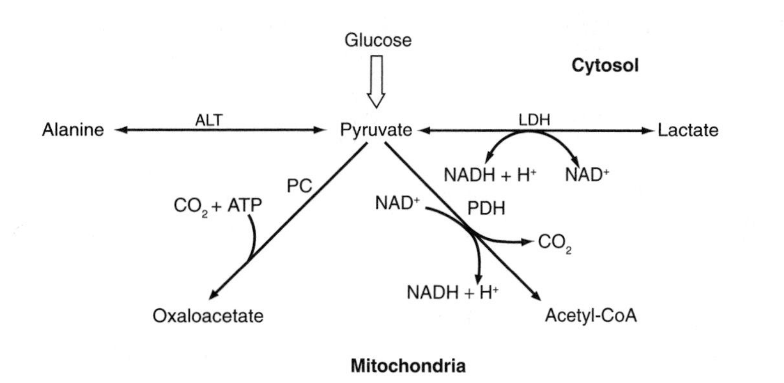

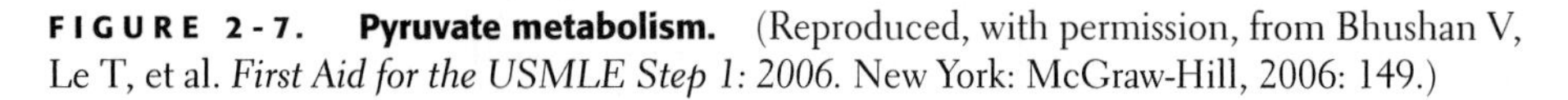
FIGURE 2-7. Pyruvate metabolism. (Reproduced, with permission, from Bhushan V, Le T, et al. *First Aid for the USMLE Step 1: 2006*. New York: McGraw-Hill, 2006: 149.)

▶ Case 11

A 5-month-old girl is brought to her pediatrician by her parents, both of whom are Jewish. Although the baby girl was developing normally for the first 4 months of her life, she can no longer roll over by herself. In addition, while she often smiled at 3 months of age, she no longer does so. Funduscopic examination reveals a "cherry-red" spot on her macula.

▪ **What is the most likely diagnosis?**	Tay-Sachs disease.
▪ **What is the biochemical defect in this condition?**	This disease, one of the sphingolipidoses, is caused by a deficiency of **hexosaminidase A.** This enzyme is present within the lysosomes of central nervous system cells and helps degrade a lipid called GM2 ganglioside. GM2 ganglioside accumulation within the neurons leads to progressive neurodegeneration. Children become blind and deaf before paralysis ultimately sets in. Children with Tay-Sachs disease usually die by age 3 years.
▪ **How is this gene responsible for this condition inherited?**	Tay-Sachs disease is inherited in an autosomal recessive fashion. Fabry's disease is the only one of the sphingolipidoses that is inherited differently; it is X-linked.
▪ **What other conditions present with similar findings on physical examination?**	**Niemann-Pick disease,** which is caused by a deficiency of sphingomyelinase, also presents with a cherry-red spot in the macula in about 50% of cases. These patients often present with anemia, fever, and neurologic deterioration. The prognosis of Niemann-Pick disease is poor as well, with most patients dying by age 3 years.
▪ **Which of the other sphingolipidoses also has a higher prevalence among Ashkenazi Jews?**	**Gaucher's disease,** which is caused by a deficiency of β-glucocerebrosidase, also has a much higher incidence in this population.

▶ Case 12

A 36-year-old homeless man presents to a community health clinic complaining of increasing shortness of breath. On questioning, the man admits to an extensive history of alcoholism. A review of systems reveals he has also experienced tingling and burning in his legs for the past several weeks. Physical examination reveals that he is tachycardic (heart rate 122/min), has rales bilaterally, and has bilateral pitting edema. He also has decreased sensation in his feet and is hyporeflexive in his lower extremities. An x-ray of the chest shows an enlarged cardiac silhouette and bilateral pulmonary congestion.

■ **What is the most likely diagnosis?**	Vitamin B_1 (thiamine) deficiency.
■ **What clinical manifestations are commonly present in this condition?**	This patient has the symptoms of both wet and dry beriberi. Patients with **wet beriberi** present with high-output congestive heart failure and dilated cardiomyopathy. Patients with **dry beriberi** present with peripheral neuropathy consisting of muscular atrophy and diminished sensation and reflexes.
■ **The deficient factor in this condition serves as a cofactor for which enzymes?**	Thiamine is part of thiamine pyrophosphate (TPP). This acts as a cofactor for transketolase (an enzyme in the HMP shunt) (see Figure 2-8A below), pyruvate decarboxylase (a component of the pyruvate dehydrogenase complex), and α-ketoglutarate decarboxylase (a component of the α-ketoglutarate dehydrogenase complex) (see Figure 2-8B below).
■ **What other pathologies are commonly seen with this vitamin deficiency?**	**Wernicke's encephalopathy** is the central nervous system manifestation of thiamine deficiency. This disease classically consists of nystagmus, ophthalmoplegia, and cerebellar ataxia. When the additional symptoms of confusion/psychosis and confabulation are seen, the disease is known as **Wernicke-Korsakoff syndrome.**
■ **What are the most likely findings on MRI?**	Although degenerative changes are often seen in the cerebellum, brain stem, and diencephalon, atrophy of the mammillary bodies is most commonly noted.

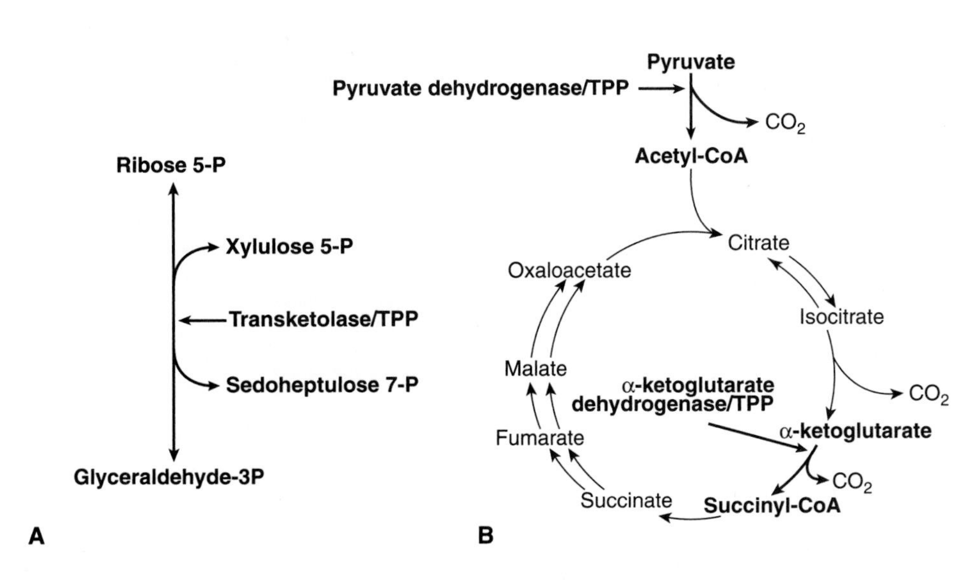

FIGURE 2-8. (A) Thiamine in HMP shunt; (B) Thiamine in TCA cycle.

► Case 13

A 6-month-old girl is brought to her pediatrician because of a 5-month history of restlessness, vomiting, and sweating. Her parents brought her in today after she had a seizure. On questioning, the parents note that the infant's symptoms most commonly occur between meals and subside after feeding. On physical examination, the baby is determined to be small for her age with a protuberant abdomen and xanthomas on the buttocks. Ultrasound shows hepatomegaly and bilaterally enlarged kidneys. Relevant laboratory values are as follows:

Serum glucose: 20 mg/dL
Anion gap: 35
Lactic acid: 9 mg/dL

- **What is the most likely diagnosis?**

von Gierke's disease (type I glycogen storage disease).

- **What is the biochemical defect in this condition?**

This is a glycogen storage disease resulting from glucose-6-phosphatase deficiency. While the liver is able to create and store glycogen, it is unable to break it down into glucose, because glucose-6-phosphatase (which catalyzes the final step of this process) is deficient (see Figure 2-9). The result is the absence of the normal buffering capacity provided by glycogen metabolism, resulting in marked fasting hypoglycemia.

- **What are the most likely findings on liver biopsy?**

Glycogen lipid droplets and significant steatosis are most likely to be found on microscopy.

- **What complications are commonly associated with this condition?**

- Gout can develop as a result of hyperuricemia.
- Hyperlipidemia—especially hypertriglyceridemia—is also common and can lead to xanthoma formation and pancreatitis.
- Platelet dysfunction is common as well and presents as easy bruising and epistaxis.
- Over time, patients may develop liver adenomas that occasionally undergo malignant transformation.
- Nephropathy often develops from the accumulation of glycogen in the kidney.

- **What is the most appropriate treatment for this condition?**

The most appropriate treatment consists of frequent meals to prevent hypoglycemia. Some patients make cornstarch a central part of their diet because it is absorbed slowly and provides a steady glucose supply. Allopurinol is often used for gout. Liver transplantation is curative.

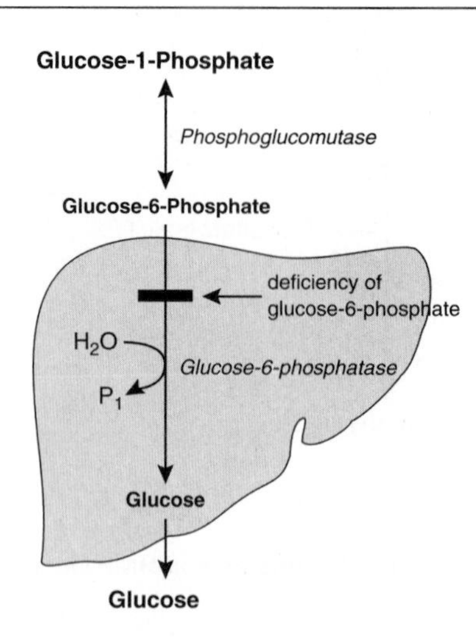

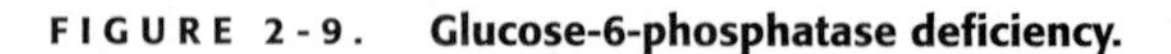
FIGURE 2-9. Glucose-6-phosphatase deficiency.

Microbiology and Immunology

▶ Case 1

A pathologist is sent a poorly labeled sample; it resembles some kind of fluid, but the source is unknown. Gram staining reveals the microorganism in the fluid is a filamentous, gram-positive rod forming long branching filaments, resembling fungi.

What are the two most likely causative bacterial microorganisms?	*Actinomyces* and *Nocardia* would both fit this description. Although they resemble fungi on Gram stain, they are both actually bacteria, not fungi. They appear as characteristic gram-positive rods with long, branching filaments.
How are these two microorganisms differentiated microscopically?	When viewed under the microscope, a slide of *Actinomyces israelii* is non–acid-fast and will have "sulfur granules" (as shown on the gross specimen in Figure 3-1 below). *Nocardia*, on the other hand, is weakly acid-fast. Additionally, while *Actinomyces* is anaerobic, *Nocardia* is an aerobic microorganism.
After paging the intern, the pathologist discovers the sample provided was drained from an oral abscess. Now which of these two microorganisms is more likely?	*Actinomyces* is part of the **normal oral flora** and can cause abscesses in the mouth or gastrointestinal tract after trauma. *Nocardia* is most often found in **lung abscesses** and in patients presenting with symptoms resembling pneumonia. It can also cause brain abscesses.
If this microorganism were found in a sputum sample that stained weakly acid-fast, what would this indicate about the patient's immune status?	This description fits *Nocardia*, and *Nocardia* is most often found in immunocompromised patients. Note this presentation is clinically similar to that of tuberculosis in this high-risk group, and this is a common misdiagnosis in these patients.
What treatment is most appropriate for each of these microorganisms?	*Nocardia* should be treated with trimethoprim-sulfamethoxazole. *Actinomyces* is best treated with penicillin G.

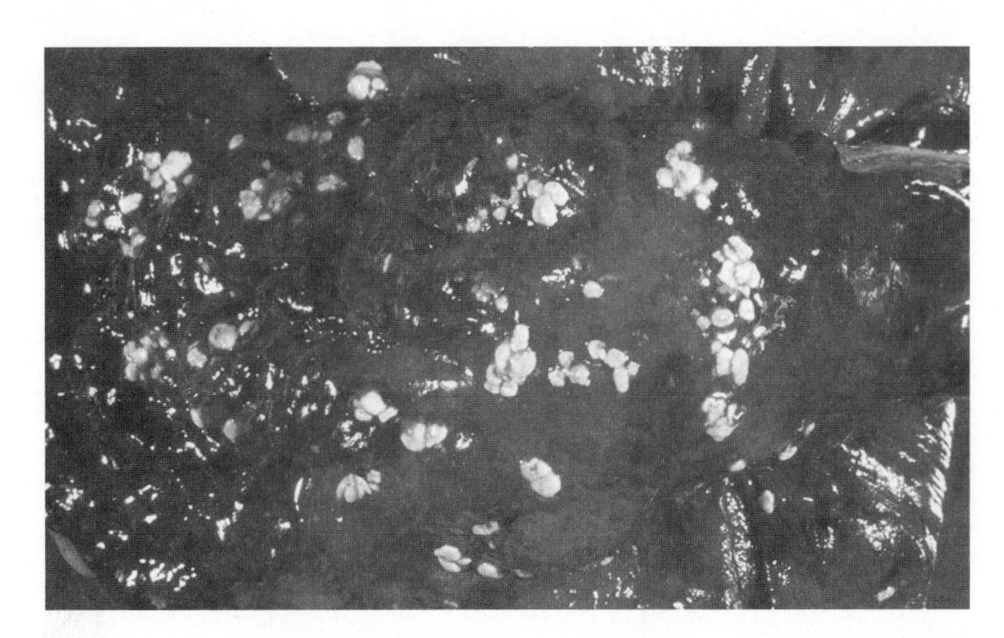

FIGURE 3-1. Gross specimen of *Actinomyces israelii* showing "sulfur granules." (Reproduced with permission of the Pathology Education Instructional Resource Digital Library (http://peir.net) at the University of Alabama, Birmingham.)

▶ Case 2

A local craftsman who makes garments from the hides of goats visits his physician because over the past few days, he has developed several black lesions on his hands and arms (see Figure 3-2 below). The lesions are not painful, but he was alarmed by their appearance. He is afebrile and his physical examination is unremarkable.

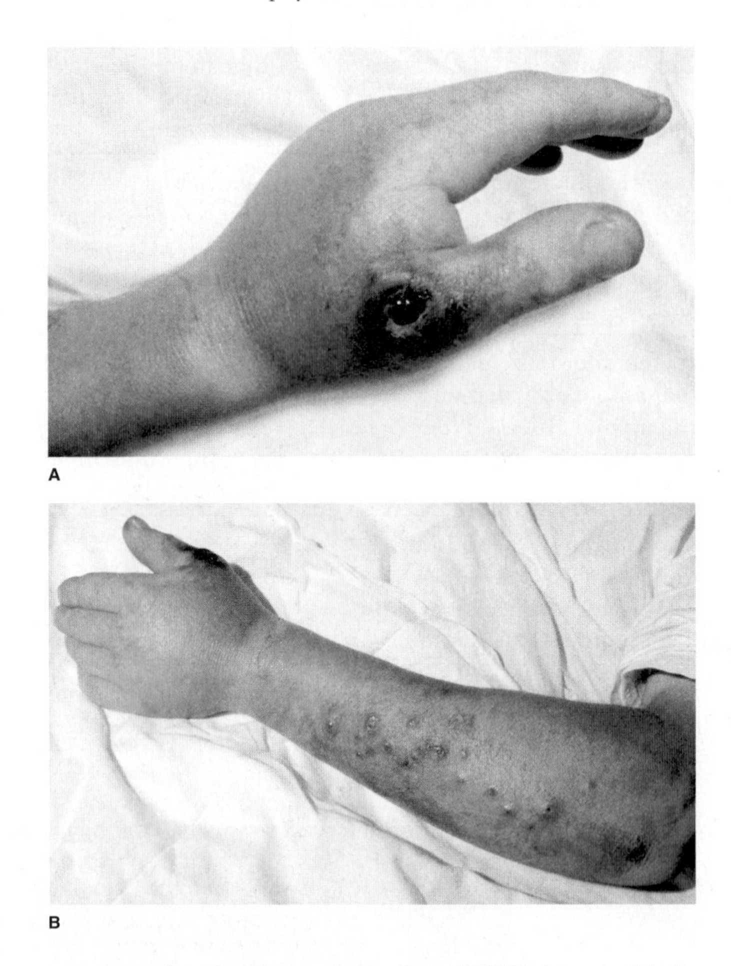

FIGURE 3-2. (Reproduced, with permission, from Wolff K, Johnson RA, Suurmond D. *Fitzpatrick's Color Atlas & Synopsis of Clinical Dermatology*, 5th ed. New York: McGraw-Hill, 2005: 631.)

▪ **What is the most likely diagnosis?**	Cutaneous anthrax, caused by *Bacillus anthracis*.
▪ **How would the causative microorganism appear on Gram staining?**	*B. anthracis* is a gram-positive rod.
▪ **Describe the capsule of this microorganism.**	*B. anthracis* is the only bacterium with a protein capsule. The capsule is composed of poly-D-glutamic acid.
▪ **What property of this microorganism makes it a feared bioterrorism agent?**	This microorganism forms spores that are resistant to many chemical disinfectants, heat, ultraviolet light, and drying.
▪ **What is the other main manifestation of this infection?**	Inhaled anthrax spores reach the alveoli and are taken up by macrophages and carried to mediastinal lymph nodes, where they cause hemorrhage (**woolsorter's disease**). This is not a true pneumonia but is due to mediastinal hemorrhage and can also cause a bloody pleural effusion.

▶ Case 3

A 48-year-old woman from Alabama presents with diffuse, colicky abdominal pain in addition to sharp, intermittent, right upper quadrant pain and decreased frequency of bowel movements. She has noticed a weight loss of about 4.5 kg (10 lb) over the past month, without any change in her diet or behavior. She has not experienced fever, nausea, or vomiting. She had a screening colonoscopy 3 months prior to presentation, which was negative. CT of the abdomen reveals an inflamed gallbladder. A complete blood count demonstrates mild anemia and increased eosinophils. Liver function tests are significant for an alkaline phosphatase level of 150 U/L and a total bilirubin level of 4 mg/dL. A stool sample reveals rough-surfaced eggs.

What is the most likely diagnosis?	Ascariasis, caused by *Ascaris lumbricoides*, a nematode (roundworm) found in the southern United States as well as tropical climates. It is the most common helminthic infection worldwide.
How is this organism transmitted, and how does it cause illness?	Fecal-oral transmission allows the eggs to hatch in the small intestine. Hatched larvae pass through the intestinal wall to enter the bloodstream. They settle in the lungs by entering alveoli and ascending the respiratory tree, causing inflammation and possibly pneumonitis. If the larvae pass from the trachea to the pharynx, they then can enter the gastrointestinal (GI) tract and mature. From the GI tract, adult worms can migrate into the bile ducts and pancreas, causing obstruction. These worms may be quite long.
What signs and symptoms are associated with this condition?	Infection can be asymptomatic, but it can also cause pneumonia and malnutrition. Complications of infection include several worms causing intestinal occlusion, and biliary obstruction caused by one worm traveling up the biliary tree.
What tests can be used to confirm the diagnosis?	Analysis of a stool sample will show eggs with a knobby, rough surface.
What treatments are most appropriate for this condition?	Mebendazole or albendazole is the primary drug, although pyrantel pamoate may also be useful.

▶ Case 4

A 54-year-old man with a history of tobacco use and corticosteroid-treated chronic obstructive pulmonary disease (COPD) presents to the emergency department because of severe shortness of breath. The patient had a COPD exacerbation 3 weeks prior to admission and began taking oral corticosteroids at that time. His symptoms resolved and he had returned to his usual state of health until 1.5 weeks later, when he again began experiencing cough and shortness of breath. He developed hemoptysis 1 week prior to admission. The patient was started on prophylactic antibiotics and underwent bronchoalveolar lavage, which revealed the presence of 45°-branching septate hyphae (see Figure 3-3 below).

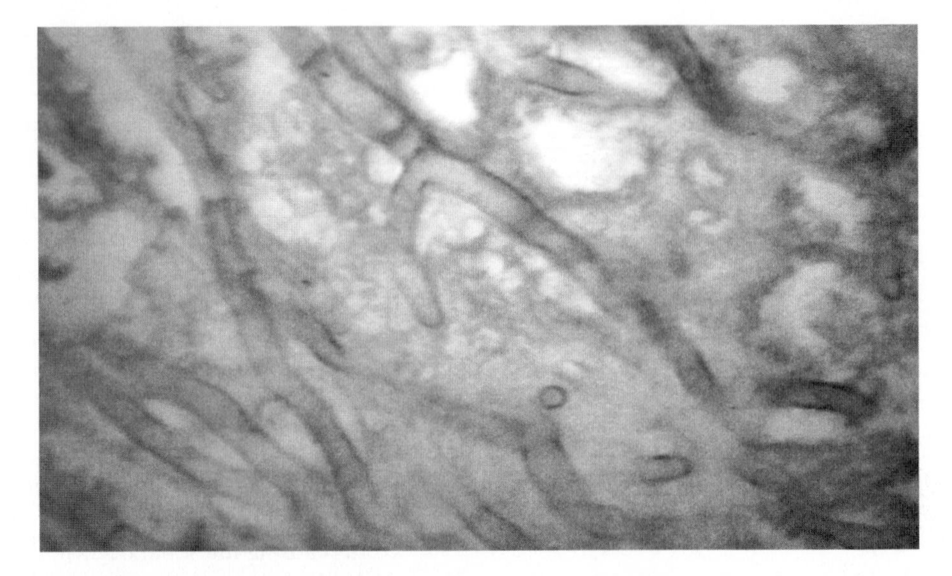

FIGURE 3-3. (Reproduced with permission of the Pathology Education Instructional Resource Digital Library (http://peir.net) at the University of Alabama, Birmingham.)

■ **What is the most likely diagnosis?**	This presentation, plus findings on lavage, indicate *Aspergillus* infection. *Candida* should also be considered, but would appear microscopically as pseudohyphae and budding yeasts.
■ **What are the likely findings on x-ray of the chest?**	*Aspergillus* can appear as a "fungus ball" within preexisting cavitary lesions in the lungs. This form of *Aspergillus* infection is called an **aspergilloma.**
■ **The patient is treated with amphotericin B. What is the drug's mechanism of action and adverse effects?**	Amphotericin B works by binding to ergosterol, disrupting the integrity of the cell membrane. It can cause fever, chills, kidney damage, hypotension, and arrhythmias.
■ **The patient's symptoms improve, and he is discharged several days later. However, he returns to the hospital 3 months later with worsened respiratory function, chest pain, and decreased urine output. Could these symptoms be sequelae of the condition that caused his previous admission?**	The patient could be suffering from **invasive aspergillosis,** which is the result of hematogenous spread of his infection to his kidneys, pericardium, and elsewhere, causing these diffuse symptoms.
■ **Why is this patient particularly prone to these complications?**	The corticosteroids that the patient takes for his COPD render his immune system less effective at fighting the infection, despite treatment with amphotericin B. Patients with <500 neutrophils/mm^3 (eg, transplant recipients and patients with leukemia) are especially susceptible to invasive aspergillosis.

▶ Case 5

A patient with diabetes presents to her physician with an adherent white, flaky substance on the skin under her breasts. Another patient, a woman who has just completed a course of oral antibiotics, presents with itching and a copious vaginal discharge that resembles "cottage cheese." A third patient, with acquired immunodeficiency syndrome (AIDS), presents with a white exudate on his oral mucosa and soft palate. The physician diagnoses the same causative microorganism for all three cases.

What is the most likely diagnosis?	The fungus *Candida albicans* can result in systemic or superficial fungal infection (candidiasis). Oral thrush, vaginitis (yeast infection), and diaper rash are common manifestations of local candidiasis.
Where is the microorganism that causes this condition normally found?	*C. albicans* is part of the normal flora of mucous membranes of the gastrointestinal tract, respiratory tract, and female genital tract. Overgrowth, especially in warm, moist areas such as the skin under the breasts, causes candidiasis.
What laboratory tests can help confirm the diagnosis?	A potassium hydroxide preparation (**KOH mount**) is used for skin or tissue scrapings. **Pseudohyphae** and **budding yeast** (see Figure 3-4 below) are observed in the tissues. Pseudohyphae are seen in culture at 20°C, and germ tube formation is seen at 37°C. For systemic disease (rare), blood cultures are positive for the fungus.
What treatments are most appropriate for this condition?	Fluconazole or nystatin is used for superficial infections, and amphotericin B or fluconazole can be used for systemic infections.
What populations are most at risk for this condition?	**Immunocompromised hosts** are at highest risk: neonates, patients taking steroids, those with diabetes, and those with AIDS. These patients are also at higher risk for developing more serious forms of candidal infection such as esophagitis and systemic infection. **Intravenous drug users** are at higher risk for candidal endocarditis. Women who have just completed a course of **antibiotics** are at higher risk for vaginitis.

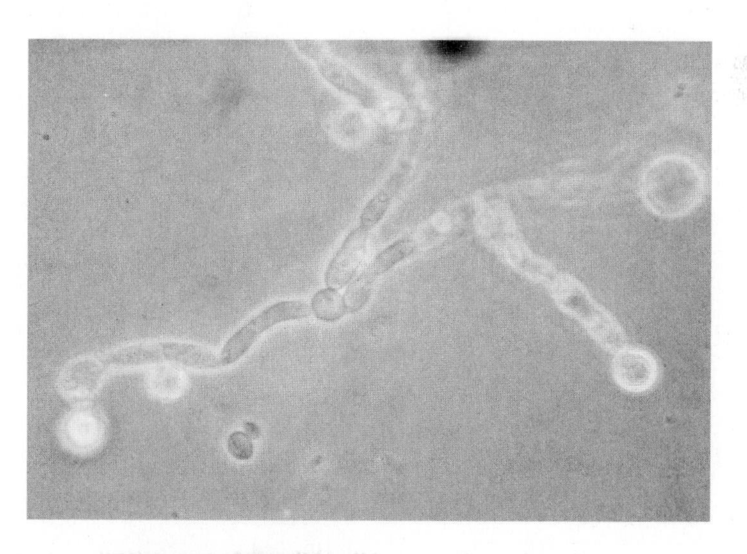

FIGURE 3-4. KOH mount of *Candida albicans*. (Reproduced, with permission, from Wolff K, Johnson RA, Suurmond D. *Fitzpatrick's Color Atlas & Synopsis of Clinical Dermatology*, 5th ed. New York: McGraw-Hill, 2005: 717.)

▶ Case 6

A 49-year-old woman who recently immigrated to the United States from Nicaragua presents to the clinic with difficulty swallowing, constipation, and abdominal pain. She says she has gone more than a week without having a bowel movement. Physical examination reveals she is tachycardic and her abdomen is distended. An electrocardiogram shows Mobitz type I heart block.

▪ **What is the most likely diagnosis?**	Chagas' disease, or American trypanosomiasis, caused by the protozoan *Trypanosoma cruzi*.
▪ **What is the vector of the responsible protozoan?**	The reduviid bug, also known as the "kissing bug."
▪ **Where in the world is this condition found?**	Southern United States, Mexico, Central and South America (ie, only in the Western hemisphere).
▪ **What is the pathophysiology of this condition?**	This woman is experiencing chronic Chagas' disease, most often characterized by heart block, ventricular tachycardia, and dilated cardiomyopathy. Dilatation of the esophagus and colon (toxic megacolon) can cause the presentation outlined above. The acute phase of the disease can be characterized by a hard red area called a **chagoma** at the parasite's site of entry into the host, fever, and meningoencephalitis. In endemic areas, the acute phase is seen more frequently in children.
▪ **What treatment is most appropriate for this condition?**	Nifurtimox and benznidazole are used to treat acute cases. However, there is no effective treatment for chronic Chagas' disease. For chronic heart disease, supporting measures for congestive heart failure, antiarrhythmics for tachycardia, and pacemaker implantation for heart block are used. For gastrointestinal disease, dilation of the esophageal sphincter, changes in diet, the use of laxatives and/or enemas, and in some cases eventual resection of the megacolon are used.

► Case 7

A 24-year-old American man is traveling in rural India during the monsoon season. During the course of a few hours, he develops severe watery diarrhea. Over the course of 30 hours he has approximately one episode per hour of liquid stools that appear clear with little white flecks of mucus. In addition, he has occasional episodes of vomiting. He quickly becomes very lethargic and generally ill and complains of crampy abdominal pain, but is afebrile. He attempts to rehydrate himself during the course of the illness, and the symptoms resolve within approximately 48 hours.

What is the most likely diagnosis?	This patient has cholera, caused by *Vibrio cholerae*. This microorganism is a gram-negative, curved, motile rod that resembles "shooting stars" on Gram stain. Symptomatic cholera usually manifests in epidemics, and it is endemic to developing countries such as Africa, Asia, South and Latin America, and recently the Middle East.
How does the microorganism exert its effect on the gastrointestinal tract?	Cholera is ingested through fecally contaminated water. It secretes an exotoxin (cholera toxin) that binds to the surface of intestinal epithelium. This toxin increases cyclic adenosine monophosphate within the intestinal mucosa, which causes increased chloride secretion and decreased sodium absorption. This leads to a massive loss of fluids and electrolytes.
What are the clinical manifestations of this condition?	The hallmark of cholera is **rice-water stools,** so described because the little white flecks of mucus look like rice. The onset of this diarrhea typically occurs from 1–3 days after infection. Many *V. cholerae* infections are asymptomatic, but severe cholera can lead to extreme dehydration that can result in death within hours. Vomiting and abdominal cramping are common, while fever (cholera is not invasive) and abdominal pain are rare.
What are some of the severe potential consequences of this condition?	The consequences of cholera result from extreme volume loss as well as the excretion of large amounts of sodium, potassium, chloride, and bicarbonate. The volume depletion can lead to renal failure, and the potassium loss can lead to hypokalemia, which in turn can cause arrhythmias, ileus, and cramps. The bicarbonate loss can lead to a metabolic acidosis. Left untreated, symptomatic cholera leads to death in 50%–70% of cases, and children are 10 times more likely to die than adults.
What is the most appropriate treatment for this condition?	The mainstay of cholera treatment is administration of **oral rehydration solution** (ORS), which has reduced mortality rates from 50% to <1%. ORS takes advantage of the fact that glucose facilitates sodium absorption from the gut, which allows for the concurrent absorption of water. A typical preparation of ORS contains glucose, potassium chloride, sodium chloride, and sodium bicarbonate. If patients become so ill they cannot drink, **intravenous fluid replacement** can be used. Antibiotics are of limited use in stopping the diarrhea, although early use of doxycycline has been shown to reduce the volume of diarrhea and decrease the duration of bacteria excretion by 1 day.

▶ Case 8

A 5-year-old girl is brought to the clinic with a 3-month history of worsening vision and behavioral difficulty in school. She emigrated with her mother and a younger sibling 2 years previously from Guatemala. Her mother received no prenatal care and, through a translator, reports the patient was delivered without complication at home. As an infant, the girl had a "wart-like" maculopapular rash around her mucous membranes, and three or four recurrent right-sided ear infections. Physical examination reveals the girl is in the 30th percentile for weight and 35th percentile for height. Also, the fundi were notable for nummular keratitis, and there was prominent notching of her upper two incisors and molars, as well as outward bowing of the tibia bilaterally.

- **What is the most likely diagnosis?**

Congenital syphilis. This infection is one of the so-called **ToRCHeS** infections (**To**xoplasmosis, **R**ubella, **C**ytomegalovirus, **He**rpes, **S**yphilis), which are the most common causes of congenital infection.

- **What is the causative microorganism in this condition?**

Treponema pallidum.

- **What symptoms are commonly found in patients with this condition?**

- Bone abnormalities (osteochondritis and periostitis)
- Eczematoid skin rash
- Fissures (lips, nares) and mucous patches
- Frontal bossing (ie, a prominent forehead)
- Hemolytic anemia
- Hepatosplenomegaly
- Interstitial keratitis
- Jaundice
- Pigmented retinopathy
- Snuffles (nasal discharge, often bloody)
- Tooth abnormalities (Hutchinson incisors, mulberry molars)

- **In the newborn, what tests can help confirm the diagnosis?**

- **Serum rapid plasma reagin (RPR) test:** umbilical cord blood may show false-positive results due to maternal titers
- **Radiography of long bones:** very poor sensitivity, difficult to obtain in the newborn
- Lumbar puncture, cerebrospinal fluid samples for **Venereal Disease Research Laboratory (VDRL) testing:** pleocytosis and elevated protein level suggest infection

- **What tests can be used to detect infection in the patient's mother?**

- Serologic testing
- VDRL and RPR for screening
- Positive results on fluorescent treponemal antigen-antibody absorption (FTA-ABS) test

- **What treatments are most appropriate for this condition?**

Benzathine penicillin G for 10–14 days. Because of the signs of tertiary involvement, congenital infection is highly likely; however, a social worker should be involved in any case there is a question of sexual abuse as a possible route of transmission. The mother and younger sibling should both receive testing and/or treatment as well. Additionally, long bone radiographs of the patient should be taken, and MRI can rule out neurologic involvement. A cerebrospinal fluid sample should be obtained for measuring cell counts and protein content and for VDRL testing. Also, the patient's auditory, visual, and dental issues need evaluation.

► Case 9

A pathologist is performing an autopsy on a 56-year-old male university professor who suffered a rapid demise from an undiagnosed neurologic disease. Approximately 1 year previously, the patient presented to a psychiatrist with symptoms of psychosis. Shortly thereafter, his symptoms advanced to include unsteadiness and involuntary movements, and the patient ultimately became immobile and unable to speak. A sample of brain tissue shows many vacuoles in the grey matter and a great deal of neuronal loss (see Figure 3-5 below).

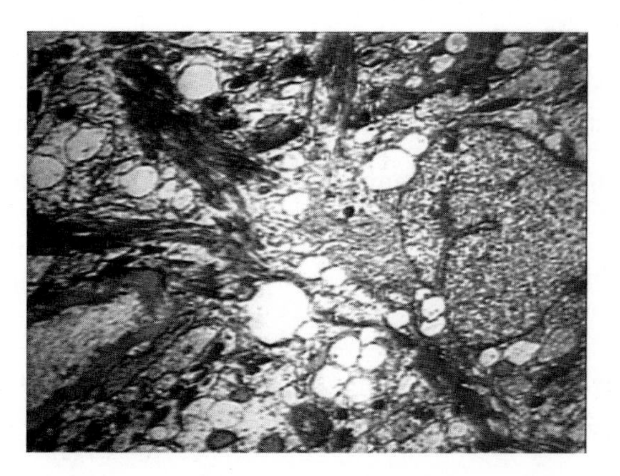

FIGURE 3-5. (Reproduced with permission of the Pathology Education Instructional Resource Digital Library (http://peir.net) at the University of Alabama, Birmingham.)

▪ **What is the most likely diagnosis?**	Creutzfeldt-Jakob disease (CJD) due to abnormal prions.
▪ **How does the causative microorganism in this condition differ from other pathogens?**	Prions do not contain RNA or DNA; they are composed only of protein.
▪ **How is this condition transmitted?**	Disease can be transmitted by central nervous system (CNS) tissue containing prions. Prion disease can also be inherited.
▪ **What other condition is associated with this type of pathogen?**	Prions cause two degenerative CNS diseases in humans: CJD and **kuru,** a slowly progressive, fatal disease found among tribes in Papua, New Guinea, who practice cannibalism and thus may ingest neurologic tissue of an infected person.
▪ **How does the structure of normal prions differ from that of pathologic prions?**	Normal prions have α-helix conformations, while pathologic prions are composed of an abnormal isoform of β-pleated sheets.
▪ **What treatment is most appropriate for this condition?**	Unfortunately there is no known treatment for CJD.
▪ **What diseases are caused by so-called "slow viruses"?**	**Slow virus** refers to the tempo of disease progression, not the growth rate of the virus. The slow viruses exist in patients for months to years before causing disease. For example, the **measles** virus can cause subacute sclerosing panencephalitis, which is a progressive demyelinating CNS disease most often seen in young people, who present with seizure, ataxia, and focal neurological symptoms. Reactivation of the **JC virus,** which causes disease in immunocompromised hosts, can cause progressive multifocal leukoencephalopathy. This is the result of progressive demyelination of oligodendrocytes.

▶ Case 10

A 32-year-old man with acquired immunodeficiency syndrome (AIDS) presents to the emergency department with complaints of worsening headache, fever, and a stiff neck. Lumbar puncture is performed, and analysis reveals an elevated opening pressure, increased protein level, and decreased glucose level. Special staining of the spinal fluid reveals budding yeast.

What is the most likely diagnosis?	Cryptococcal meningitis is the most common fungal cause of meningitis, and is prevalent among patients with AIDS.
What microorganism causes this disease, and what is its morphology?	*Cryptococcus neoformans* is a heavily encapsulated yeast. It is only found as a yeast; it is not a dimorphic microorganism.
How is the microorganism transmitted, and how does it cause illness?	*C. neoformans* is found in pigeon droppings, and is also found in soil. When inhaled, the yeast causes local infection in the lung that can be asymptomatic or result in pneumonia. Hematogenous spread to the central nervous system can result in meningitis and brain abscesses.
What laboratory tests can help confirm the diagnosis?	**India ink** will stain the heavy polysaccharide capsule and reveal budding yeast (see Figure 3-6 below). **Serology** is most commonly used: latex agglutination detects polysaccharide capsular antigen. The microorganism can also be cultured on **Sabouraud's agar.**
What treatment is most appropriate for this condition?	Patients who are not immunocompromised can be treated sufficiently with amphotericin B and flucytosine for the meningitis. Patients with AIDS require lifetime suppression with fluconazole after induction with amphotericin B and flucytosine, without which the illness will relapse.

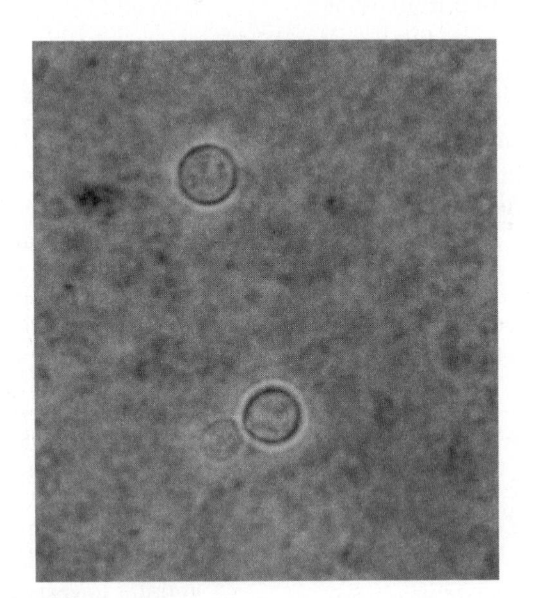

FIGURE 3-6. ***Cryptococcus neoformans.***

► Case 11

A 42-year-old woman who works in a pork processing plant presents to her physician with new-onset seizures and bilateral lower extremity weakness. CT of the head reveals several calcified regions, but no mass lesion or evidence of bleeding. A complete blood count reveals mild anemia and a WBC count of 78,000/mm^3, with 12% eosinophils.

▪ **What is the most likely diagnosis?**	Cysticercosis, caused by *Taenia solium* (pork tapeworm), which is a cestode (tapeworm).
▪ **How is this organism transmitted, and how does it cause illness?**	Ingestion of undercooked pork allows for introduction of larvae from pig muscle into the human gastrointestinal (GI) system. These larvae mature in the small intestine. Eggs from the adult worms are released into the feces. Fecal-oral contact then allows eggs in the GI tract to hatch into onchospheres. The onchospheres then penetrate the intestinal wall and migrate into the blood and tissues.
▪ **What signs and symptoms are associated with this condition?**	Infection can be asymptomatic, or cause malnutrition and abdominal discomfort. Cysticercosis can be found anywhere in the body, including the brain and eye, leading to seizures, focal neurological symptoms, and blindness.
▪ **What tests can help confirm the diagnosis?**	Intestinal infection is revealed by eggs in stool. Calcified cysticerci can be observed on CT when cysticercosis occurs in the brain (see arrow in Figure 3-7 below). X-ray films may reveal calcified cysticerci in other parts of the body, such as muscle.
▪ **What treatments are most appropriate for this condition?**	Praziquantel or albendazole is used for cysticercosis. In addition, steroids and anticonvulsants may be given for neurocysticercosis. Asymptomatic patients are rarely treated.

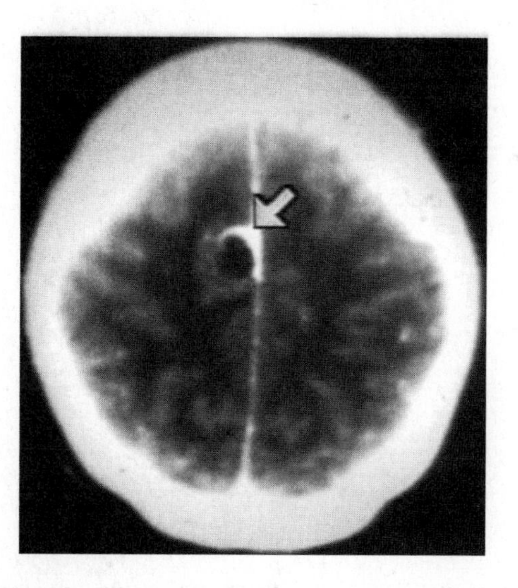

FIGURE 3-7. Cysticercosis. (Reproduced with permission of the Pathology Education Instructional Resource Digital Library (http://peir.net) at the University of Alabama, Birmingham.)

▶ Case 12

A 7-year-old girl is brought to her primary care physician because of a sore throat and fever of 38.3° C (101° F). Physical examination reveals a grayish membrane covering her pharynx, as well as cervical lymphadenopathy. The child was born in Africa and did not receive all of her childhood vaccinations.

What is the most likely diagnosis?	The child most likely has diphtheria caused by *Corynebacterium diphtheriae*.
How does this microorganism cause this presentation?	Exotoxin A is an enzyme that blocks protein synthesis by inactivating elongation factor EF-2 by adenosine phosphate ribosylation. This results in decreased mRNA translation and protein synthesis. Note that *Pseudomonas* toxin has a similar mechanism.
What growth media is used to identify this microorganism, and how does it appear on culture?	Potassium tellurite agar and Loeffler's coagulated blood serum media are the media to use for isolating this microorganism. *C. diphtheriae* is a gram-positive rod. In culture, it often appears in clumps described as **"Chinese characters."**
Which vaccine would have prevented this child's illness?	The inactivated form, or toxoid, is a component of the DPT vaccine (**D**iphtheria, **P**ertussis, **T**etanus).
What treatment is most appropriate for this condition?	Antitoxin can inactivate circulating toxin that has not yet reached its target tissue. Penicillin or erythromycin can be given to prevent further bacterial growth and exotoxin release, thus making the patient noncontagious. The patient also needs cardiac monitoring with electrocardiography and telemetry to monitor for myocarditis; treatment of any heart failure or arrhythmias; monitoring of neurologic function for motor deficits; and supporting care to ensure a secure airway and to avoid aspiration pneumonia.

▶ Case 13

A 32-year-old man presents with extreme swelling of his legs (see Figure 3-8 below) and scrotum. The skin associated with the swollen areas is thick and scaly. The patient admits to an episode of fever associated with enlarged inguinal lymph nodes some time ago, but did not think much of it. His travel history is significant for spending 9 months in the tropics approximately 2 years prior to presentation.

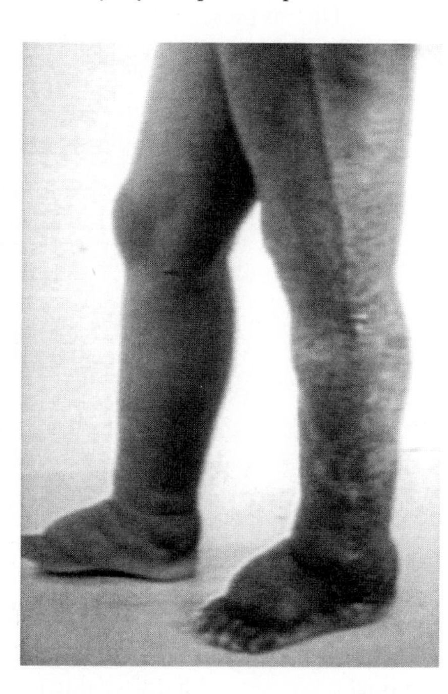

FIGURE 3-8. (Reproduced with permission of the Pathology Education Instructional Resource Digital Library (http://peir.net) at the University of Alabama, Birmingham.)

■ **What is the most likely diagnosis?**	Elephantiasis, caused by the nematode (roundworm) *Wuchereria bancrofti.*
■ **How is this organism transmitted, and how does it cause illness?**	The organism is transmitted by the bite of a female mosquito. Larvae are released into the bloodstream and travel to the lymphatics of the lower extremities and genitals, where they mature. Approximately 1 year later, adult worms, which reside in lymph nodes, trigger an inflammatory response.
■ **What signs and symptoms are associated with this condition?**	Inflammation resulting from the presence of adult worms causes fever and swelling of lymph nodes. Repeated infections cause repeated bouts of inflammation, resulting in fibrosis around the dead adult worms in the lymph nodes. This fibrosis can obstruct lymphatic drainage and lead to edema and scaly skin.
■ **What test can be used to confirm the diagnosis?**	Blood cultures reveal larvae (**microfilariae**). Interestingly, as larvae usually emerge at night, drawing blood in the evening is preferred.
■ **What is the most appropriate treatment for this condition?**	Diethylcarbamazine is effective in killing the larvae, but is not effective against the adult worms.

▶ **Case 14**

A previously healthy 24-year-old man goes to see his doctor with complaints of significant weight loss, flatulence, and foul-smelling stools. He reports feeling fatigued since his return from Peru 3 months previously, and has suffered abdominal cramping and intermittent loose, nonbloody stools since then. The patient's stool ova and parasite studies demonstrated characteristic trophozoites on two separate occasions (see Figure 3-9 below). He was prescribed a course of drug therapy and warned that consumption of alcohol during treatment could lead to nausea and vomiting.

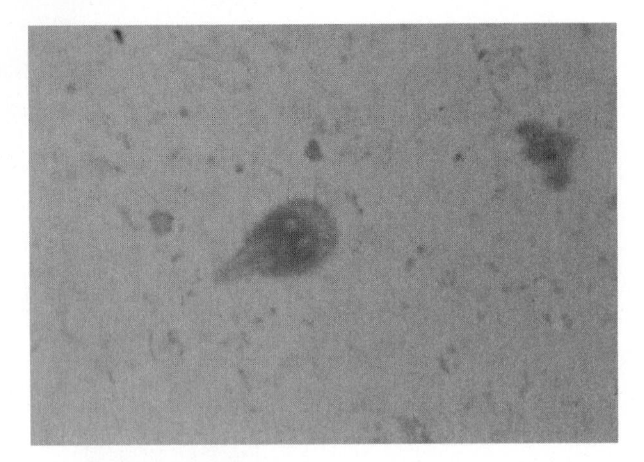

FIGURE 3-9. (Reproduced, with permission, from Bhushan V, Le T, et al. *First Aid for the USMLE Step 1: 2006*. New York: McGraw-Hill, 2006: Color Image 5.)

■ **What is the most likely diagnosis?**	Giardiasis due to *Giardia lamblia* infection. *Giardia* appear as both a flagellated, motile, dinucleated trophozoite and as a round cyst.
■ **What is another less likely infecting microorganism?**	*Entamoeba histolytica* can also cause a similar spectrum of symptoms, although there is debate over whether *E. histolytica* can in fact cause nondysenteric diarrhea. Amebic dysentery would present with bloody diarrhea in addition to the above clinical spectrum.
■ **What is the most appropriate treatment for this condition?**	Metronidazole. The described effects of concurrent alcohol use with metronidazole is a "disulfiram-like effect," in reference to the use of disulfiram to discourage alcohol consumption in situations of alcohol addiction. Metronidazole interferes with the effect of aldehyde dehydrogenase in ethanol metabolism, which increases serum acetaldehyde levels and thus leads to nausea, vomiting, flushing, thirst, palpitations, vertigo, and chest pain.
■ **What is the mechanism of action of this antibiotic?**	Metronidazole is effective specifically against anaerobic microorganisms. It diffuses across the cell membrane of microorganisms and is reduced in the mitochondria of obligate anaerobes to cytotoxic intermediates. These intermediates cause DNA strand breakage and generate free radicals to consequently damage the cell. Furthermore, the reduction of metronidazole creates a concentration gradient that leads to further uptake of the drug.
■ **What are other uses of this antibiotic?**	Metronidazole is used to treat *Clostridium difficile* infection in pseudomembranous colitis, amebic dysentery, bacterial vaginitis, and *Trichomonas* vaginitis, and as a component of triple therapy for *Helicobacter pylori* eradication. Broadly, it is effective against most anaerobic bacteria as well as various protozoa.

▶ Case 15

A 3-year-old boy is brought to the pediatrician by his mother. The mother states that 2 days ago, the child started refusing solid foods, preferring his bottle and applesauce. Today, the mother noticed a rash on her son's hands and feet (see Figure 3-10 below), and found that he was also running a low-grade fever, which prompted her to bring him to the doctor.

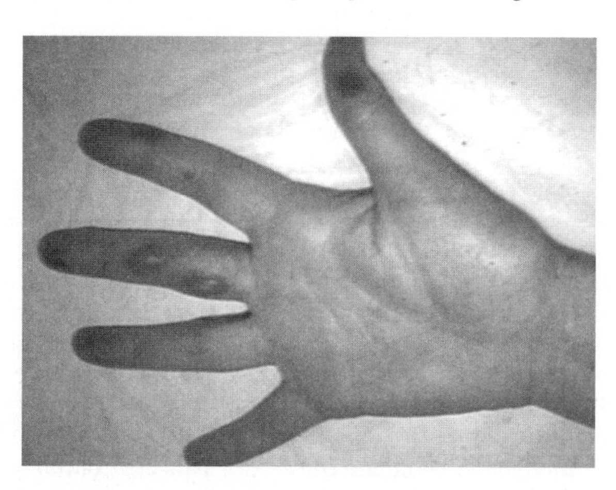

FIGURE 3-10. (Reproduced with permission of the Pathology Education Instructional Resource Digital Library (http://peir.net) at the University of Alabama, Birmingham.)

- **What is the most likely diagnosis?**

This is a case of hand, foot, and mouth syndrome, caused by coxsackie A virus (a picornavirus). This syndrome presents with a tender rash on the palms, soles, and often the buttocks, in addition to painful vesicles on the oral mucosa. This patient's avoidance of solid food strongly suggests involvement of the oral mucosa.

- **What other microorganisms are included in this family, and what are their characteristics?**

The picornavirus family are Enteroviruses (they infect intestinal epithelia and lymphoid cells), and includes

- Poliovirus
- Echovirus
- Hepatitis A virus
- Coxsackie viruses
- Rhinovirus

The pico**RNA**viruses all have a single-stranded, positive polarity, linear, **RNA** genome in a nonenveloped icosahedral capsid.

- **What other illnesses can this particular microorganism cause?**

Coxsackie A virus may also cause **herpangina,** which presents with sore throat, red vesicles on the back of the throat, pain with swallowing, and fever. Herpangina is a mild, self-limited disease that presents in children and usually results in complete recovery. Less commonly, coxsackie A virus can cause petechial and purpuric rashes, which may also have a hemorrhagic component.

- **What illnesses may be caused by the group B coxsackie viruses?**

The coxsackie B virus may cause aseptic meningitis, myocarditis, pericarditis, orchitis, and pleurodynia (fever, headache, spasms of the chest wall muscles, and pleuritic pain). Nephritic syndrome may also occur after a coxsackie B virus infection.

- **What type of immune response would this infection elicit?**

Because this is a viral infection, it will elicit a cell-mediated and antibody-mediated immune response. As the virus infects cells, viral particles will be presented by class II MHC, activating $CD4^+$ cells. These cells will release cytokines that subsequently activate both cytotoxic T cells ($CD8^+$) and B cells, which will synthesize immunoglobulin.

▶ Case 16

A 9-year-old girl is brought to a public clinic by her mother. The family immigrated from Guatemala 3 years previously. Her mother reports the girl seems very small for her age and has been continually lethargic for quite some time. Physical examination reveals a small girl with a thin, scaphoid abdomen. Relevant laboratory findings are as follows:

Hematocrit: 36%
Mean corpuscular volume: 83 fL
WBC count: 11,000/mm^3
Differential: 35% segmented cells, 1% bands, 33% lymphocytes, 21% eosinophils

---

- **What is the most likely diagnosis, and what test can be used to confirm this?**

The patient's eosinophilia points to a possible parasitic infection, therefore, a stool ova and parasite study should be the next step. The patient's recent immigration from Guatemala increases the risk of a parasitic infection.

- **The test demonstrates the patient is infected with the hookworm *Ancylostoma duodenale*. What are the characteristic findings of this infection?**

A. *duodenale* presents as characteristic small, round eggs and occasional worms approximately 1 cm in size. The ova and parasite examination can differentiate between the helminthic causes of eosinophilia. The stool exam is only useful in chronic hookworm infections.

- **Describe how this infection causes disease in humans.**

Percutaneous infection occurs most commonly through the soles of the feet. The larvae pass into the lungs, and 8–21 days later they cross the pulmonary vasculature and enter the airways. They ascend to the pharynx and are swallowed. By the time they reach the small intestine, the larvae have become adult worms. The adults attach to the mucosa and feed with the help of an orally secreted factor X inhibitor, and females produce eggs that are passed through the stool and deposited in the soil.

- **What are the signs of both acute and chronic infection?**

Acute symptoms:

- Cutaneous tracks of larval migration under the skin (less common)
- Diarrhea
- Flatulence
- Nausea
- Postprandial abdominal pain
- Pruritic maculopapular eruption at the site of entry (less common)
- Vomiting

Chronic hookworm infection:

- Failure to thrive
- Iron deficiency anemia

This patient has symptoms of chronic hookworm infection. Chronic hookworm infection leads to the high morbidity of the disease in countries where hookworm infection is prevalent.

- **What treatments are most appropriate for this condition?**

Mebendazole. Alternatively, pyrantel pamoate and albendazole can be used.

▶ **Case 17**

A 46-year-old woman visits her physician complaining of "feeling poorly," with fever, chills, muscle aches, dry cough, and sore throat. She has had these symptoms for several days with no significant improvement. She works as a secretary and says these symptoms have been "going around the office." Physical examination reveals small, tender cervical lymphadenopathy, swollen nasal mucosa, and an erythematous pharynx.

■ **What is the most likely diagnosis?**	Infection with influenza virus.
■ **Describe the microorganisms that can cause this condition.**	Orthomyxoviruses are helical, enveloped, negative single-stranded RNA viruses.
■ **Even though the patient has had a similar infection, why isn't her immune system protecting her from this illness?**	Because of a phenomenon known as **antigenic drift.** This is the result of random small mutations causing changes in the antigenic structure of the virus. These mutations result in antigen structures that are only partially recognized by the host immune system.
■ **What characteristic of this microorganism's genome makes deadly epidemics possible?**	Influenza A virus infects diverse species including birds, horses, and swine; in contrast, influenza B and C only infect man. With its segmented genome, influenza A can swap segments of RNA between animal and human strains, leading to new human strains with novel surface antigens not recognized by the immune system. This type of change is termed **antigenic shift.**
■ **What pharmacologic agents can be used as prophylaxis against this infection?**	Amantadine and rimantadine can be used to treat the symptoms of influenza A infection. Zanamivir and oseltamivir can be used to treat both influenza A and B infections. These need to be started in the first 2 days of symptom onset to be most effective. The vaccine should be given in October or November, prior to the start of flu season. It takes about 2 weeks for the body to make antibodies to the viruses.

▶ Case 18

A 43-year-old man with human immunodeficiency virus (HIV) infection presents to the HIV clinic with multiple, reddish-purple plaques, in addition to a few papules of the same color, distributed across the skin (see Figure 3-11 below). The patient says he feels fine, and denies fever, chills, malaise, or headache. A complete blood count reveals his CD4+ T cell count is 350 cells/μL.

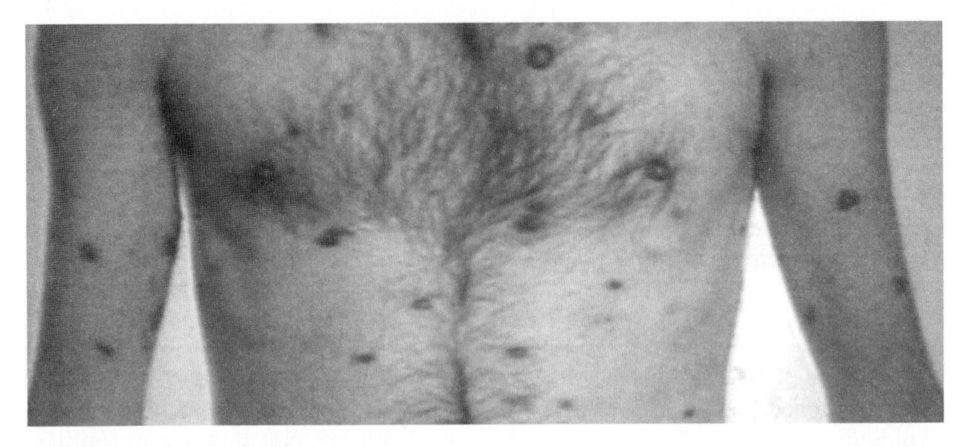

FIGURE 3-11. (Reproduced with permission of the Pathology Education Instructional Resource Digital Library (http://peir.net) at the University of Alabama, Birmingham.)

- **What is the most likely diagnosis? What important alternative diagnosis must be ruled out?**

This is Kaposi's sarcoma, a neoplasm prevalent in HIV-positive patients. Kaposi's sarcoma is caused by human herpes virus-8 (HHV-8), a member of the herpes virus family. Members of the herpes family are DNA viruses with a double-stranded, linear genome in an enveloped, icosahedral capsid. An important alternative diagnosis for such skin lesions is bacillary angiomatosis (BA), which typically presents with systemic symptoms such as fever, chills, and malaise. Because BA is caused by *Bartonella* bacteria, however, it can readily be treated with antibiotics.

- **How does the microorganism cause the characteristic discolored skin lesions?**

HHV-8 has a tropism for endothelium cells, and is thought to induce vascular endothelial growth factor (VEGF), which causes irregular vascular channels to develop in the skin. RBCs extravasate into these spaces, causing the characteristic purple-red skin lesions as seen in Figure 3-11 (above).

- **What other diseases are associated with this microorganism?**

Kaposi's sarcoma is not limited to the skin; the gastrointestinal tract, oral mucosa, lungs, lymph nodes, and other visceral organs may be infected. HHV-8 also infects B lymphocytes, and has been linked to **body-cavity B-cell lymphoma** (a non-Hodgkin's lymphoma subtype) and to **Castleman's disease** (a lymphoproliferative disorder that may progress to lymphoma).

- **What other patient population is at increased risk for developing this infection?**

Transplant patients, who, like patients with HIV, are chronically immunosuppressed have a higher incidence of infection than the general public.

- **What treatments are most appropriate for this condition?**

Daunorubicin and doxorubicin. Both drugs cause DNA breaks by two mechanisms: (1) intercalating into the DNA double helix, and (2) creating oxygen free radicals that damage DNA. A major adverse effect of their use, however, is cardiotoxicity. In HIV-positive patients, the first goal is to boost immunity by starting highly active antiretroviral therapy, which often leads to improvement of the disease.

▶ Case 19

A 64-year-old man with a past history of smoking and well-controlled diabetes mellitus, presents to the emergency department with a 3-day history of low-grade fevers, mild diarrhea, and nonproductive cough. He works as a maintenance worker in a local apartment complex. Workup includes a Gram stain of sputum, which shows prominent polymorphonuclear leukocytes, but no microorganisms. X-ray of the chest reveals diffuse, patchy bilateral infiltrates (see Figure 3-12 below). Relevant laboratory findings are as follows:

Hemoglobin: 14 g/mL
Hematocrit: 40%
Platelets: 200,000/mm^3
WBCs: 15,000/mm^3
Blood urea nitrogen: 16 mg/dL
Creatinine: 1.2 mg/dL
Urinalysis: 2+ proteinuria; no glucose, ketones, or blood

Sodium: 128 mEq/L
Chloride: 90 mEq/L
Potassium: 4.2 mEq/L
Bicarbonate: 17 mEq/L
Glucose: 110 mg/dL

The patient is treated empirically with a β-lactam antibiotic, with no clinical improvement.

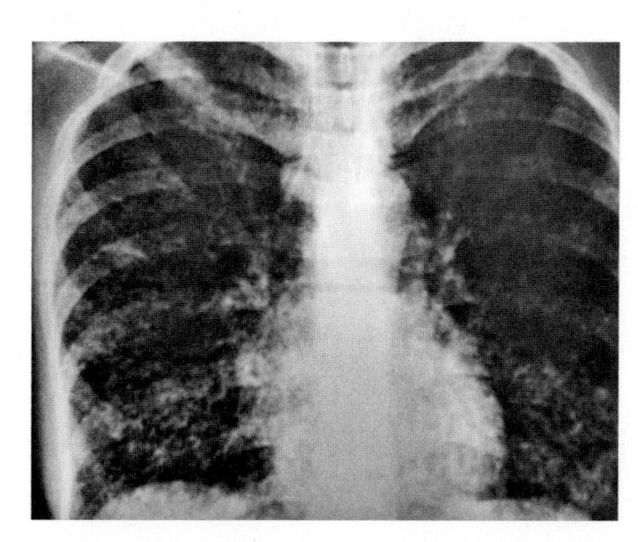

FIGURE 3-12. (Reproduced, with permission, from Bhushan V, Le T, et al. *First Aid for the USMLE Step 1: 2006*. New York: McGraw-Hill, 2006.)

- **What are the abnormal laboratory findings? Based on all the data, what is the most likely diagnosis?**

The patient's laboratory studies reveal hyponatremia, a low bicarbonate level, and leukocytosis. Diarrhea, when prolonged and severe, can cause hyponatremia. *Legionella* infection, a common source of community-acquired pneumonia (CAP), is also associated with hyponatremia. The leukocytosis suggests an immune response to some type of pathogen. The patient's subacute clinical presentation, relatively benign chest x-ray findings, and laboratory abnormalities suggest an atypical CAP such as that caused by *Mycoplasma*, *Chlamydia*, or *Legionella*.

- **An astute intern orders a commonly used urinary antigen test for CAP, which comes back positive. What does this test measure, and can it explain the patient's symptoms?**

The urinary antigen test described is likely a *Legionella* antigen test, which measures *Legionella* serotype 1. *Legionella*, as discussed above, is a possible source of the patient's symptoms.

▪ **What risk factors does the patient have for developing this condition?**	The patient's history of diabetes and smoking predisposes him to *Legionella* infection. Given his occupation as a maintenance man, he may work with air conditioning systems. As this microorganism grows in infected water sources, the patient's occupation places him at risk.
▪ **What is the best way to Gram stain and culture this microorganism? Why does it not show up when traditional Gram staining methods are used?**	*Legionella* is a gram-negative rod that can be identified using a **silver stain.** *Legionella* is primarily intracellular, which explains its poor staining characteristics. It is cultured on charcoal yeast extract agar, supplemented with iron and cysteine.
▪ **What treatments are most appropriate for this condition?**	*Legionella* responds best to antibiotics that can achieve a high intracellular concentration, such as the newer aminoglycosides (examples include erythromycin, clarithromycin, and azithromycin), quinolones, and tetracyclines. *Legionella* produces β-lactamase, and therefore cephalosporins and penicillins are ineffective.

▶ Case 20

A 41-year-old woman who is a recent immigrant from Mexico presents to a local clinic complaining of "white spots" on her body. The woman says she first noticed the lesions about 1 month ago and thought they were from the sun, but they have gradually increased in number and did not seem to improve despite her new job indoors. Physical examination reveals multiple, asymmetrically distributed, circular, hypopigmented lesions on the patient's arms, abdomen, and back (see Figure 3-13 below). The lesions are sharply demarcated, with raised, erythematous borders and atrophic, scaly centers. The lesions are anesthetic, and there is no hair growth within any of the hypopigmented areas. Biopsy of the lesions demonstrates granuloma formation within the dermal nerves of the forearm.

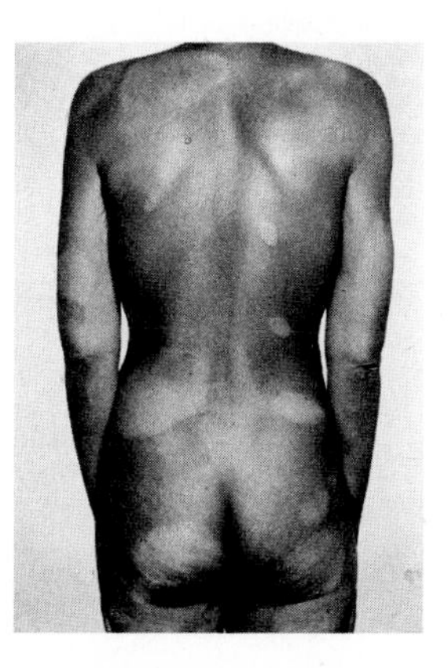

FIGURE 3-13. (Reproduced, with permission, from Wolff K, Johnson RA, Suurmond D. *Fitzpatrick's Color Atlas & Synopsis of Clinical Dermatology*, 5th ed. New York: McGraw-Hill, 2005: 657.)

▪ **What is the most likely diagnosis?**	The lesions described are characteristic for tuberculoid leprosy. Lesions in this disease typically evolve from hypopigmented, well-demarcated macules to fully developed lesions that are anesthetic and devoid of hair follicles or sweat glands.
▪ **What conditions should be included in the differential diagnosis of these lesions?**	▪ Leishmaniasis ▪ Lupus vulgaris ▪ Lymphoma ▪ Sarcoidosis ▪ Syphilis ▪ Yaws However, the biopsy findings here are pathognomonic for leprosy. Sarcoidosis causes granuloma formation around peripheral nerves, but the finding here of granulomas within the nerves is diagnostic of leprosy.
▪ **Describe the microorganism that causes this condition.**	Both lepromatous and tuberculoid leprosy are caused by *Mycobacterium leprae*, an acid-fast bacillus that cannot be grown in vitro. *M. leprae* is an obligate intracellular bacillus that, like other mycobacteria, contains mycolic acid in its cell wall. *M. leprae* grows best in cooler temperatures (skin, peripheral nerves, testes, upper respiratory tract).

How does this patient's condition differ from the more severe form?	Tuberculoid leprosy is a disease largely confined to the skin (hypopigmented macules) and peripheral nerves. Cell-mediated immunity is intact, and patients' T cells recognize *M. leprae* (positive lepromin skin test). Lepromatous leprosy holds a much worse prognosis because patients have ineffective cell-mediated immunity (negative lepromin skin test). Skin lesions and nerve involvement are much more extensive than in the tuberculoid form, and there may be involvement of the testes, upper respiratory tract, and anterior chamber of the eye.
What treatment is most appropriate for this condition?	Both tuberculoid and lepromatous leprosy can be treated with a course of oral dapsone. The tuberculoid form is reliably cured by a short course of this medication. Patients with lepromatous leprosy have an exceptionally high bacterial load and may require an extended or even lifelong course of chemotherapy. Alternate therapies for leprosy include rifampin or a combination of clofazimine and dapsone.

▶ Case 21

The mother of a 1-week-old female infant calls her pediatrician because the infant has been fussy all morning. The infant's temperature is 39° C (102.2° F), and the mother is asked to bring the infant to the hospital for further workup and treatment. The workup includes cerebrospinal fluid (CSF) analysis, hematology studies, and cultures. Empiric antibiotic therapy is initiated. Later, upon microscopic examination of the CSF, microorganisms with tumbling end-over-end motility are visualized.

- **What is the most likely diagnosis?**

  Meningitis due to *Listeria* infection. This microorganism, identifiable by its classical tumbling motility, is a gram-positive rod.

- **What findings are most likely on laboratory testing?**

  The WBC count would likely be elevated. The WBC differential would show predominantly neutrophils and/or monocytes. Protein levels may be elevated, and glucose levels should be normal or decreased. The microorganisms visualized in the CSF are bacteria. Compare this CSF profile to CSF profiles seen in fungal or viral CSF infections (see Table 3-1 below).

- **What microorganisms should empiric antibiotic therapy target?**

  Group B streptococcus, *Escherichia coli*, and *Listeria monocytogenes* are the most common causes of sepsis and bacterial meningitis in infants <1 month old. Other notable causes of sepsis/meningitis in this age group include *Streptococcus pneumoniae*, *Haemophilus influenzae*, *Staphylococcus aureus*, *Neisseria meningitidis*, and *Salmonella*.

- **How does this microorganism evade the host immune response?**

  L. monocytogenes is a facultative intracellular bacterium able to survive in the macrophages of neonates and immunosuppressed patients. In an immunocompetent host, activation of macrophages will destroy phagocytosed *Listeria*.

- **What treatment is most appropriate for this condition?**

  Ampicillin and gentamicin. Ampicillin disrupts cell wall synthesis, resulting in increased uptake of gentamicin into bacterial cells.

TABLE 3-1. CSF Findings in Meningitis

	PRESSURE	CELL TYPE	PROTEIN	SUGAR
Bacterial	↑	↑ PMNs	↑	↓
Fungal/TB	↑	↑ lymphocytes	↑	↓
Viral	Normal/↑	↑ lymphocytes	Normal	Normal

Reproduced, with permission, from Bhushan V, Le T, et al. *First Aid for the USMLE Step 1: 2006.* New York: McGraw-Hill, 2006: 200.

GENERAL PRINCIPLES

MICROBIOLOGY & IMMUNOLOGY

▶ Case 22

A 49-year-old man comes to the clinic complaining of vertigo and fatigue for the past day. He has no chronic health conditions, and enjoys walking several miles a day in the park for exercise. Physical examination reveals a bull's-eye-shaped rash on the patient's left shoulder, as depicted in Figure 3-14 below.

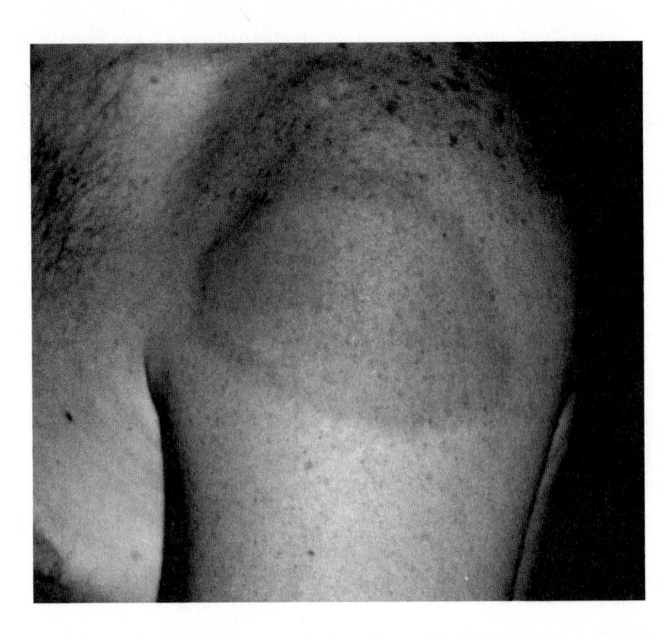

FIGURE 3-14. (Reproduced, with permission, from Wolff K, Johnson RA, Suurmond D. *Fitzpatrick's Color Atlas & Synopsis of Clinical Dermatology*, 5th ed. New York: McGraw-Hill, 2005: 679.)

■ **What is the most likely diagnosis?**	Lyme disease. This disease is caused by *Borrelia burgdorferi*, a spirochete that is a gram-negative, corkscrew-shaped bacterium too small to be visualized under light microscopy. They are better visualized using **dark-field microscopy,** immunologic staining, or silver stains.
■ **How are human beings infected?**	The ***Ixodes*** **tick** can transmit *B. burgdorferi* from white-footed mice, other small rodents, and white-tailed deer to man by attaching to a person **for at least 24 hours.** Checking for ticks at least once a day can prevent infection resulting from a tick bite.
■ **What is the name for the rash on the patient's shoulder?**	**Erythema chronicum migrans.** This name describes the ring of erythema that migrates outward (over time) from the site of the tick bite.
■ **What organs are affected in the early disseminated stage of infection?**	■ Heart (heart block, myocarditis) ■ Musculoskeletal system (arthritis) ■ Nervous system (encephalitis, Bell's palsy, peripheral neuropathy) ■ Skin (erythema chronicum migrans)

■ **In the detection of anti-*B. burgdorferi* antibodies, some protocols recommend using enzyme-linked immunosorbent assays (ELISA) first. If anti-*B. burgdorferi* antibodies are found using ELISA, then a Western blot is performed. What can be inferred about the sensitivity and specificity of these two tests?**	Since ELISA is used as a screen, it must be a relatively sensitive test. However, Western blots must be more specific, since it is used to confirm the presence of the antibody in question.
■ **What treatment is most appropriate for this condition?**	Doxycycline or amoxicillin is used for primary infection. For disseminated infection (ie, cardiac or central nervous system involvement), ceftriaxone is preferred. Doxycycline or azithromycin is used for arthritis.

▶ **Case 23**

While doing a rotation in Ghana, a medical student encounters a patient who has been having nearly continuous high-grade fever with occasional chills and sweats. Physical examination reveals a palpable spleen. A drop of the patient's blood placed in a copper sulfate solution reveals the patient is anemic. Over the next few days, while waiting for medication to arrive, the patient's level of consciousness waxes and wanes, and the patient is somnolent at times.

▪ **What is the most likely diagnosis?**	Malaria, most likely due to *Plasmodium falciparum*. The symptoms give a clue as to the species. This patient's continuous fever and irregular chills and sweats are characteristic of *P. falciparum* malaria. In contrast, *P. vivax* and *P. ovale* cause episodes of fever, chills, and sweats every 48 hours. With *P. malariae*, these episodes occur every 72 hours. The patient's altered mental status may support a diagnosis of *P. falciparum* malaria, since this is the only strain that has cerebral involvement.
▪ **What phase of the microorganism's life cycle results in the development of anemia?**	RBC lysis occurs during the erythrocytic cycle, when the products of asexual replication inside the RBCs (the **merozoite** form) are released. The immune response to the merozoites, and resultant cytokine release, is responsible for the fever, chills, and sweats.
▪ **What would be the likely findings on peripheral blood smear (PBS)?**	A PBS is likely to show ring-shaped trophozoites inside the RBCs (see Figure 3-15 below), and there may be several trophozoites per RBC. More rarely, **schizonts**, the large, multinucleated cell formed from the trophozoite by multiple cycles of nuclear division, may be visible in the erythrocytes. Outside the RBCs, oblong **gametocytes** may also be visible.
▪ **In an area without drug-resistant microorganisms, what is the drug of choice for treating this condition?**	Chloroquine is the drug of choice in areas where there is no resistance. Its major mode of action against *Plasmodium* is inhibition of the enzyme responsible for polymerizing heme. This results in the accumulation of free heme, which is toxic to the protozoan.
▪ **In areas where drug resistance is high, what are the drugs of choice for treating this condition?**	Quinidine plus tetracycline or doxycycline or pyrimethamine/sulfadoxine and mefloquine plus malarone may be used in areas where resistant *P. falciparum* is endemic.

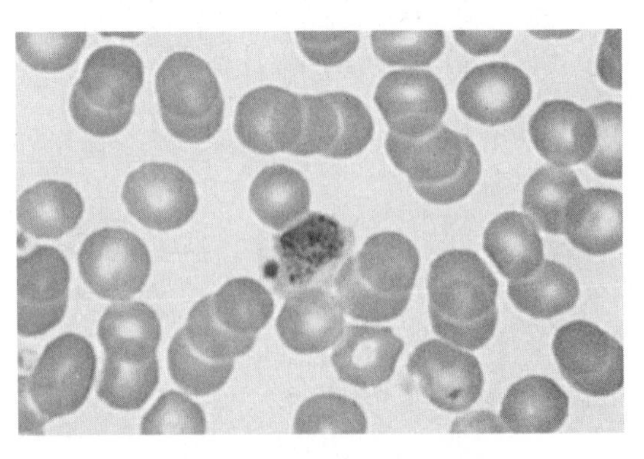

FIGURE 3-15. Trophozoite in RBC in malaria. (Reproduced, with permission, from Lichtman MA, Beutler E, Kipps TJ, et al. *Williams Hematology*, 7th ed. New York: McGraw-Hill, 2006: Plate I-11.)

► Case 24

A 4-year-old girl is brought to her pediatrician by her mother because she has been experiencing flulike symptoms. The child is pale and febrile, and her respiratory rate is 25/min. Her buccal mucosa has multiple blue-gray spots, and she has a maculopapular rash. Upon questioning, the mother admits the child's immunizations are not up to date. The physician orders that the girl stay home from preschool and avoid all unvaccinated contacts in the family.

What is the most likely diagnosis?	Measles, one of the most transmissible viral infections.
What microorganism causes this disease, and how does it cause illness?	Measles is caused by an RNA virus that is a member of the genus *Morbillivirus* and the family Paramyxoviridae. Respiratory droplets from the host breech respiratory tract epithelium, resulting in viremia. Spread to the mucosa, dermis, respiratory tract, and brain causes the illnesses' clinical presentation.
What signs and symptoms are associated with this condition?	Clinical presentation includes flulike symptoms, **Koplik's spots** (bluish-gray spots on the buccal mucosa), and a maculopapular rash that starts at the head and moves to the feet (as shown in an older patient in Figure 3-16 below). Respiratory tract involvement causes rhinorrhea and cough. Involvement of the brain can result in meningitis or encephalitis. A variant form of measles called subacute sclerosing panencephalitis (SSPE) causes slowly progressive neurological disease, which eventually leads to death.
What tests can help confirm the diagnosis, and which clinical findings are pathognomonic for the condition?	Diagnosis can be confirmed by isolating virus from nasopharyngeal secretions, blood, or urine. Koplik's spots on the mucosa and/or **Warthin-Finkeldey cells** (multinucleated giant cells with inclusion bodies in the nucleus and cytoplasm) in the respiratory secretions are pathognomonic.
What treatment is most appropriate for this condition?	No treatment is available for active infection. Vaccination with the live attenuated measles virus in the MMR (measles-mumps-rubella) vaccine is available.

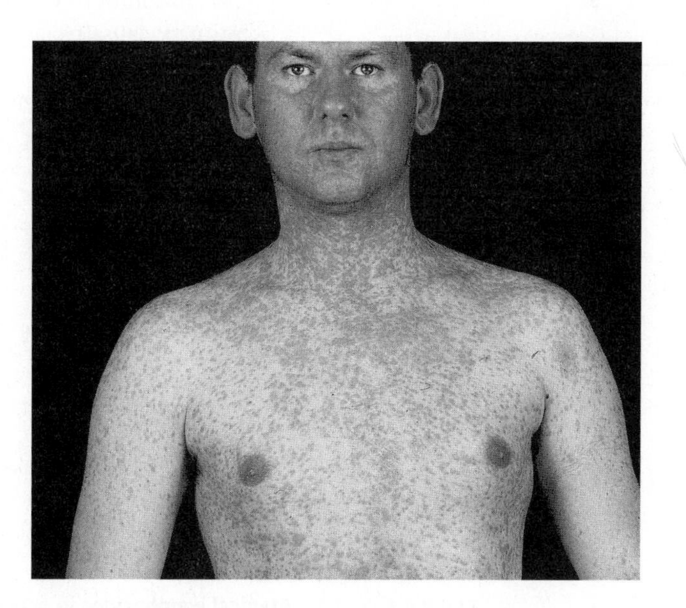

FIGURE 3-16. Measles rash. (Reproduced, with permission, from Wolff K, Johnson RA, Suurmond D. *Fitzpatrick's Color Atlas & Synopsis of Clinical Dermatology*, 5th ed. New York: McGraw-Hill, 2005: 788.)

▶ **Case 25**

A 19-year-old college sophomore comes to the university health clinic complaining of a worsening sore throat, headache, and fatigue of 1 week's duration. The young man has a slightly elevated temperature of 37.7° C (99.8° F). Physical examination reveals enlarged, tender cervical lymph nodes and a palpable spleen. His throat is notable for a gray-green tonsillar exudate.

▪ **What is the most likely diagnosis?**	Infectious mononucleosis, caused by Epstein-Barr virus (EBV).
▪ **To confirm the clinical diagnosis, a Monospot test is performed. What is the basis of this test?**	When infected with EBV, many people synthesize antibody that is cross-reactive with a surface antigen on sheep RBCs called **heterophile antibody.** The Monospot test uses serum from the patient added to sheep RBCs. A positive test results in agglutination of the RBCs. This test is the most sensitive and specific available for confirming EBV infection.
▪ **What would be the likely findings on peripheral blood smear (PBS)?**	**Atypical lymphocytes** are the hallmark finding on PBS during acute infectious mononucleosis (see Figure 3-17 below). These cells are activated T lymphocytes with a large amount of cytoplasm. However, it should be noted that atypical lymphocytes may also be found with other infections (eg, cytomegalovirus, rubella, toxoplasmosis), some malignancies, and as a result of drug reactions.
▪ **Describe the infective microorganism in this case.**	EBV is an enveloped, double-stranded, linear DNA virus (like cytomegalovirus, varicella zoster, and herpes simplex virus). EBV preferentially infects B lymphocytes—the virus adheres to the C3d complement receptor found on the surface of B cells.
▪ **Infection with this microorganism has been associated with which two major malignancies?**	▪ **Burkitt's lymphoma** affects children in central Africa. EBV is believed to be a cofactor for the malignancy, as children in other parts of the world infected with EBV rarely develop Burkitt's lymphoma. The disease is a B-cell lymphoma and often presents with a tumor of the jaw. ▪ **Nasopharyngeal carcinoma** is one of the most common cancers in southern China, where evidence supports EBV as the primary causative agent in this neoplasm.

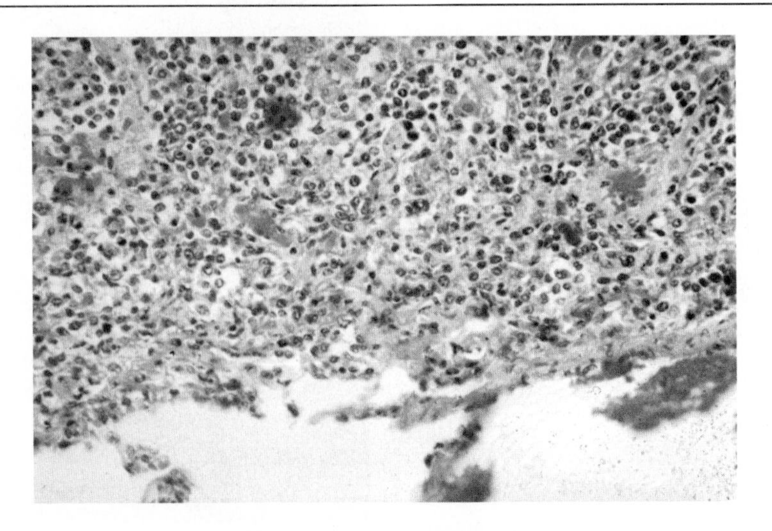

FIGURE 3-17. Atypical lymphocytes in acute infectious mononucleosis. (Reproduced with permission of the Pathology Education Instructional Resource Digital Library (http://peir.net) at the University of Alabama, Birmingham.)

► Case 26

A 21-year-old man from Guatemala presents to the physician with a 2-day history of painful unilateral testicular swelling. The patient admits to minimal fever and myalgias about a week earlier. Physical examination reveals the parotid glands are swollen and painful. No vaccination history is available, but the patient does not believe that he received any shots when he was younger.

▪ **What is the most likely diagnosis?**	Mumps. In rare instances, the orchitis described above can affect both testes. This can lead to sterility.
▪ **What microorganism causes this disease, and how does it cause illness?**	The mumps virus is a member of the Paramyxoviridae family, which are single-stranded RNA viruses. The virus breeches the 2- to 3-week incubation period; infection results in painful enlargement (inflammation and edema) of glandular tissues including the parotid gland, testes, and ovaries.
▪ **What other clinical syndrome can result from infection with this microorganism?**	If the viral infection spreads to the meninges, **aseptic meningitis** may develop. This virus, along with coxsackievirus and echovirus, is one of the three most common causes of aseptic meningitis. However, as a result of the mumps vaccination program in the United States, coxsackievirus and other enteroviridiae cause substantially more cases of aseptic meningitis than does the mumps virus.
▪ **What tests can help confirm the diagnosis?**	The virus can be detected in the saliva, serum, urine, or cerebrospinal fluid.
▪ **What treatment is most appropriate for this condition?**	The treatment is supportive and directed at reducing pain. Analgesics and compression of the parotid gland can be useful. The live attenuated rubella virus (found in the MMR—measles-mumps-rubella) vaccine is used to prevent disease.

► Case 27

An 18-year-old college freshman is brought to the university health center by his dormitory roommate. The patient complains of 2 days of fever, several episodes of vomiting, and joint and muscle pain. His temperature is 38.9° C (102° F). Physical examination reveals nuchal rigidity, a petechial rash on the lower extremities, and photophobia.

■ **What is the most likely diagnosis?**	*Neisseria meningitidis* meningitis.
■ **What test can confirm the diagnosis?**	Lumbar puncture would show gram-negative, bean-shaped diplococci, an elevated WBC count (with mainly polymorphonuclear cells), decreased glucose levels, and normal to high protein levels.
■ **What laboratory test can confirm the pathogen involved?**	Culture of meningococcus from cerebrospinal fluid or blood on Thayer-Martin media (chocolate agar with antibiotics to kill competing bacteria) can positively identify *N. meningitidis*. Additionally, *Neisseria* is oxidase positive.
■ **What are some of the most important virulence factors of this microorganism?**	■ **Pili:** involved in attachment to nasopharyngeal epithelial cells that serve as both reservoir site and inoculation site ■ **IgA protease:** cleaves lysosome-associated membrane protein 1, which promotes survival within epithelial cells ■ **Endotoxin:** lipopolysaccharide in the cell wall that induces sepsis and hemorrhage (causes the characteristic petechial rash seen in meningococcemia) ■ **Capsule:** polyanionic polysaccharides that serve as physical protection from host defense factors such as complement and phagocytosis; serogrouping is possible based on immunochemical differences in the capsule ■ No exotoxins!
■ **What treatment is most appropriate for this condition?**	Penicillin G or ceftriaxone. Contacts of the index case may be given rifampin as prophylaxis.

▶ Case 28

A 35-year-old woman is seen in a clinic in a riverside South American village. She complains of itchy, hyperpigmented skin and nodules on her right cheek. Visual testing reveals she has decreased visual acuity of her right eye. Fundoscopic examination reveals the movement of a microorganism in the sclera of her right eye.

What is the most likely diagnosis?	Onchocerciasis (river blindness), which is caused by *Onchocerca volvulus*. This organism is a nematode (roundworm), and is found near rivers.
How is this organism transmitted, and how does it cause illness?	The bite of a female black fly transmits larvae (microfilariae) into the host's skin. The larvae become adults, and subsequent fibrosis around the adult worms results in subcutaneous nodules. From within the nodule, mating and release of new larvae can occur. The movement of larvae through subcutaneous tissue induces an inflammatory response.
What signs and symptoms are associated with this condition?	Inflammation of subcutaneous tissue causes itching, thickening, and hyperpigmentation of the skin. If the larvae reach the eye, the inflammation can cause blindness.
What tests can help confirm the diagnosis?	A skin biopsy reveals larvae. Nodules will contain adult roundworms.
What treatments are most appropriate for this condition?	Ivermectin is effective against the larvae (microfiliarae). Surgical removal of subcutaneous nodules is effective in eliminating adult worms.

▶ Case 29

A 30-year-old man presents to the emergency department with complaints of extreme throbbing pain in his right shin, in addition to chills and myalgias. He was previously healthy but did undergo surgery to the knee 3 weeks prior. His temperature is 40° C (104° F), blood pressure is 130/80 mm Hg, and heart rate is 80/min. Physical examination reveals his right leg is red, tender, warm, and swollen over the right anterior tibia just below the knee. X-ray of the extremity demonstrates periosteal elevation and changes consistent with soft tissue swelling adjacent to the tibia. The patient is admitted, and blood and bone biopsy cultures are pending.

▪ **What is the most likely diagnosis?**	Osteomyelitis. *Staphylococcus aureus* is responsible for about 90% of pyogenic osteomyelitis. S. *aureus* expresses receptors for the bone matrix, thus allowing it to adhere to bone and produce a focus of infection. Affected adults usually have a previous history of a compound fracture or surgery. Children may develop osteomyelitis secondary to hematogenous spread.
▪ **If this man has a history of intravenous drug use, which pathogen should be considered?**	Osteomyelitis in the context of intravenous drug use is often caused by *Pseudomonas* infection, but S. *aureus* is still more common in this population.
▪ **What type of malignant tumor is this man at higher risk for developing?**	**Sarcomas** can be derived from bone, as well as other mesenchymal tissue such as muscle.
▪ **How does a subperiosteal abscess lead to accelerated bone necrosis?**	A subperiosteal abscess separates the bone from its blood supply in the periosteum, thus leading to ischemic injury and necrosis.
▪ **A history of sickle cell disease would place this patient at increased risk of infection from which pathogen?**	Patients with sickle cell disease have an increased risk of developing *Salmonella* osteomyelitis.
▪ **What are the typical findings on imaging?**	Periosteal elevation is often found on radiography. This finding, however, can lag the onset of the infection by days to weeks.

► Case 30

A 4-year-old boy is brought to the pediatrician because of perianal itching, which is worse at night. He attends preschool during the day, where he shares toys and play areas with other children. The patient's mother recalls her son playing with another child who had been "scratching his backside" and wonders if there is a connection.

■ **What is the most likely diagnosis?**	Pinworm infection caused by *Enterobius vermicularis,* a nematode (roundworm).
■ **How is this organism transmitted, and how does it cause illness?**	Fecal-oral ingestion allows eggs to hatch in the small intestine. Adults mature in the ileum and large intestine and mate in the colon. Females exit the rectum at night to lay eggs in the perianal area.
■ **What symptom is commonly associated with this condition?**	Perianal itching, especially at night, when the worm exits the anus to lay its eggs.
■ **What test can help confirm the diagnosis?**	The **Scotch tape test:** The physician places adhesive tape over the perianal area and removes it. The presence of eggs under light microscopy is indicative of pinworm infection.
■ **What treatments are most appropriate for this condition?**	Mebendazole or albendazole is first-line therapy. Pyrantel pamoate can also be helpful.

▶ Case 31

A 52-year-old woman with acquired immunodeficiency syndrome (AIDS) presents to her physician with difficulty breathing. She has experienced a slowly worsening dry cough in addition to dyspnea for about 1 week prior to presentation. Her most recent $CD4^+$ T cell count is 175 cells/μL. In the office, her oxygen saturation is 92%. The patient relates she is not currently taking any medications because she is "tired of taking pills."

▪ **What is the most likely diagnosis?**	*Pneumocystis jiroveci* (formerly *carinii*) pneumonia. *P. jiroveci* causes interstitial pneumonia in certain patient populations. Once thought to be a protozoan, it is now recognized to be a fungus (yeast).
▪ **What patients are most at risk for developing clinical infection with this microorganism?**	Most individuals are exposed to *P. jiroveci* during childhood, but develop no symptoms. However, immunocompromised patients (including patients with AIDS who have low CD4+ cell counts) and malnourished infants may develop severe clinical disease.
▪ **What would be the likely findings on x-ray of the chest?**	**"Ground glass"** bilateral infiltrates are commonly seen on x-ray of the chest (see Figure 3-18 below). In these patients, hypoxia (characterized by decreased arterial oxygen pressure) is often out of proportion to the radiographic findings.
▪ **What tests can help confirm the diagnosis?**	Sputum samples, bronchoalveolar lavage, or lung biopsy treated with **silver stain** will demonstrate cysts and dark oval bodies contained within the cyst **(sporozoites).**
▪ **What treatment is most appropriate for this condition?**	Treatment is trimethoprim-sulfamethoxazole, pentamidine, or clindamycin-primaquine. In immunocompromised patients, trimethoprim-sulfamethoxazole or dapsone may be used as prophylaxis when CD4+ cell counts fall below 200 cells/μL.

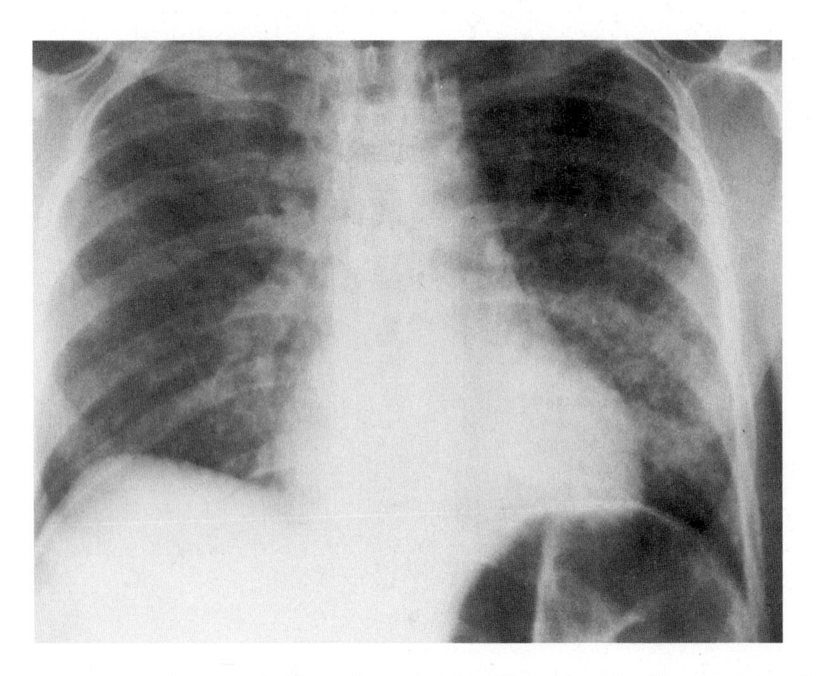

FIGURE 3-18. *Pneumocystis jiroveci* pneumonia. (Reproduced, with permission, from Kasper DL, Braunwald E, Fauci AS, Hauser SL, Longo DL, Jameson LJ, Isselbacher KJ [eds]. *Harrison's Principles of Internal Medicine*, 16th ed. New York: McGraw-Hill, 2005: 1195.)

► Case 32

A 20-year-old woman returns from a day hike in a densely wooded area, and develops a rash that evening. The next day she presents to her physician. The patient has never had a similar rash, and the area is one of her favorite hiking spots. Physical examination reveals the rash (see Figure 3-19 below) is mostly on the legs, arms, and hands, areas the patient says "were not covered by clothing." The patient has no significant past medical history. She is afebrile.

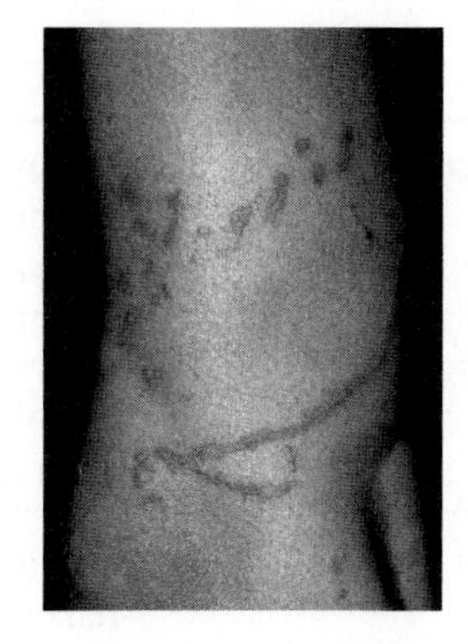

FIGURE 3-19. (Reproduced, with permission, from Wolff K, Johnson RA, Suurmond D. *Fitzpatrick's Color Atlas & Synopsis of Clinical Dermatology*, 5th ed. New York: McGraw-Hill, 2005: 29.)

▪ **What is the most likely diagnosis?**	Poison ivy. This rash is characterized by vesicles, fluid-filled domes <5 mm in diameter. The leaves of poison ivy brush across the skin in a linear path; thus, the typical poison ivy rash consists of lines of vesicles, as seen in the image above.
▪ **What are the four types of hypersensitivity reactions?**	▪ **Type I:** Anaphylactic and atopic ▪ **Type II:** Cytotoxic ▪ **Type III:** Immune complex/serum sickness/arthus reaction ▪ **Type IV:** Delayed/cell-mediated
▪ **Which type of hypersensitivity reaction is occurring in this patient?**	Type IV hypersensitivity (delayed, or cell-mediated) includes contact hypersensitivity from poison ivy, transplant rejection, hypersensitivity pneumonitis, granulomatous hypersensitivity reactions, and the tuberculosis skin test. Type IV reactions are also important in the control of mycobacterial and fungal infections.
▪ **Which cells mediate the immune response in this condition?**	**Type 1 T-helper cells** and **CD8** cytotoxic T cells are the mediators of this immune response.
▪ **Why is this rash occurring now, when she has hiked the area many times previously without developing this rash?**	A key feature of type IV hypersensitivity is that the patient must be sensitized to the antigen prior to development of hypersensitivity on subsequent exposure. The tuberculin skin test, another example of type IV hypersensitivity, relies on the principle of prior sensitization to assess for previous exposure to tuberculosis.
▪ **The oil that causes the skin reaction in this patient's condition (urushiol or pentadecacatechol) can bind to antibodies, but cannot elicit an adaptive immune response on its own. It must be linked to a protein to elicit an adaptive immune response. What term describes this type of molecule?**	A **hapten** is a small molecule that is not immunogenic by itself, but can become so when attached to a carrier protein.

► **Case 33**

A 27-year-old graduate student who recently returned from working in sub-Saharan Africa presents to the clinic complaining of paralysis of his lower extremities. He says he had a mild fever about 2 weeks previously, then several days ago the fever recurred and he experienced nuchal rigidity, followed by paralysis of both legs. The student was not born in the United States and his vaccination history is unknown. Physical examination demonstrates 0/5 strength and hyporeflexia (without sensory loss) of the lower extremities.

▪ **What is the most likely diagnosis?**	Poliovirus can cause subclinical infection, aseptic meningitis, or poliomyelitis. **Poliomyelitis** results in the classis flaccid paralysis secondary to destruction of anterior horn cells of the spinal cord.
▪ **This microorganism is a member of which family?**	Poliovirus is a member of the Picornavirus family. Other members include echovirus, rhinovirus, coxsackievirus, and hepatitis A virus.
▪ **Describe the morphology of this microorganism.**	Poliovirus is a single-stranded, positive-sense RNA virus with naked icosahedral symmetry.
▪ **How is this condition transmitted?**	Via the fecal-oral route. The virus has a tropism for Peyer's patches of the intestine and motor neurons, explaining its transmission and pathology.
▪ **What treatments are available to prevent this illness, and how do they differ?**	▪ Salk vaccine: formalin-killed virus leads to an IgG response. ▪ Sabin vaccine: oral attenuated poliovirus leads to an IgG response as well as an IgA response in the gastrointestinal tract. This vaccine should not be given to immunocompromised individuals.

▶ Case 34

An 18-year-old man with cystic fibrosis and a history of multiple respiratory infections is brought to the emergency department after recent onset of cough productive of purulent sputum, dyspnea, and chills. His mother reports he has been lethargic, and recorded his temperature at 39° C (102.2° F). Physical examination reveals a poorly responsive man in moderate respiratory distress. Laboratory studies are notable for a WBC count of $17,000/mm^3$, with a left shift on the differential. Sputum culture yields gram-negative, non–lactose-fermenting bacilli.

- **What is the most likely diagnosis?**

Pseudomonas aeruginosa infection. This bacterium is an opportunistic pathogen, and causes infection in patients with impaired defense mechanisms, especially immunocompromised individuals and burn victims. It commonly lives in water or wet environments and can be particularly problematic for patients on ventilators. Additionally, it is the major cause of respiratory failure in patients with cystic fibrosis.

- **What are some common consequences of infection with this microorganism?**

Community-acquired infections:
- Endocarditis (in intravenous drug users)
- Osteomyelitis
- Otitis externa after swimming in freshwater
- Peritonitis
- Pneumonia (especially in patients with human immunodeficiency virus infection or cystic fibrosis)

Nosocomial *Pseudomonas* infections:
- Bacteremia in neutropenic patients
- Burn sepsis
- Lung infection associated with ventilator use
- Neonatal sepsis
- Urinary tract infection from indwelling Foley catheters

- **What is the pathology of chronic respiratory infection with this microorganism in patients with cystic fibrosis?**

Pseudomonas can colonize the lungs of patients with cystic fibrosis, where it may survive for up to 40 years. During this time, the patient's immune response leads to a chronic inflammatory state that eventually results in progressive loss of pulmonary function.

- **What virulence factors contribute to acute infection with this microorganism?**

Pseudomonas has a host of virulence factors that contribute to pathology in acute infection. These include pili and a flagellum for host invasion; lipopolysaccharide (endotoxin); exotoxins A, S, and U; elastase; and various cytotoxins.

- **What treatments are most appropriate for this condition?**

Pseudomonas is frequently resistant to multiple drug regimens. In addition to its intrinsic resistance to many antibiotics, it is able to acquire resistance rapidly during treatment. Potentially useful antibiotic regimens include ceftazidime, ciprofloxacin, aztreonam, or imipenem plus an aminoglycoside, piperacillin-tazobactam plus tobramycin, and the fourth-generation cephalosporin cefepime. Colistin is a drug of last resort for severe cases of multidrug-resistant *Pseudomonas* infection.

► **Case 35**

A 15-year-old boy is camping with his family in the Adirondack Mountains when he is bitten on his leg by a raccoon. His family cuts the vacation short and brings the boy to the nearest emergency department.

■ **What disease is this boy at risk of contracting?**	Rabies. If left untreated, rabies results in a nearly 100% mortality rate. It causes, at most, a few deaths per year in the United States, but is a much bigger concern in countries with unvaccinated animals. (In India, rabies-infected dog bites cause tens of thousands of deaths each year.)
■ **What microorganism is the cause of this disease, and what are its characteristics?**	Rhabdoviridae are single-stranded RNA viruses enveloped by a bullet-shaped capsid, which is covered by glycoprotein "spikes." The spikes bind to acetylcholine receptors and thus contribute to virulence.
■ **How is this microorganism transmitted, and how does it cause illness?**	Animals transfer the virus to humans via bites. The virus remains local for a period of days to months, then binds to acetylcholine receptors to enter the peripheral nervous system. The virus then travels to the central nervous system (CNS); the starting distance of the inoculate from the CNS determines incubation time. In the CNS, the virus infects neurons, including Ammon's horn cells of the hippocampus.
■ **What signs and symptoms are commonly associated with this disease?**	Spasms of the pharyngeal muscles cause dysphagia (buildup of saliva causes "foaming at the mouth"); the dysphagia causes hydrophobia. As rabies travels via axons to various organs and multiplies in the CNS, many symptoms result: confusion, agitation, hallucinations, sensitivity to bright light, and focal neurological deficits such as cranial nerve palsies. Encephalitis can give rise to seizures and eventually leads to coma then death.
■ **How is the disease diagnosed, and what kinds of treatment are available?**	Identification of cytoplasmic inclusions called **Negri bodies** in infected cells, polymerase chain reaction for viral RNA, and serology are diagnostic. Treatment includes washing the wound and administering **human diploid cell vaccine,** a live, attenuated virus that is used after a bite. **Human rabies immune globulin** is used to confer passive immunity, and immunization of domesticated animals is used to prevent the disease. Unfortunately, once symptoms appear, no treatment is effective.

▶ Case 36

A 30-year-old man who recently joined a gym complains of itching between his toes. Physical examination reveals pustules on the fingers of both hands, and white macerated tissue between the toes (see Figure 3-20 below). The patient says the pustules have been quite itchy, and appeared about a week after the itching between the toes began.

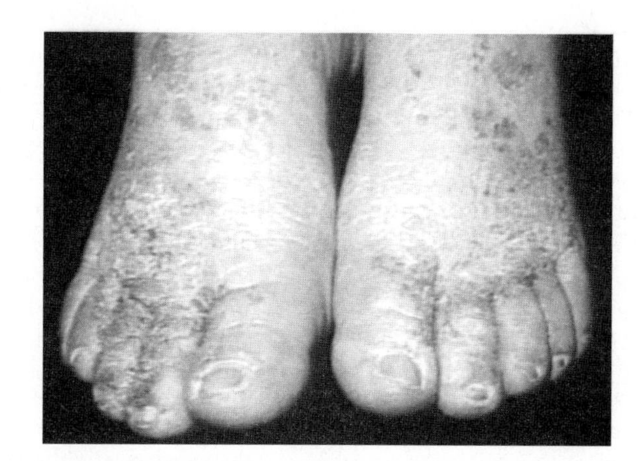

FIGURE 3-20. (Reproduced with permission of the Pathology Education Instructional Resource Digital Library (http://peir.net) at the University of Alabama, Birmingham.)

What is the most likely diagnosis?	Ringworm (tinea pedis) infection. Each dermatophytosis is named after the region of the body it is infecting: tinea cruris (creases of inner thigh, "jock itch"), tinea pedis ("athlete's foot"), tinea capitis (scalp), tinea unguium (nails), and tinea corporis (body).
What are the three microorganisms that are often responsible for this presentation?	*Microsporum*, *Trichophyton*, and *Epidermophyton* are three filamentous fungi that cause dermatophytosis.
How is the microorganism transmitted, and how does it cause illness?	After contact with an infected host, the keratinized epithelium of warm, moist skin is colonized. The infection expands radially, and is characterized by curvy (worm-like) borders. Thus, it is termed "ringworm," despite the fact that the microorganism is actually a fungus.
What tests can help confirm the diagnosis?	Branched hyphae are observed on potassium hydroxide preparation **(KOH mount).** This fungus is not dimorphic. However, the pustules on this patient's hand will not reveal any microorganisms. They are the result of fungal antigens (not the actual fungus) diffusing systemically, resulting in hypersensitivity reactions (such as pustules) at remote sites.
What treatment is most appropriate for this condition?	Topical azoles (butenafine, terbinafine), fluconazole, or griseofulvin.

▶ Case 37

In the month of January, a 2-year-old girl is brought to her pediatrician by her parents because of a 3-day history of watery, nonbloody diarrhea, nausea, vomiting, and abdominal pain. Physical examination reveals the child is slightly tachycardic, and has sunken eyes and poor skin turgor.

What is the most likely diagnosis?	Rotavirus infection is the most common infectious cause of diarrhea in infants and young children, and it is a major cause of acute diarrhea in the United States during the winter. It is also the most important cause of gastroenteritis in infants globally.
How does the microorganism cause illness?	The microorganism is transmitted via the fecal-oral route and infects villus cells of the proximal small intestine. The virus replicates intracellularly and eventually causes host cell lysis. Cell destruction results in decreased absorption, which leads to vomiting and watery diarrhea. Rotavirus does not cause inflammation, so the stool is nonbloody.
Describe the characteristics of this microorganism.	Rotavirus belongs to the Reoviridae family, which also contains the reoviruses and orbiviruses. These naked viruses are the only RNA viruses that are double stranded (think: "repeato"-viridae). The viruses contain 10 or 11 segments of dsRNA, allowing for frequent gene reassortment.
How is this condition diagnosed, and how is it treated?	The virus can be identified by enzyme-linked immunosorbent assay of a stool specimen. Treatment is supportive via rehydration.
In what age group is this condition usually seen?	Infection is not commonly seen before 6 months of age, as the child has passive immunity from IgA passed from the mother's breast milk. By age 3 years, most individuals worldwide have developed lifelong immunity from prior infection.

► Case 38

A 21-year-old woman presents to the clinic with fever, hives, headache, weight loss, and cough. She reports doing field research in Africa with a professor from her university over the summer. When the patient is asked about previous fresh water exposure, she recalls an intense itching reaction within minutes of wading into a river while she was in Africa. Physical examination reveals lymphadenopathy and hepatosplenomegaly.

■ **What is the most likely diagnosis?**	Schistosomiasis, caused by a type of trematode (fluke), likely acquired from contact with contaminated water. The three main flukes are *Schistosoma japonicum* (in East Asia), *S. mansoni* (in South America and Africa), and *S. haematobium* (in Africa).
■ **What is the intermediate host of this organism, and what are the reservoirs?**	Snails are the intermediate host for all trematodes. Reservoirs include primates (*S. mansoni* and *S. haematobium*) and domesticated animals (*S. japonicum*).
■ **These organisms are found in which human organs?**	*S. japonicum* and *S. mansoni* reside in the intestines, where organisms mate in the mesenteric veins and release eggs into the feces. *S. haematobium* resides in the bladder, where organisms mate in the vesicular (bladder) veins and deposit eggs in the urine.
■ **How is this condition diagnosed?**	Examination of the urine (*S. haematobium*) and stool (all three species), or rectal biopsy, will reveal eggs.
■ **What are the acute and chronic manifestations of this condition?**	An immediate manifestation of schistosomiasis is **swimmer's itch,** a dermatitis that occurs as the organism initially penetrates the skin. Manifestations 4–8 weeks after infection include **Katayama fever,** which occurs as the adult organisms lay eggs. Chronic manifestations include granulomas, fibrosis, and inflammation at the sites of egg deposition. Complications include portal hypertension (*S. japonicum, S. mansoni*), pulmonary artery hypertension, chronic abdominal pain, and central nervous system injury. *S. haematobium* can increase the risk for developing bladder cancer.
■ **What treatment is most appropriate for this condition?**	Praziquantel is the treatment of choice.

▶ **Case 39**

A 59-year-old woman complains of fatigue and a "burning" pain on her scalp for the 2 previous days. Her temperature is 38° C (100.4° F). Physical examination indicates her pain is localized to the left parietal-occipital scalp, and extends down to include the skin of the left side of her neck. She denies any recent rash in the area, headaches, mental status changes, or recent infections.

- **Which sensory nerve root is implicated in this patient's condition?**

Nerves from the right C2 root innervate the parietal-occipital scalp. C3 innervates the neck, and C4 innervates the superior surface of the shoulder.

- **What laboratory process can be used to help detect the presence of a suspected pathogen's genome in a sample?**

Polymerase chain reaction (PCR) can be used to amplify and aid in the detection of the double-stranded DNA of herpes virus. Key steps in this process include:

1. **Denaturing** the DNA with heat to separate complementary paired strands
2. Cooling to allow DNA primers to **anneal** to denatured strands of DNA
3. Extending the DNA sequence from the DNA primers by heat-stable **DNA polymerase**
4. Repeating steps 1–3 to achieve the desired level of amplification

- **Four days later, the patient develops an erythematous vesicular rash in the same area (see Figure 3-21 below). What are the likely findings on histologic examination of these vesicles?**

A **Tzanck smear** may demonstrate multinucleated giant cells, which are typical for varicella and herpes simplex and zoster.

- **What treatments are most appropriate for this condition?**

Acyclovir is activated by viral thymidine kinase to inhibit viral DNA polymerase. Valacyclovir and famciclovir have a similar mechanism and longer half-lives. These drugs target herpes virus and may provide relief, speed recovery, and prevent post-herpetic neuralgia.

- **What type of vaccine is the varicella vaccine, and what branches of the immune system does it stimulate?**

A **live attenuated vaccine** is used for prevention of initial varicella infection (chickenpox). Live attenuated vaccines induce both humoral and cell-mediated immunity.

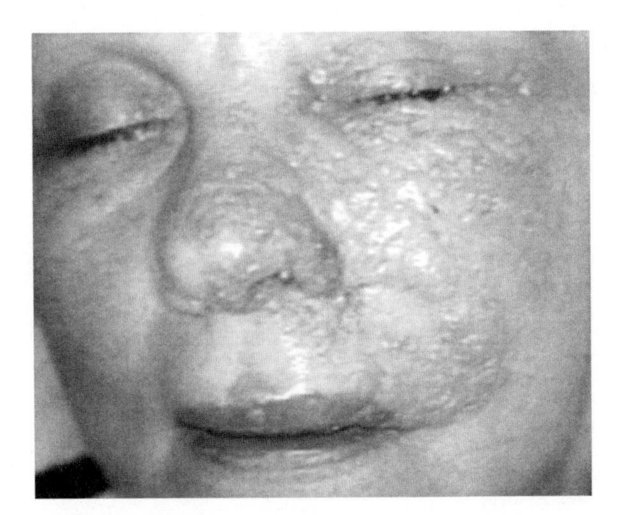

FIGURE 3-21. Shingles. (Reproduced with permission of the Pathology Education Instructional Resource Digital Library (http://peir.net) at the University of Alabama, Birmingham.)

► Case 40

A 36-year-old woman from Georgia presents with abdominal pain and diarrhea of 3 days' duration. She does not complain of nausea, vomiting, or fever. She has no sick contacts or significant travel history. A complete blood count is performed, and results are normal except for elevated eosinophils at 13%. A stool sample is obtained, which reveals larvae. Further questioning reveals that the woman frequently gardens in her backyard while barefoot.

What is the most likely diagnosis?	Strongyloidiasis, caused by *Strongyloides stercoralis*, a nematode (roundworm).
How is this agent transmitted, and how does it cause illness?	Larvae in the soil penetrate the skin, usually the sole of the foot (fecal-cutaneous transmission). Local itching at the entry site promotes scratching, which aids larvae entry into the bloodstream. Once in the blood, the larvae settle in the respiratory tree and can make their way up the trachea into the pharynx to be swallowed. They enter the small intestine, where the larvae mature into adults. Female adults invade the intestinal wall and lay eggs, which hatch into larvae and cause inflammation.
What other two organisms demonstrate the same life cycle in humans?	*Necator americanus* (New World hookworm), and *Ancylostoma duodenale* (Old Worm hookworm).
What signs and symptoms are commonly associated with this condition?	Disease can range from asymptomatic, to mild pneumonitis, to gastroenteritis with malabsorption. Infection/inflammation in the intestinal wall causes pain and diarrhea. Exit of feces in diarrhea facilitates release of larvae into the soil/environment. The **hyper-infection syndrome**, caused by rapid cycles of autoinfection, can result in increased parasitic burden and widely disseminated disease. This is more common in individuals with defective cellular immunity, such as those with acquired immunodeficiency syndrome.
What tests can help confirm the diagnosis?	Stool sample would reveal larvae (not eggs as in hookworm infection). Blood samples will reveal eosinophilia. A **string test** can be performed to test for the presence of organisms in the duodenum. With this test, the patient is asked to swallow a long string, which is then removed to extract larvae.
What treatments are most appropriate for this condition?	Ivermectin or thiabendazole.

▶ **Case 41**

A 13-year-old girl is brought into the physician's office by her mother. Her mother says the girl had a sudden onset of fever (39.4° C, or 103° F), lightheadedness, nausea, vomiting, and watery diarrhea. Physical examination reveals a desquamating rash of her palms and soles. She has no sick contacts, and there is no evidence of ingestion of unsafe food. Upon questioning, the patient says she began menstruating a little over a month ago.

■ **What is the most likely diagnosis?**	Toxic shock syndrome (TSS).
■ **What microorganism is the most likely cause of this condition?**	*Staphylococcus aureus* is the most common cause, although β-hemolytic group A streptococci can cause a similar presentation. The most common niduses of infection are tampons and cutaneous wounds.
■ **What are the distinguishing characteristics of the responsible microorganism?**	*S. aureus* is a gram-positive coccus. It is catalase and coagulase positive, and produces an enterotoxin. Figure 3-22 on the following page shows a useful laboratory algorithm for differentiating the gram-positive bacteria.
■ **What is the pathophysiology of this condition?**	The exotoxin (TSST-1) acts as a "superantigen" and is responsible for this presentation. Superantigens activate large numbers of T cells at once by binding directly to T-cell receptors and MHC molecules. Activated T cells then release large amounts of inflammatory cytokines, which are responsible for the manifestations of TSS.
■ **What other conditions should be considered in the differential diagnosis?**	■ Gram-negative sepsis (rare in healthy, nonhospitalized individuals) ■ Meningococcemia (associated with petechial rash) ■ Pneumococcal sepsis ■ Rocky Mountain spotted fever (associated with rash on palms and soles)
■ **What treatment is most appropriate for this condition?**	Removal of the infected wound dressing or tampon is the first step, followed by supportive care. Antibiotics that cover both *Staphylococcus* and *Streptococcus* will kill these bacteria and stop the production of additional exotoxin. However, it is the toxin, not the bacteria, that is responsible for the symptoms. In severe cases, intravenous immunoglobulin is also given.

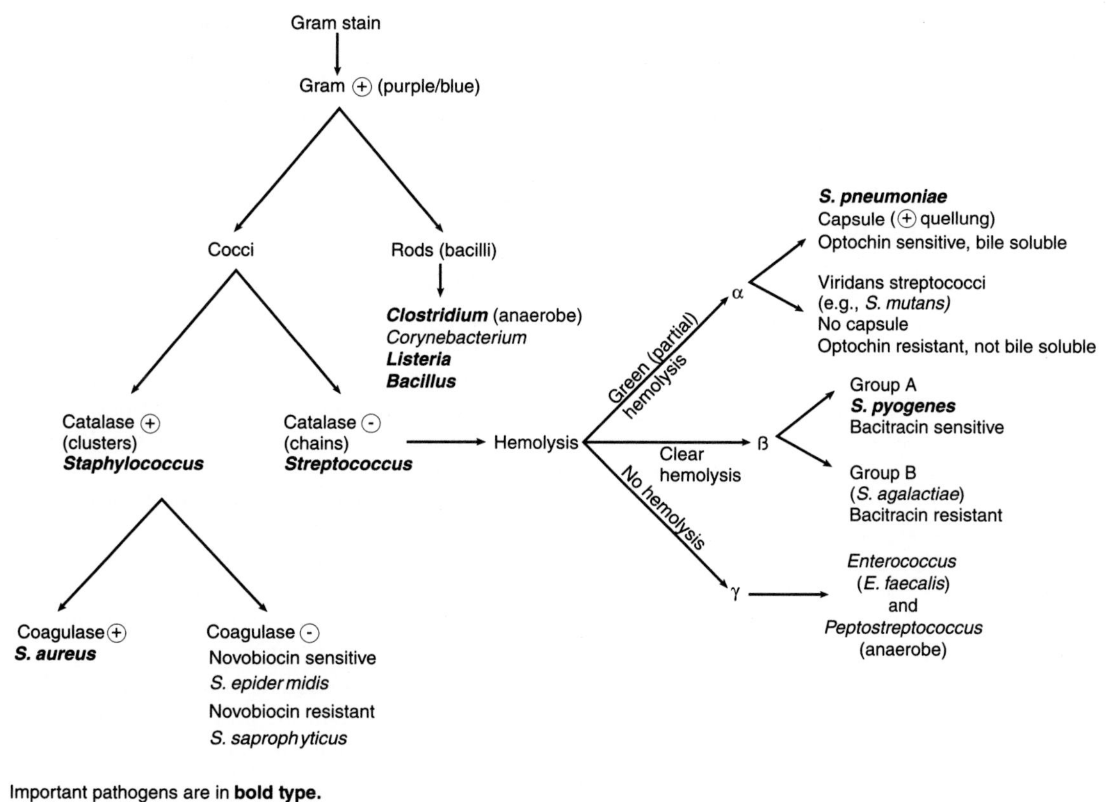

FIGURE 3-22. Algorithm for differentiating gram-positive bacteria. (Reproduced, with permission, from Bhushan V, Le T, et al. *First Aid for the USMLE Step 1: 2006*. New York: McGraw-Hill, 2006: 134.)

▶ Case 42

A 52-year-old man from Ohio presents with worsening cough, fever, chills, and pleuritic chest pain. He has also noted multiple, ulcerated sores on his skin, which began as pimple-like lesions. X-ray of the chest reveals segmental consolidation. Biopsy of a skin lesion reveals big, broad-based, budding yeast.

▪ **What is the most likely diagnosis?**	Blastomycosis, one of the systemic mycoses.
▪ **To what areas are the systemic mycoses endemic?**	▪ **Coccidioidomycosis** (also called desert bumps, San Joaquin valley bumps, or "valley fever") is specific to the Southwestern United States. ▪ **Histoplasmosis** is endemic to the Mississippi and Ohio River valleys, and is found in bird and bat droppings. ▪ **Blastomycosis** is found east of the Mississippi River (and in Central America). ▪ **Paracoccidioidomycosis** is found in rural Latin America.
▪ **What tests can help confirm the diagnosis?**	Culture on **Sabouraud's agar** at multiple temperatures. Systemic mycoses are caused by dimorphic fungi, which grow as mold in the cold (eg, in the soil) and as yeast at higher temperatures (eg, in tissue at 37° C). The exception is coccidioidomycosis, which is a spherule in tissue. In addition, a tissue biopsy revealing **b**road-**b**ased **b**udding yeast is diagnostic for **b**lastomycosis. Tissue biopsy demonstrating yeast cells within macrophages is diagnostic of histoplasmosis.
▪ **What are the typical findings on x-ray of the chest?**	These diseases can mimic tuberculosis, forming **granulomas,** which show up as small calcium deposits on x-ray films.
▪ **What treatment is most appropriate for this condition?**	Systemic infection is treated with itraconazole or amphotericin B.

▶ Case 43

A 54-year-old man with human immunodeficiency virus (HIV) infection presents to the emergency department after suffering a grand mal seizure. He has no known personal or family history of seizures. He is afebrile and his vital signs are stable. Fundoscopic examination reveals yellow cotton-like lesions on his retina. Findings on physical examination are otherwise unremarkable. A CT scan of the head demonstrates multiple ring-enhancing lesions in the cerebral cortex. Laboratory studies reveal a $CD4^+$ cell count of 153 μL.

What is the most likely cause of this patient's seizure?	*Toxoplasma gondii* infection.
How did this patient likely become infected with this microorganism?	It is likely that this man (like most individuals) has been latently infected with this protozoan for many years. However, his immunocompromised status has resulted in disease reactivation. Humans are most often infected by ingestion of cysts in undercooked meat, or by ingestion of food contaminated by cat feces.
In what other patient population is infection with this microorganism particularly dangerous?	Primary infection with *T. gondii* in a pregnant woman can result in parasites crossing the placenta. This leads to congenital problems in the newborn, including mental retardation, microcephaly, chorioretinitis, intracerebral calcifications, and blindness.
Given this patient's ring-enhancing lesions on CT, what other conditions should be included in the differential diagnosis?	This patient is also at an increased risk of lymphoma and tuberculosis, which can also cause seizures and appear as ring-enhancing lesions on CT.
What treatment is most appropriate for this condition?	First-line treatment is a regimen of pyrimethamine and sulfadiazine.

▶ Case 44

A 34-year-old nurse complains to her physician of occasional rust-colored sputum and fever of 6 months' duration. She also notes her clothes fit more loosely than they used to. Her only medication is an oral contraceptive. X-ray of the chest is shown in Figure 3-23 below.

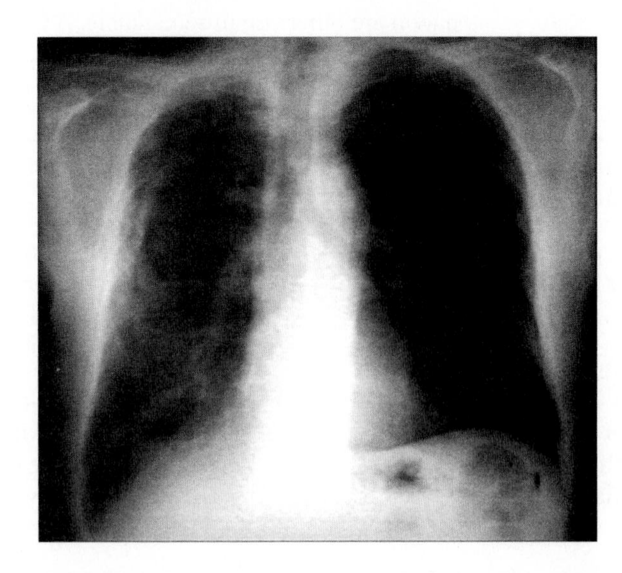

FIGURE 3-23. (Reproduced with permission of the Pathology Education Instructional Resource Digital Library (http://peir.net) at the University of Alabama, Birmingham.)

What is the most likely diagnosis?	Her symptoms and x-ray of the chest suggest tuberculosis (TB). Associated findings include a positive purified protein derivative test, granulomatous inflammation in the upper lobes of the lung, positive culture, and/or positive staining.
Where are the lesions in this condition usually located?	As seen in this chest x-ray, TB lesions are usually seen in the apical and posterior portions of the upper lobes. The hilar lymph nodes may also be involved. Primary lesions are usually found in the lower lobes, while secondary lesions are usually in the upper lobes.
How is the microorganism that causes this condition cultured? How is it stained?	*Mycoplasma tuberculosis* is cultured on **Lowenstein-Jensen agar.** It is an acid-fast bacterium, and therefore, stains with **Ziehl-Neelsen stain.**
What treatment is most appropriate for this condition?	The standard treatment lasts for 6 months. **R**ifampin, **I**soniazid, **P**yrazinamide, and **E**thambutol (**RIPE**) are used for the initial phase of therapy (usually 2 months), followed by rifampin and isoniazid for an additional 4 months. Susceptibility testing is also done to guide the choice of agents.
What are the main adverse events associated with this treatment?	▪ Rifampin colors urine, feces, sweat, and tears a reddish-orange color. It also upregulates the P450 system, increasing the metabolism of many drugs, including oral contraceptives. If the patient stays on her current dose of birth control pills and remains sexually active, she is more likely to become pregnant while taking rifampin. ▪ Isoniazid causes peripheral neuropathies and hepatitis. It is given with vitamin B_6 to reduce these adverse events. ▪ Pyrazinamide is associated with liver toxicity. ▪ Ethambutol can cause impaired color vision.

► Case 45

A man visiting rural Argentina develops fever, headache, pain in his knees and back, and nausea and vomiting. After 3 days these symptoms resolve, and the man decides not to seek medical help. However, 2 days later, the symptoms return, and he develops epigastric pain and yellowing of his skin, and his vomitus becomes dark in color.

■ What is the most likely diagnosis?

Yellow fever, which is endemic in South America and parts of Africa. It is characterized by an initial febrile illness, during which time serum aspartate aminotransferase and alanine aminotransferase levels may begin to rise, followed by a remission of symptoms. About 15% of those infected will experience a return of symptoms 2–3 days later, developing further liver dysfunction (resulting in jaundice, coagulopathy), renal damage, and myocardial damage.

■ What other microorganisms are in the same family?

The yellow fever virus is a Flavivirus, a family that also includes the following:

- Dengue fever virus
- St. Louis encephalitis virus
- Japanese encephalitis virus
- Hepatitis C virus
- West Nile virus

These viruses have positive, single-stranded RNA genomes in icosahedral, enveloped capsids.

■ How do viruses with this type of genome replicate?

Viruses with positive-stranded RNA genomes have genetic material that is equivalent to host mRNA. Thus, after the viral particle adsorbs to the surface of the host cell, enters the cell by endocytosis, and uncoats, the RNA is translated using host enzymes and ribosomes into structural proteins, including an RNA-dependent RNA polymerase. The viral genome is replicated by a host RNA polymerase that creates a negative strand copy. This acts as a template from which the RNA-dependent RNA polymerase makes multiple copies of positive-stranded genome. The resulting structural proteins and RNA are assembled into virions, which are then released by exocytosis.

■ What are the most likely findings on liver biopsy?

The characteristic finding on liver biopsy is mid-zone hepatocellular death, with sparing of cells bordering the central vein and portal tracts. **Councilman bodies** are found in the affected hepatocytes; these are eosinophilic inclusions that represent condensed chromatin. Typically, there is no inflammatory response. Liver biopsies are usually not done in patients because of their concomitant coagulopathy.

■ Enzyme-linked immunosorbent assay (ELISA) may be useful in confirming the diagnosis. How does ELISA work?

ELISA is a technique often used for serologic testing. It involves the coating of a surface with the desired antigen (in this case, yellow fever viral particles), then placing the patient's serum on the surface, followed by a secondary antibody (anti-human antibody), which is linked to an enzyme. If the patient's serum has antibody to the antigen, the secondary antibody will bind, creating a color reaction via a colorimetric agent, which can be quantified by spectroscopy.

NOTES

Pharmacology

▶ Case 1

A 20-year-old woman is brought to the emergency department by her roommate, who found the woman lethargic and covered in vomit. The roommate explains that the woman appeared normal the day before but adds that she had been depressed and had started a new antidepressant 1 week earlier. On examination, the patient is sweaty and lethargic with marked right upper quadrant tenderness. Her transaminase values are elevated, with an aspartate aminotransferase (AST) level of 1245 U/L. A urine toxicity screen is sent.

What is the most likely diagnosis?	Acetaminophen overdose. At therapeutic doses, a small quantity of acetaminophen is metabolized by hepatic cytochrome P450 into a hepatotoxic intermediate, N-acetyl-p-benzoquinoneimine (NAPQI) (see Figure 4-1A below). Glutathione rapidly conjugates with NAPQI to form nontoxic compounds. At toxic doses, more NAPQI is formed and exceeds glutathione storage, leading to hepatic damage (see Figure 4-1B below).
What is the antidote and its mechanism of action?	N-acetylcysteine (NAC), the antidote, works via several pathways. In general, NAC enhances the conjugation of NAPQI into nontoxic compounds. Notably, NAC increases glutathione stores to allow for more conjugation and detoxification of NAPQI. NAC can also directly conjugate with, and detoxify, NAPQI. Other benefits of NAC include anti-inflammatory, antioxidant, and vasodilatory effects.
Why is it important to ask about this patient's history of alcohol use?	Lower doses of acetaminophen may be toxic in a patient with a history of chronic alcohol use. Chronic alcohol exposure upregulates cytochrome P450, thereby speeding the production of NAPQI. Chronic alcohol ingestion can also lead to depletion of glutathione stores.
What changes in bilirubin levels are characteristic of this condition?	Total bilirubin increases, primarily as a result of increased indirect (unconjugated) bilirubin levels and impaired conjugation of bilirubin in the liver.
What vital organs are directly damaged by this condition?	The liver and the kidneys are both damaged by NAPQI by similar mechanisms. Indirect effects result from damage to these organs, including coagulation disorders and hepatic encephalitis.

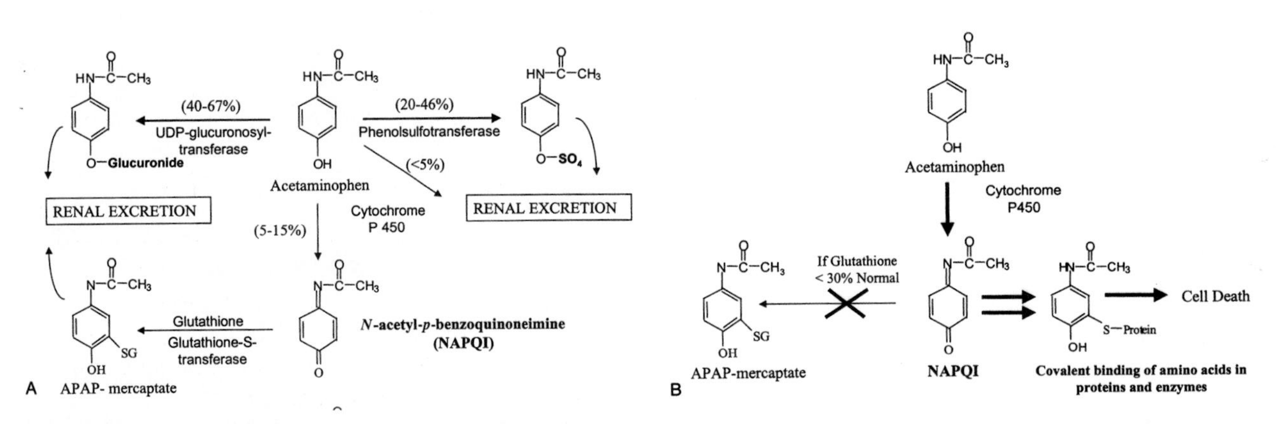

FIGURE 4-1. (A) and (B): Acetaminophen metabolism. (Reproduced, with permission, from Tintinalli JE, Kelen GD, Stapczynski JS, Ma OH, Cline DM. *Tintinalli's Emergency Medicine: A Comprehensive Study Guide*, 6th ed. New York: McGraw-Hill, 2004: 1089.)

► Case 2

A 45-year-old woman is brought to the emergency department by the police for unusual and disruptive behavior. She is muttering to herself, does not make eye contact, and does not answer any of the physician's questions but is otherwise cooperative. The patient's temperature is 38° C (100.4° F). A throat examination yields the findings shown in Figure 4-2 below. Her urine screen is negative for drugs and alcohol, and she is found to be HIV-negative. Relevant laboratory findings are as follows:

WBC count: 2000/mm^3
- Neutrophils: 1%
- Monocytes: 15%
- Eosinophils: 8%
- Basophils: 2%

Hemoglobin: 12 g/dL
Lymphocytes: 74%
Platelet count: 270,000/mm^3

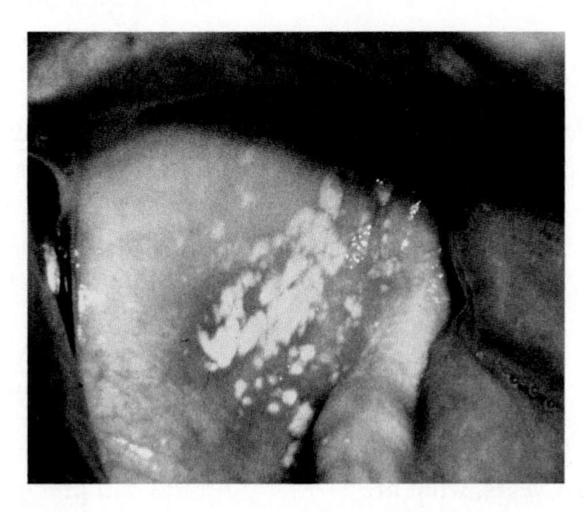

FIGURE 4-2. (Reproduced, with permission, from Knoop KJ, Stack LB, Storrow. *Atlas of Emergency Medicine*, 2nd ed. New York: McGraw-Hill, 2002.)

■ **What is the most likely diagnosis?**	Oral candidiasis (thrush); Figure 4-2 shows the characteristic whitish plaques on the buccal mucosa. The lymphoreticular disorders in this patient suggest agranulocytosis.
■ **Given her laboratory functions, this patient is most susceptible to which types of pathogens?**	This can be determined by looking at her WBC differential, which shows neutropenia. Patients with neutropenia often present clinically with recurrent bacterial and fungal infections.
■ **Given this patient's presentation, what medication is she likely to be taking?**	She is likely taking clozapine. This patient is acutely psychotic and suffering from agranulocytosis. Clozapine, an antipsychotic, causes agranulocytosis in 1%–2% of patients.
■ **What treatment would help restore her neutrophil count?**	Iatrogenic agranulocytosis usually resolves within 1 month after discontinuation of the offending drug.
■ **What is the most appropriate treatment for her throat condition?**	Oral thrush is treated with nystatin "swish and swallow."
■ **What are two mechanisms by which drugs can lead to the development of this condition?**	■ **Direct toxicity:** Drugs can be directly toxic to granulocytic precursors and neutrophils (eg, cyclophosphamide). ■ **Autoimmune destruction of neutrophils:** Drugs may lead to autoimmune destruction of neutrophils by binding to neutrophil membranes and acting as haptens.

► **Case 3**

A 36-year-old man is brought to the emergency department after his wife finds him in a confused and drowsy state. Questioning reveals he has a chronic anxiety disorder and has taken his entire anxiolytic prescription in a suicide attempt. He is found to have a decreased respiratory rate and his blood pressure is 100/65 mm Hg. He is ataxic and his speech is slurred.

Which class of drug did this patient likely ingest?	A benzodiazepine (eg, lorazepam, alprazolam, diazepam).
What is the mechanism of action of this class of drugs?	Benzodiazepines bind to **γ-aminobutyric acid** (GABA) receptors of the central nervous system, enhancing the affinity of GABA for the receptor and thus increasing the conductance of the associated chloride channel. This results in hyperpolarization of the neuron and inhibition of firing (see Figure 4-3 below).
What is the antidote and its mechanism of action?	Flumazenil may be given in benzodiazepine overdose. Flumazenil acts as a competitive inhibitor at the GABA receptor, interrupting the GABA-benzodiazepine complex. Because the half-life of flumazenil is much shorter than that of benzodiazepines, it must be administered frequently. One must also be aware that flumazenil may decrease the seizure threshold by blocking GABA. If it is given to a patient who has ingested a substance that induces seizure activity, seizure activity may result.
If the patient has been taking this anxiolytic for many years, what are some of the possible adverse effects of rapid reversal with this class of drugs?	Abrupt discontinuation of benzodiazepines after chronic high doses can precipitate withdrawal symptoms, including confusion, agitation, gastrointestinal upset, and anxiety. If the benzodiazepine is being given for seizure control, flumazenil may precipitate seizure.
For what other conditions is this class of drugs commonly used?	■ **Panic disorders** ■ **Status epilepticus:** Diazepam is the drug of choice ■ **Sleep disorders**, including insomnia ■ **Alcohol withdrawal:** Diazepam is the drug of choice

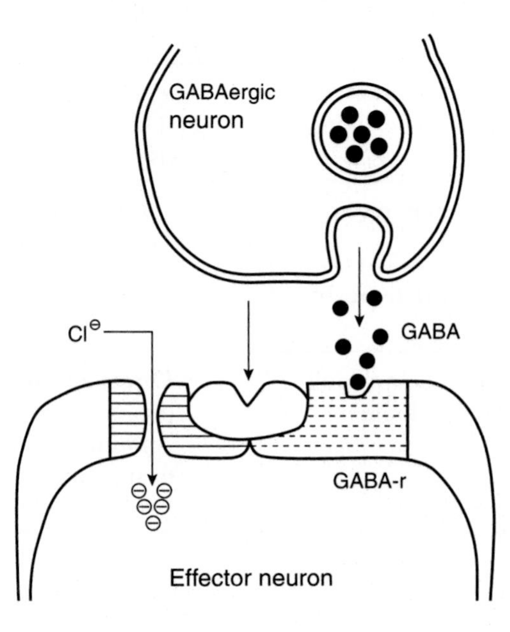

FIGURE 4-3. GABA receptors at work.

GENERAL PRINCIPLES

PHARMACOLOGY

► Case 4

A 32-year-old woman with a history of asthma begins to have difficulty breathing. She has forgotten her inhaler, and is brought to the emergency department, where she is noted to be in moderate respiratory distress. She is using her accessory muscles, and her oxygen saturation is 96%. She is becoming anxious, because it is becoming more and more difficult for her to breathe. She is immediately given an albuterol treatment.

- **On what type of receptor does this drug act?**

Albuterol is a β_2-adrenergic agonist that causes bronchodilation. Other β_2 agonists include terbutaline, metaproterenol, and ritodrine.

- **In what other locations can this subset of receptors be found?**

β_2 receptors are also found:

- on blood vessels, where they induce vasodilation
- on bronchioles, where they facilitate bronchodilation
- in pancreatic α cells, where they stimulate glucagon release
- in the central nervous system
- on parietal cells of the gastric mucosa, where they stimulate acid secretion
- in the uterine myometrium, where they cause uterine relaxation

- **What second-messenger system does stimulation of these receptors activate?**

All adrenergic receptors, including α- and β-adrenergic receptors (see Table 4-1 below), are G protein-linked receptors, and β_2 receptors are linked to the S class of G proteins.

- **What is the mechanism of action for this subclass of G receptors?**

The G_s protein activates adenyl cyclase, which converts ATP to cAMP, which in turn activates protein kinase A (PKA). In uterine myometrial cells, the activated PKA phosphorylates other proteins; this leads to a reduction in intracellular Ca^{2+} concentration and hence to decreased activity of myosin light-chain kinase and diminished contractility of the uterine muscle cells.

- **What other classes of receptors are linked to this particular subclass of G receptors?**

Other receptors linked to G_s include β_1, D_1, H_2, and V_2 receptors. Activation of any of these receptors leads to activation of G_s and adenyl cyclase.

TABLE 4-1. G Protein–Linked Second Messengers

	G_i receptor	G_s receptor	G_q receptor
Action	Adenyl cyclase → ↓ cAMP → ↓ PKA	Adenyl cyclase → ↑ cAMP → ↑ PKA	PLC → PIP_2 → IP_3 → ↑ Ca^{2+}
Types of receptors	α_2 M_2 D_2	β_1, β_2, β_3 H_2 D_1 V_2	α_1 M_1, M_3 H_1 V_1

▶ Case 5

A small biotechnology company has developed a new drug that holds promise for the treatment of osteoarthritis. Currently, it is being tested on a group of 100 patients with osteoarthritis, some of whom are receiving placebo.

In which stage of testing is this drug?	The drug is in **phase 2** of clinical testing. Phase 2 entails enrolling a small group of patients, usually between 100 and 300. These trials are usually single-blinded and compare the new product to placebo as well as to an older drug that has already been proven effective. However, they can also be double-blind and placebo-controlled only.
What stages of testing has the drug already been through?	Before a drug reaches clinical trials, it must first be extensively evaluated in animal models and in vitro systems such as cell and tissue cultures. Information about acute toxicity, chronic toxicity, teratogenicity, carcinogenicity, and mutagenicity must then be obtained from these trials before testing is conducted on humans. The first step of clinical testing, **phase 1**, involves nonblinded testing on a small group (20–30) of healthy volunteers (see Figure 4-4 on the following page). The goals in this phase are to determine if humans have significantly different responses to the drug than do animals, as well as to determine the effects of the drug as a function of dose. Phase 2, discussed above, follows.
What are the next stages of testing?	**Phase 3** involves evaluating the drug in a large group of patients (between hundreds and thousands). The trial is usually double-blinded and aims to further show efficacy and safety. If phase 3 testing is successful, the company will submit a New Drug Application to the FDA, which will include preclinical and clinical data. The FDA will then review this material in a process that may take several years. If the drug is approved for market, phase 4 starts. **Phase 4** entails monitoring of the drug as it is used in real conditions with large numbers of patients. This phase is important for discovering low-incidence toxicities that would not be uncovered in clinical trials. Phase 4 continues indefinitely.
What is a double-blind study, and why are such studies the gold standard for drug testing?	A **double-blind** study means that neither the patients being treated nor the physicians administering the drug know who is receiving medication or who is receiving placebo. Masking this information eliminates both observer and subject bias.
If this drug passes all stages of testing, when will a generic form become available?	A drug patent lasts 20 years after the filing of a New Drug Application, after which time generics become available. However, the evaluation of the new drug application by the FDA may take several years. Up to 5 years of the review time may be added back to the patent.

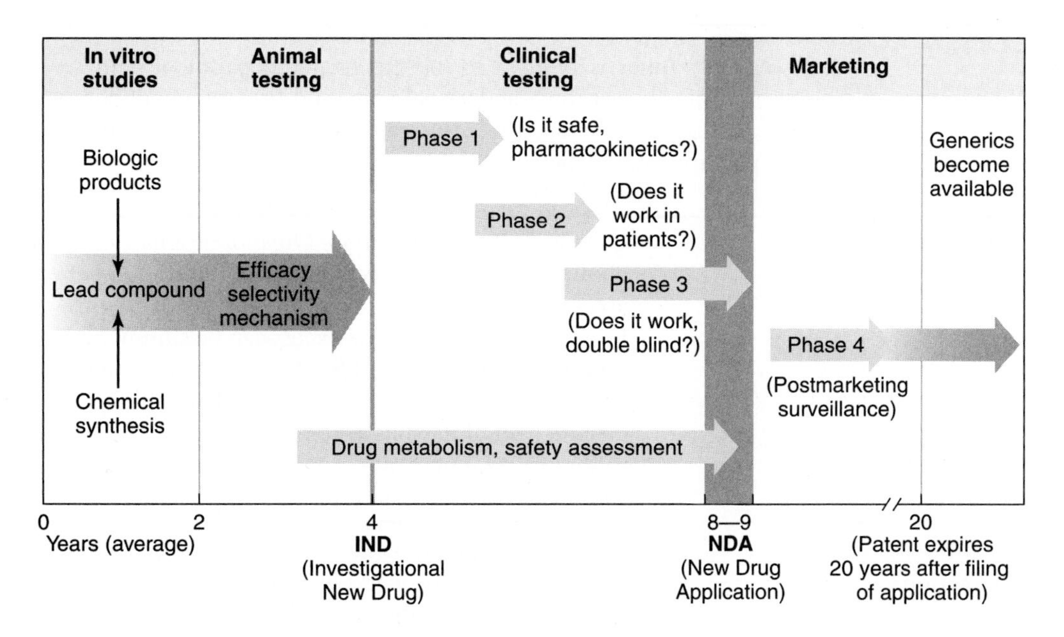

FIGURE 4-4. Phases of FDA review process. (Adapted, with permission, from Katzung BG, Trevor AJ. *Pharmacology: Examination & Board Review*, 5th ed. Stamford, CT: Appleton & Lange, 1998: 365.)

▶ Case 6

A 30-year-old farmer is brought to the emergency department with severe diarrhea, shortness of breath, sweating, abdominal pain, and urinary incontinence. The patient appears confused and his speech is slurred. His brother reports having seen the farmer drink liquid from an unlabeled bottle approximately 1 hour earlier.

What is the most likely diagnosis?	Organophosphate ingestion. Organophosphates, which are cholinesterase inhibitors commonly found in insecticides, cause an excess of acetylcholine in the synapse. Symptoms resulting from this parasympathetic excess can be summarized by the mnemonic **DUMBBELSS:** **D**iarrhea, **U**rinary incontinence, **M**iosis, **B**ronchospasm, **B**radycardia, **E**xcitation of skeletal muscle and central nervous system, **L**acrimation, **S**weating, and **S**alivation. Central nervous system effects, such as confusion or slurred speech, are common.
What are the antidotes and their mechanism of action?	Atropine and pralidoxime (2-PAM) can reverse organophosphate poisoning. Atropine works by inhibiting muscarinic receptors, thereby decreasing the effect of acetylcholine. 2-PAM works by inhibiting the binding of organophosphates to acetylcholinesterase. A schematic of neuromuscular blockade is shown in Figure 4-5 below.
What adverse events are associated with this treatment?	Atropine poisoning can lead to sympathomimetic adverse effects, including pupillary dilation, decreased gastrointestinal motility, increased body temperature, rapid heart rate, dry mouth, dry skin, constipation, and disorientation.
If this patient had a thymectomy in the past, what other adverse events might be seen?	Thymectomy can be therapeutic in myasthenia gravis. Anticholinesterases such as pyridostigmine and neostigmine are common treatments for myasthenia gravis. Toxic levels of these agents can also result in symptoms of parasympathomimetic excess.

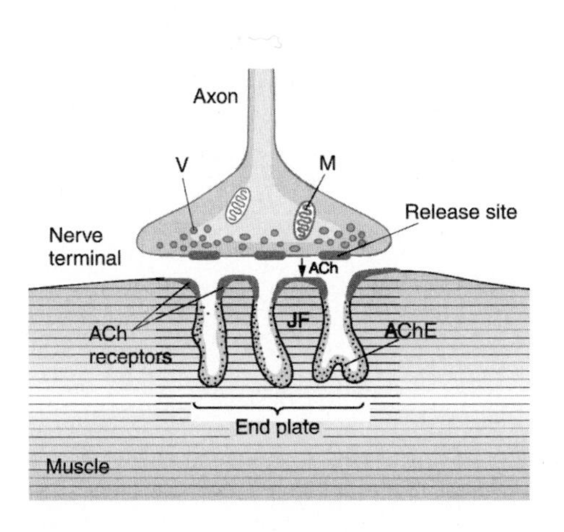

FIGURE 4-5. Neuromuscular blockade. (Modified, with permission, from Drachman DB. Myasthenia gravis. *N Engl J Med* 1978;298:135.)

▶ Case 7

The kinetics of a new pharmaceutical drug are being tested in an animal model. A dose of 50 mg of the substance is injected intravenously into a rat. The concentration of the substance in the animal's blood is measured every 30 minutes thereafter for the next 10 hours. The concentration of the drug plotted against time produces the graph shown in Figure 4-6A below.

- **Is this substance being metabolized by first-order or zero-order kinetics?**

The shape of the graph shows that the drug is being eliminated by **first-order kinetics** (see Figure 4-6A below), meaning that a constant **fraction** of the substance is eliminated per unit of time. As a result, the rate of elimination is proportional to the concentration of the drug. In contrast, **zero-order kinetics** (see Figure 4-6B below) result in a constant **amount** of the substance being cleared per unit of time; the elimination rate is constant regardless of the **plasma concentration** (C_p), and the plot of C_p versus time is a straight line.

- **What is the half-life of this substance, and how does the half-life change if a dosage of 100 mg is administered?**

Half-life ($t_{1/2}$) is the time necessary to decrease the C_p of the drug by 50%. As shown in the graph below, at 5 hours the C_p of the drug is half of the initial concentration, and thus $t_{1/2}$ is 5 hours. Half-life does not depend on the size of the dose being eliminated.

- **If renal clearance is determined to be 2 mL/min, what is the volume of distribution for this substance?**

Volume of distribution (V_d) is the amount of drug in the body divided by C_p. A useful equation is the following:

$$t_{1/2} = (0.7 \times V_d)/\text{clearance}$$

From this equation, $V_d = 857$ mL. A large volume of distribution indicates that most of the drug is not in the plasma compartment.

- **Why does the volume of distribution affect the half-life of a drug?**

As indicated by the equation above, $t_{1/2}$ is directly proportional to V_d. This is because the larger the V_d, the less drug is present in the plasma compartment, and therefore the less drug is circulated through the kidneys and liver for metabolism and excretion.

- **How would the therapeutic index of this drug be determined, and why is this important?**

Therapeutic index is the ratio of a drug's toxic dose to the therapeutic dose. Safe drugs will have a high therapeutic index because this indicates a large difference between the doses used to treat patients and the dose resulting in toxicity.

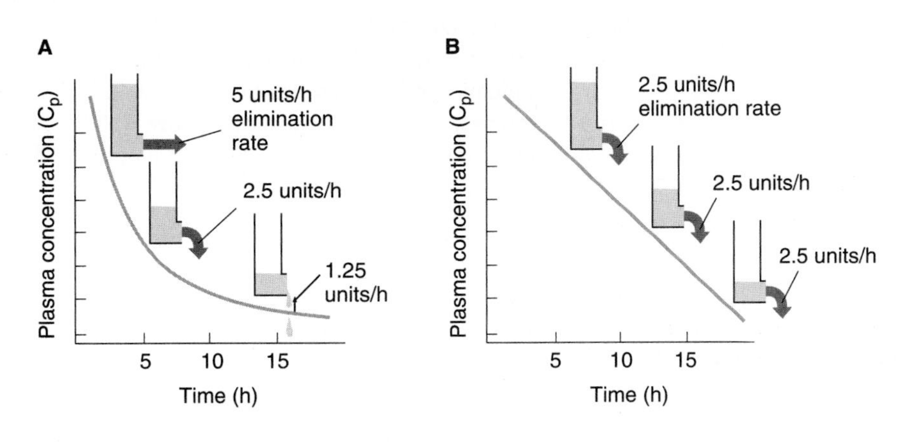

FIGURE 4-6. First-order drug elimination (A) and zero-order drug elimination (B). (Adapted, with permission, from Katzung BG, Trevor AJ. *Examination and Board Review: Pharmacology*, 5th ed. Stamford, CT: Appleton & Lange, 1998: 5.)

▶ Case 8

A 53-year-old woman presented to her primary care physician 3 months ago for a check-up, her first in 5 years. She is found to be hypertensive and was prescribed hydralazine, a β-blocker, and furosemide. The woman takes no additional prescription or over-the-counter medications. At the current follow-up visit, she complains of muscle aches, joint pain, and a rash. Physical examination reveals an erythematous, slightly scaly rash on her chest and back. The patient is febrile. The physician orders an autoantibody panel that yields the following results:

Antinuclear antibodies: positive
Anti-RNP antibodies: negative
Anti-Sm antibodies: negative
Anti-DNA antibodies: negative
Antihistone antibodies: positive

- **What is the most likely diagnosis?**

This is a case of drug-induced lupus, as suggested by the rash, arthralgias, and antihistone antibodies. Hydralazine is the causative agent in this case.

- **What other medications might cause a similar presentation?**

Drugs known to induce lupus include procainamide, chlorpromazine, isoniazid, methyldopa, minocycline, penicillamine, and diltiazem.

- **What underlying metabolic defect is likely contributing to the patient's reaction?**

Drug-induced lupus develops more frequently in people who have polymorphisms in the genes that participate in acetylation reactions of drug metabolism. In these individuals, acetylation occurs more slowly, and thus drugs have a longer half-life during which they may be converted to toxic metabolites. This in turn induces antibody formation and the lupuslike syndrome.

- **How are lipid-soluble medications metabolized?**

Lipid-soluble medications are metabolized by the liver in phase I and phase II reactions (see Figure 4-7 on the following page). **Phase I reactions** convert lipophilic drugs into more polar molecules, which may increase, decrease, or have no effect on the drug's activity. Many phase I reactions involve the P450 system; other reactions include amine oxidation, hydrolysis, and dehydrogenation. **Phase II reactions** are conjugation reactions that make the molecules even more water-soluble for excretion in the kidney. The drug may be conjugated to glucuronic acid, sulfuric acid, an amino acid, or an acetyl group, among others.

- **What is the mechanism of action of the causative agent?**

Hydralazine is a direct vasodilator that acts on arteries and arterioles more than on venous circulation. One result of its vasodilating effects is reflex tachycardia and stimulation of the renin-angiotensin-aldosterone pathway. Thus, hydralazine is almost always administered with a β-blocker and a diuretic.

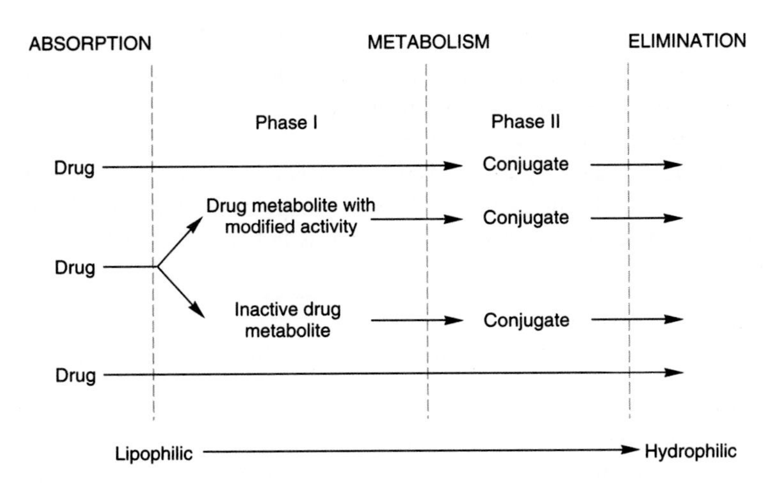

FIGURE 4-7. Phase I and phase II reactions. (Reproduced, with permission, from Katzung BG. *Basic & Clinical Pharmacology*, 9th ed. New York: McGraw-Hill, 2004: 52.)

► Case 9

Several new drugs are being tested for their effects on β_2-adrenergic receptors. The investigator plots an S-shaped curve of the activity of adenylate cyclase versus drug dose in response to drug A. When the response of drug D is similarly plotted, D is found to have a lower median effective dose (ED_{50}) and a lower maximal response than A. In the presence of drug A plus drug B, the curve has the same shape but is now shifted to the right. In the presence of drug A plus drug C, the curve is not shifted, but the maximal response is lower.

- **Which drug, A or D, is more efficacious?**

Efficacy refers to the maximal response a drug elicits. Thus, drug A has a higher efficacy, since it produces a higher maximal response (see Figure 4-8 below).

- **Which drug is more potent?**

Drug D is more potent (see Figure 4-8 below). **Potency** is the amount of drug required for a specified response. Typically, potency is measured by the $\mathbf{ED_{50}}$, or the dose that gives 50% of the maximal response. The lower the ED_{50}, the more potent the drug.

- **What type of antagonist is drug B?**

Drug B is a competitive antagonist—ie, it binds to the same site on the receptor as does drug A (see Figure 4-9A on the following page). It does not affect the maximal response the agonist can elicit, but it does increase the ED_{50}, requiring more agonist to achieve the same response.

- **What type of antagonist is drug C?**

Drug C is a **noncompetitive antagonist** (see Figure 4-9B on the following page). These drugs act by binding irreversibly to a site on the receptor distinct from the site of agonist binding. Noncompetitive antagonists do not affect the ED_{50} but do affect the maximal response that the agonist can elicit.

- **How can the effect of drug B be overcome?**

Since **competitive antagonists** bind at the same site as the agonist, their action can be overcome by increasing agonist dose.

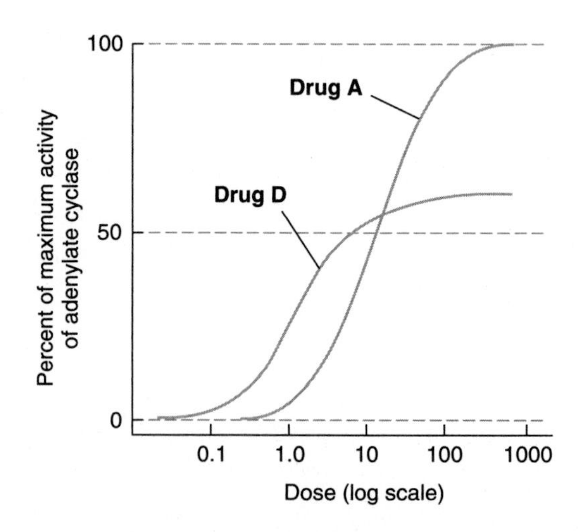

FIGURE 4-8. Dose-response curves comparing Drug A and Drug D.

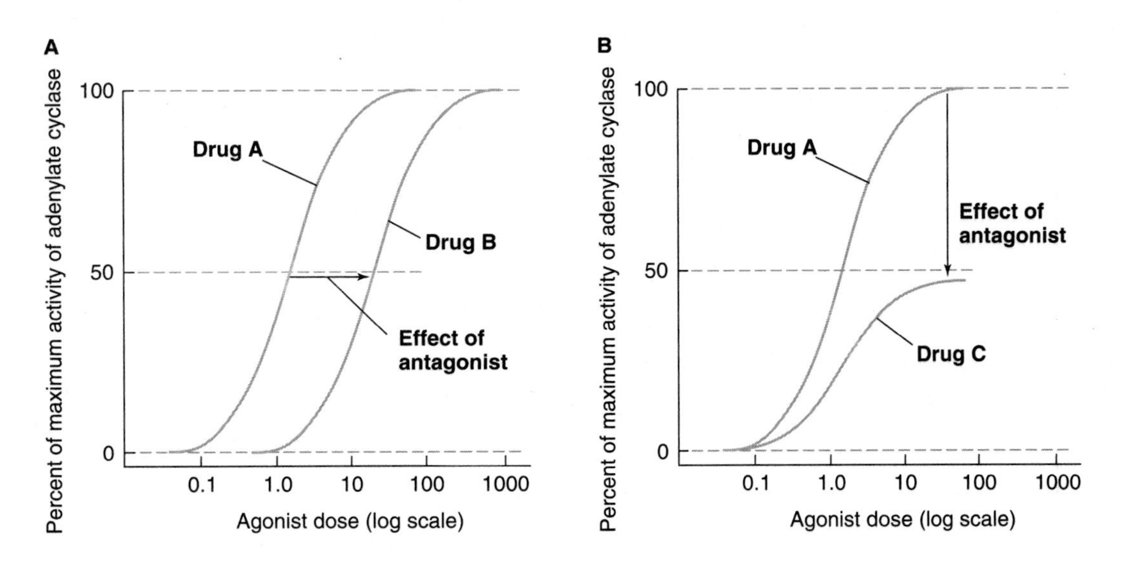

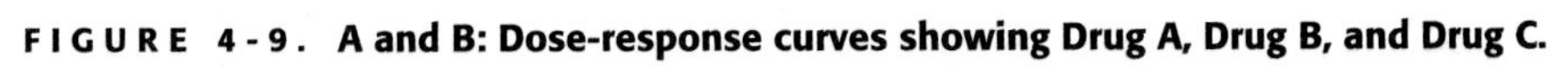

FIGURE 4-9. A and B: Dose-response curves showing Drug A, Drug B, and Drug C.

NOTES

SECTION II

Organ Systems

- Cardiovascular System
- Endocrine System
- Gastrointestinal System
- Hematology and Oncology
- Musculoskeletal System and Connective Tissue
- Neurology and Psychiatry
- Renal System
- Reproductive System
- Respiratory System

Cardiovascular System

▶ Case 1

A 75-year-old man visits his physician complaining of lower back pain. He has a history of hyperlipidemia and hypertension. On physical examination, he is obese and has moderately limited range of motion of the back. Magnetic resonance imaging studies demonstrate significant dilation of the abdominal aorta to 4 cm, 200% its expected size.

■ **What is the most likely diagnosis?**	Abdominal aortic aneurysm.
■ **What are the major branches of the aorta below the diaphragm?**	Blood flow to the major organs is of special concern with an abdominal aneurysm. The inferior phrenic arteries, celiac trunk, middle suprarenal arteries, renal arteries, superior mesenteric artery, testicular arteries, inferior mesenteric artery, lumbar arteries, and the common iliac arteries are located below the diaphragm (see Figure 5-1 below).
■ **Of what are the three layers of muscular arteries composed?**	■ The **tunica intima** is adjacent to the lumen and includes the endothelial layer and the internal elastic lamina. ■ The **tunica media** includes smooth muscle, collagen, and reticular and elastic fibers. ■ The **tunica adventitia** contains blood and lymph vessels and nerves supplying the artery.
■ **Defects in the genes coding for which proteins are associated with an increased risk of this condition?**	**Fibrillin** and **collagen.** Marfan's syndrome is linked to a mutation in the fibrillin-1 gene. Ehlers-Danlos syndrome results from various defects in collagen synthesis or structure. Each of these syndromes is associated with an increased incidence of aortic aneurysms.
■ **In which space will blood collect if the posterior wall of the aorta ruptures?**	With a rupture, blood will collect in the retroperitoneal space (see Figure 5-2 below; arrow points to site of rupture). A confined retroperitoneal bleed from a posterior rupture portends a better prognosis than does bleeding into the peritoneal cavity from a ruptured anterior wall.
■ **Once the aortic wall is disrupted, how does coagulation proceed?**	Exposure of tissue factor in the vessel wall initiates the extrinsic pathway of coagulation.

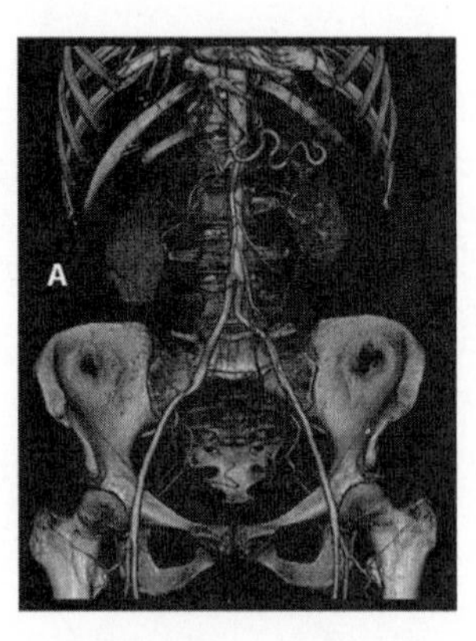

FIGURE 5-1. 3D reconstruction of CT angiogram in healthy person. (Reproduced, with permission, from Fuster V, Alexander RW, O'Rourke RA [eds]; and Roberts R, King SB II, Nash IS, and Prystowsky EN [assoc eds]. *Hurst's The Heart,* 11th ed. New York: McGraw-Hill, 2004.)

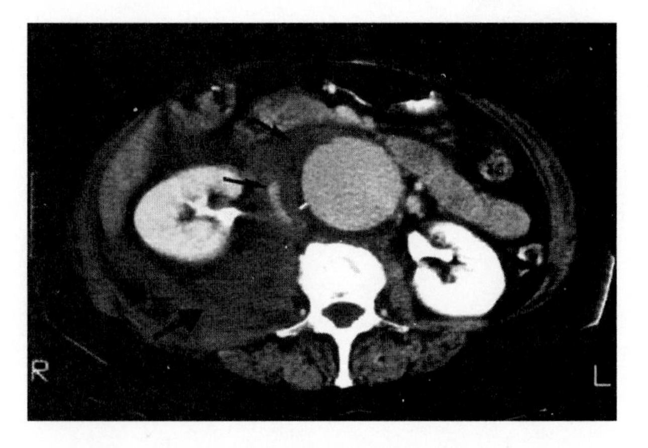

FIGURE 5-2. CT showing abdominal aortic aneurysm rupture. (Reproduced, with permission, from Dean RH, Yao JST, Brewster DC [eds]. *Current Diagnosis & Treatment in Vascular Surgery.* Stamford, CT: Appleton & Lange, 1995. Copyright © The McGraw-Hill Companies, Inc.)

▶ Case 2

A 65-year-old man presents to his cardiologist for evaluation of recurrent episodes of lightheadedness, chest pain, and shortness of breath with exertion. One week earlier, he experienced an episode of syncope while walking up the stairs of his house. Doppler echocardiography demonstrates a heavily calcified aortic valve, with a calculated valve area 40% of normal size.

■ **What is the most likely diagnosis?**	Aortic stenosis.
■ **What risk factors increase a person's likelihood of developing this condition?**	Aortic stenosis is commonly associated with older age, male gender, hypercholesterolemia, rheumatic fever, and congenital bicuspid aortic valve.
■ **What are the qualities of the murmur caused by this condition?**	The murmur of aortic stenosis is a **systolic ejection murmur** at the right upper sternal border, radiating to the neck.
■ **Which specific qualities of this murmur indicate severe illness?**	Indications of a severely stenosed valve include peaking of the murmur late in systole, a palpable delay of the carotid upstroke, and a soft second heart sound (which disappears when the valve is too stiff to open and close properly).
■ **How is this condition associated with congestive heart failure?**	Aortic stenosis implies a decreased functional area of the valve, causing a measurable obstruction of outflow. In severe stenosis (<50% of normal size), the obstruction causes a progressive pressure overload on the left ventricle. In response, there is concentric left ventricular hypertrophy, which compromises coronary blood flow during exertion, and can lead to congestive heart failure.
■ **What symptoms are associated with this condition?**	■ **Angina**—without proper intervention, half of patients who present with angina will die within 5 years ■ **Syncope**—half will die within 3 years ■ **Dyspnea** on exertion—half will die within 2 years
■ **What is the most appropriate treatment for this condition?**	**Valve replacement** is strongly recommended in patients with symptomatic severe aortic stenosis, as 10-year survival rates after replacement approach rates of the normal population. Mechanical intervention, such as **balloon valvotomy,** provides only temporary symptomatic relief for patients with calcified valves, and offers no survival benefit. In all patients with aortic stenosis, **prophylactic antibiotics** should be used to prevent infective endocarditis. Afterload reducers, including β-blockers, angiotensin-converting enzyme inhibitors, and vasodilators should **not** be used in patients with aortic stenosis, as the resulting peripheral dilation can cause the patient to go into shock.

▶ Case 3

A 58-year-old man comes to the physician complaining of occasional chest pain that occurs with strenuous activity. He is obese and has a history of hypertension and diabetes mellitus. During the physical examination, he admits to eating most of his meals at fast-food restaurants. He also reports he has little time for exercise.

▪ **What is the most likely diagnosis?**	Stable angina, characterized by chest pain with exertion, is often secondary to atherosclerosis.
▪ **What risk factors increase a person's likelihood of developing this condition?**	Hypertension, diabetes mellitus, age, gender, and hyperlipidemia are major risk factors for atherosclerosis. Family history and smoking are also risk factors. Of note, obesity and lack of exercise have not been firmly linked to increased risk for the development of atherosclerosis.
▪ **What is the pathophysiology of this condition?**	Endothelial injury resulting from various factors, including hyperlipidemia, smoking, and hypertension, can lead to monocytic and lipid infiltrates into the subendothelium (fatty streaks), release of growth factors leading to smooth muscle cell proliferation into the intima (proliferative plaque), and subsequent development of foam cells and complex atheromas with calcification and ischemia of the intima (see Figure 5-3 below).
▪ **Which arteries are most commonly affected in this condition?**	Arteries most commonly affected in atherosclerosis include the abdominal aorta, proximal coronary arteries, popliteal artery, carotid artery, arteries of the Circle of Willis, and renal artery.
▪ **What complications are most commonly associated with this condition?**	In addition to angina, other complications of atherosclerotic injury include aneurysms, myocardial infarction, stroke, ischemia, and ischemic bowel disease.
▪ **How is the patient's symptom classified?**	▪ **Stable angina:** chest pain with exertion; responds to nitroglycerine. ▪ **Unstable angina:** chest pain at rest secondary to thrombus in a branch. May not completely respond to nitroglycerine; antithrombic agents and heparin may also be required. ▪ **Prinzmetal's angina:** chest pain at rest, secondary to coronary artery spasm. Treatment includes calcium channel blockers.

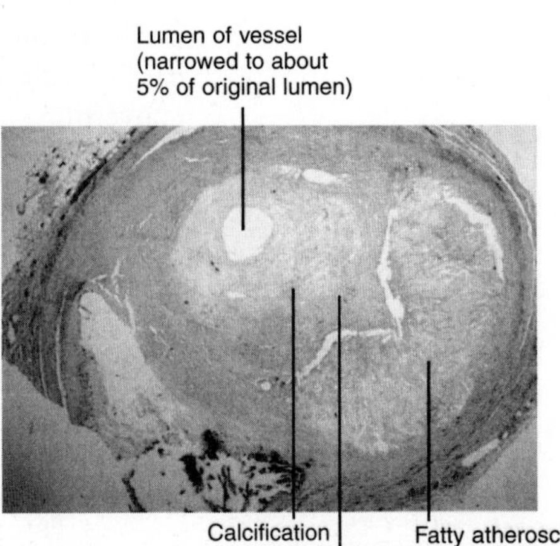

FIGURE 5-3. Cross-section of atherosclerotic coronary artery. (Reproduced, with permission, from Bhushan V, Le T, et al. *First Aid for the USMLE Step 1: 2006*. New York: McGraw-Hill, 2006.)

▶ Case 4

A 58-year-old woman comes to the physician's office complaining of feeling lightheaded for the past week. She says she can feel her heart racing in her chest. She mentions she has been staying up late for the past few weeks because of her workload at work. The medical history reveals well-controlled diabetes mellitus. Physical examination reveals an anxious woman with pallor and mild diaphoresis. Cardiac examination reveals an irregularly irregular beat. Vital signs are as follows:

Temperature: 36.1° C (97.0° F)
Respiratory rate: 22/min
Heart rate: 142/min
Blood pressure: 118/55 mm Hg
Glucose: 130 mg/dL

▪ **What is the most likely diagnosis?**	Atrial fibrillation.
▪ **What clinical and ECG abnormalities are most commonly associated with this condition?**	The patient has lightheadedness, palpitations, anxiety, pallor, and diaphoresis. Her recent late nights might indicate high caffeine intake, which is a question worth asking the patient. Her heart rate is elevated and she might have borderline hypotension, depending on her baseline blood pressure. The ECG shows an absence of P waves, irregular R-R intervals, and tachycardia (see Figure 5-4 below).
▪ **What is the most appropriate treatment for this condition?**	The patient has a high heart rate, which should be slowed down, possibly with β-blockers, calcium channel blockers, or digoxin. Metoprolol is a β_1-blocker that slows conduction through the atrioventricular node, thereby slowing heart rate. One might also consider cardioversion to a normal sinus rhythm. However, care must be taken not to promote thromboembolus formation, which might occur if cardioversion is performed more than 48 hours after the onset of atrial fibrillation. A transesophageal echocardiogram may be done to screen for a left atrial thrombus, or the patient may be given an anticoagulant like warfarin for several weeks before cardioversion is attempted.
▪ **How do heparin and warfarin work together to treat this condition?**	Given intravenously, heparin activates antithrombin III. Its effectiveness is monitored by measuring the partial thromboplastin time (which reflects activity of the intrinsic pathway). Given orally, warfarin impairs the synthesis of vitamin K–dependent clotting factors (II, VII, IX, and X). It is monitored by measuring the prothrombin time (extrinsic pathway).
▪ **Why does paradoxical coagulation sometimes occur after starting warfarin therapy?**	Warfarin also inhibits the synthesis of protein C and protein S. Because proteins C and S inhibit factors Va and VIIIa, a deficiency in these proteins promotes coagulation.

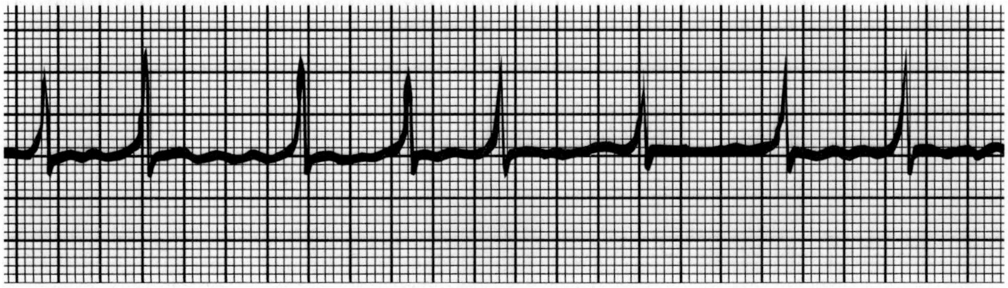

FIGURE 5-4. ECG strip in atrial fibrillation.

▶ Case 5

A 55-year-old man comes to his physician for a follow-up visit, after being hospitalized 2 weeks earlier for an inferior wall myocardial infarction. The patient has a history of coronary artery disease. His ECG is shown in Figure 5-5 below.

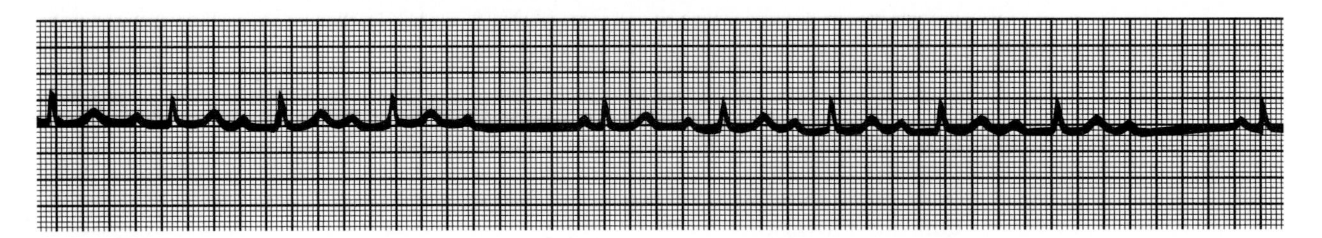

FIGURE 5-5.

▪ **What pathology does the ECG in Figure 5-5 depict?**	Second-degree atrioventricular (AV) block, also known as **Mobitz type I block** or **Wenckebach block.** As shown in Figure 5-5, note the progressive lengthening of the PR interval from one beat to the next, until finally a beat is dropped (a P wave is not followed by a QRS complex).
▪ **What is the pathophysiology of this condition?**	This occurs secondary to impaired conduction at the level of the AV node, such that atrial impulses fail to reach the ventricles. This patient's recent myocardial infarction may have compromised the conductive ability of his AV node.
▪ **How is this condition classified?**	▪ In **first-degree block,** the PR interval is prolonged but there are no missed beats (a QRS complex follows every P wave). ▪ In **second-degree block,** there is intermittent failure of AV conduction. In a **Mobitz type I block,** the PR interval progressively lengthens until a beat is dropped. In a **Mobitz type II** block, there is a sudden loss of impulse conduction without a corresponding change in PR interval. ▪ In **third-degree block** (also known as **complete heart block**), there is no conduction via the AV node; atrial impulses do not reach the ventricles, and the ventricles beat at their intrinsic pace. On an ECG, this is reflected as P waves and QRS complexes occurring independently of each other.
▪ **What is an escape rhythm?**	Cells in the AV node and His-Purkinje system are capable of generating their own inherent, pacemaking stimuli (**automaticity**), but their rhythm is normally suppressed due to the faster rhythm of the SA node (**overdrive suppression**). In cases where the SA impulse is blocked, the rhythm of the latent pacemakers "escapes" to elicit ventricular contraction. Junctional **escape rhythms** from the AV node or proximal bundle of His have a rate of 40–60/min. Ventricular escape rhythms from more distal pacemakers have rates of 30–40/min and are characterized by wide QRS complexes.
▪ **What is the most appropriate treatment for this condition?**	Often, no treatment is necessary in asymptomatic patients with a second-degree Mobitz type I block. In symptomatic patients, atropine or isoproterenol may be used, or a pacemaker may be required.

▶ Case 6

A 2-week-old baby boy is seen in the pediatrician's office for a well-baby checkup. On physical examination, the baby's femoral pulses are weak and delayed bilaterally.

- **What is the most likely diagnosis?**

Coarctation of the aorta, a condition that occurs two to five times more often in males than in females.

- **What are the two main variations of this disease?**

- **Preductal/infantile coarctation** (2% of cases) is a narrowing proximal to the ductus arteriosus. It is caused by a fetal cardiac defect that causes reduced left heart blood flow and consequent hypoplastic aortic development. **IN**fantile coarctation occurs **IN**side of the ductus.
- **Postductal/adult coarctation** (98% of cases) is a narrowing distal to the ductus arteriosus. It is likely the result of excess muscular tissue from the ductus arteriosus growing out into the aorta. At birth, when the muscular tissue of the ductus arteriosus constricts, the ectopic ductal tissue in the aorta will also constrict and create a narrowing of the aorta. Figure 5-6 below shows the anatomic features of aortic coarctation.

- **What is the characteristic finding on physical examination?**

Auscultation over the chest and/or back may reveal a midsystolic ejection murmur. Weak, delayed pulses in the lower extremities are also characteristic of coarctation.

- **What syndrome is associated with this condition?**

Preductal, or infantile, coarctation is associated with Turner's syndrome (45,XO).

- **What physical examination, ECG, and chest x-ray findings often develop over time in patients with this condition?**

- Many patients develop hypertension of the upper extremities, with weak, delayed femoral pulses. If the coarctation is proximal to the point of division of the left subclavian artery, the systolic pressure in the patient's right arm may be greater than that in the left arm.
- Left ventricular hypertrophy is a common finding on ECG.
- Chest radiographs often show an indented aorta and/or notching of the inferior surface of the ribs. This notching is the result of increased blood flow through the interthoracic and intercostal vessels, which serve as collateral circulation.

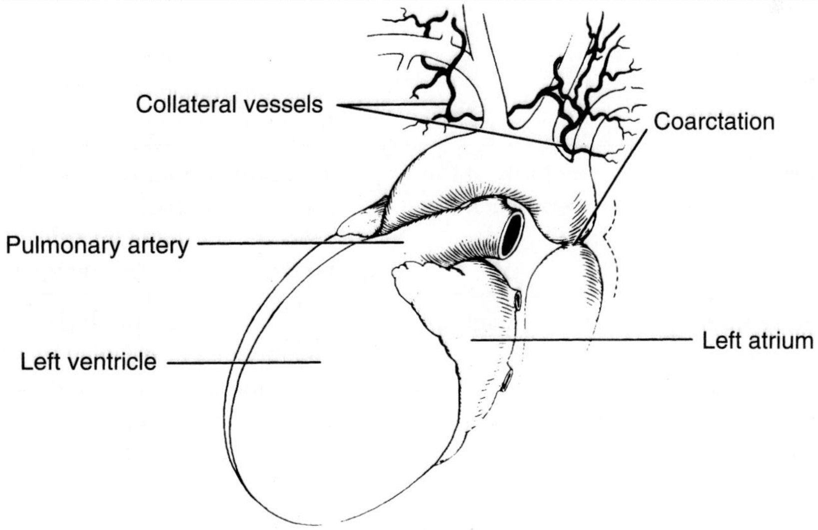

FIGURE 5-6. Anatomic features of aortic coarctation. (Reproduced, with permission, from Cheitlin M, Sokolow M, McIlroy M. Congenital heart disease. In *Clinical Cardiology*. Norwalk, CT: Appleton & Lange, 1993.)

▶ **Case 7**

At home, a 56-year-old man develops chest pressure and pain radiating to his left arm. He has a 50-pack-year history of smoking and a body mass index of 33 kg/m^2. He calls 9-1-1 and is rushed to the hospital, where his ECG shows ST elevation in the precordial leads and his creatine kinase (CK) and CK-MB fraction levels are found to be elevated. He undergoes cardiac catheterization, which reveals his left anterior descending (LAD) artery is occluded.

- **Which area of the heart is affected by this obstruction?**

The LAD runs along the anterior interventricular groove and supplies the anterior right and left ventricles, as well as the anterior interventricular (IV) septum. The LAD is the most common coronary artery to become occluded.

- **From what vessel does the LAD originate?**

The left coronary artery (LCA) arises as the left main artery, then bifurcates in most people to the LAD and the circumflex artery (see Figure 5-7 on the following page). In 20% of people, the LCA also gives rise to the **SA nodal artery,** which supplies the sinoatrial (SA) node. Most of the blood flow from the LCA goes to the LAD, which travels along the IV groove to the apex of the heart. The **circumflex artery** is a smaller branch of the LCA. The circumflex artery travels posteriorly to supply the left atrium and left ventricle. The LCA also gives rise to the **left marginal artery,** which runs along the left border of the heart and supplies the left ventricle.

- **What are the branches of the right coronary artery (RCA), and what territories do they supply?**

The **RCA** first travels in the atrioventricular groove, then wraps around the inferior border of the heart to the posterior IV groove. In 80% of people, the **SA nodal artery,** which ascends to supply the SA node, is the first branch of the RCA. Other branches of the RCA include the right marginal, posterior descending, and AV nodal arteries. The **right marginal artery** runs along the inferior margin of the heart to the apex; it supplies the right ventricle and apex. The **posterior descending artery** is the next to branch, and travels in the posterior IV groove to the apex, supplying the posterior right and left ventricles and IV septum. The **AV nodal artery** is a small branch of the RCA that arises near the terminus of the RCA to supply the AV node and bundle of His. In 90% of people the RCA provides the posterior descending artery; these people are considered right dominant. In the remainder, the circumflex artery provides the posterior descending artery; these people are considered left dominant.

- **What vessel drains the majority of the blood from the cardiac veins back into the chambers of the heart?**

The **coronary sinus** receives venous drainage from the great, middle, and small cardiac veins; the left posterior ventricular vein; and the left marginal vein. The coronary sinus lies in the posterior AV groove, and opens directly into the right atrium.

- **During which part of the contraction cycle do coronary arteries fill?**

The coronary arteries have maximum blood flow during diastole, and minimal flow during systole. This is due to their location above the cusps of the aortic valve, which obstructs flow into the coronary arteries when the valve opens during systole.

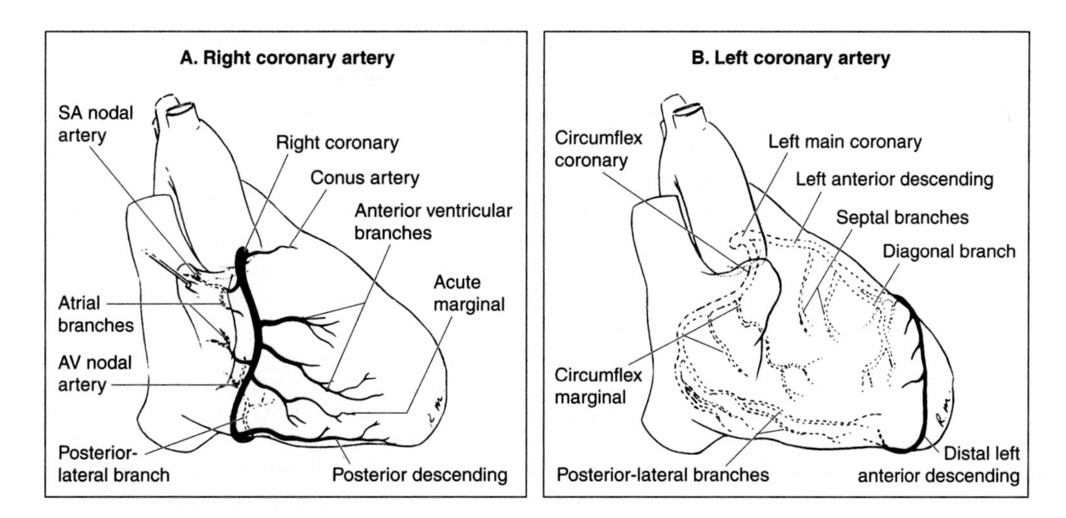

FIGURE 5-7. Arteries of the heart. (Reproduced, with permission, from Doherty GM. *Current Surgical Diagnosis and Treatment*, 12th ed. New York: McGraw-Hill, 2006: 391.)

▶ **Case 8**

A 65-year-old woman with a 60-pack-year smoking history comes to the physician because she has noticed swelling in both of her feet over the past 3 months. Until recently, she was able to walk four blocks to the grocery store without becoming short of breath; however, now she is only able to walk one block before having to stop and rest. Her sleep has also been poor recently, as she awakens many times each night with difficulty breathing. Sleeping on two pillows relieves her symptoms somewhat. Except for mild edema over her lower extremities, her physical examination is unremarkable. There is no evidence of hepatosplenomegaly or jugular venous distention.

▪ **What is the most likely diagnosis?**	Left heart failure (LHF), as evidenced by orthopnea, paroxysmal nocturnal dyspnea, dyspnea on exertion, and mild edema.
▪ **What are the common causes of this condition?**	Hypertension, myocardial infarction, valvular heart disease, myocarditis, and cardiomyopathies are associated with the development of LHF.
▪ **What symptoms help identify the anatomic source of this condition?**	Right heart failure is characterized by compromised venous return. This can manifest as ascites, significant edema of the lower extremities, jugular venous distention, and hepatosplenomegaly secondary to liver and spleen congestion.
▪ **This patient is at risk for which other conditions?**	LHF is the most common cause of right heart failure. In addition, her history of smoking places her at increased risk for chronic lung disease. This can lead to cor pulmonale, characterized by right ventricular hypertrophy and failure due to pulmonary congestion in patients with lung disease or pulmonary hypertension. Emphysema is commonly associated with cor pulmonale.
▪ **What are the likely findings on gross pathology?**	Hemosiderin-laden macrophages in the lung are commonly seen in LHF.

▶ Case 9

A 51-year-old man comes to the physician's office for a routine physical examination. At his last examination 3 years ago, he was advised to make appropriate lifestyle modifications because his blood pressure was 144/87 mm Hg. At the current visit his blood pressure is 150/95 mm Hg. The patient is overweight (body mass index 28 kg/m^2), and he has smoked one pack of cigarettes per day for the past 30 years.

What is the most likely diagnosis?	Hypertension.
What is the primary treatment for this condition?	Lifestyle modification is attempted before pharmacologic therapy is undertaken. This includes moderate dietary sodium restriction, weight reduction in obese patients, avoidance of excess alcohol intake, and regular aerobic exercise.
What is the initial pharmacologic therapy of choice for this condition?	The initial pharmacologic therapy of choice is a **thiazide diuretic** (hydrochlorothiazide, chlorothiazide, indapamide, metolazone), which are as effective as other drugs but cause fewer adverse effects. Thiazide diuretics inhibit sodium chloride reabsorption in the early distal tubule, reducing the diluting capacity of the nephron.
What is the mechanism of action and major toxicities of angiotensin-converting enzyme (ACE) inhibitors?	**ACE inhibitors,** such as captopril and enalapril, are particularly useful when comorbidities such as diabetes mellitus and cardiovascular disease coexist with hypertension. These drugs work by inhibiting ACE, thereby reducing levels of angiotensin II and preventing inactivation of bradykinin (a vasodilator). Toxicities include cough, angioedema, proteinuria, taste changes, hypotension, fetal renal damage, rash, and hyperkalemia. Angiotensin II receptor blockers such as losartan have a decreased incidence of cough as an adverse effect.
What is the mechanism of action and major toxicities of β_1-adrenergic blockers?	**β_1-selective blockers** (acebutalol, betaxolol, esmolol, atenolol, and metoprolol) are particularly useful in decreasing mortality after ischemic events. They work by blocking β-adrenergic receptors, slowing the heart rate, and decreasing blood pressure. While β_1-specific antagonists have fewer respiratory adverse effects than nonspecific β-blockers (such as propranolol), major adverse effects include bradycardia, congestive heart failure, atrioventricular block, sedation, sleep alteration, and impotence.
What is the mechanism of action and major toxicities of calcium channel blockers?	**Calcium channel blockers** such as nifedipine (which is more specific for vasculature than verapamil and diltiazem) block voltage-dependent L-type calcium channels of smooth and cardiac muscle, thus reducing muscle contractility. They are particularly useful when hypertension is not adequately controlled with the above agents. Major toxicities include cardiac depression, peripheral edema, flushing, dizziness, and constipation.

▶ **Case 10**

A 30-year-old man is evaluated in the emergency department for complaints of difficulty breathing, chills, and chest pain for the past 24 hours. He denies any previous history of medical problems. On physical examination, he appears ill. His temperature is 40° C (104° F), his blood pressure is 90/50 mm Hg, and his heart rate is 110/min. Cardiac examination reveals a 3/6 diastolic murmur; however, the patient denies any history of a murmur. ECG results are normal. Gram stain of a peripheral blood smear is shown in Figure 5-8 below.

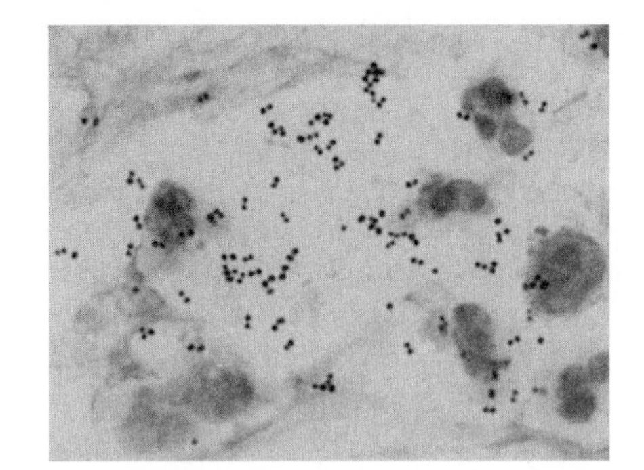

FIGURE 5-8. (Reproduced, with permission, from Bhushan V, Le T, et al. *First Aid for the USMLE Step 1: 2006*. New York: McGraw-Hill, 2006.)

▪ **What is the most likely diagnosis?**	Acute endocarditis caused by *Staphylococcus aureus*. The man's new heart murmur suggests a possible valvular lesion as the source of infection. In this case, a Gram stain which demonstrates gram-positive organisms in clusters is suggestive of staphylococci.
▪ **Which valvular structure is most commonly affected in this condition?**	In the general population, endocarditis most frequently involves the mitral valve. Common organisms include staphylococcal species and *Candida*. In intravenous drug users, however, the tricuspid valve is most commonly involved. In these cases, venous blood contaminated by nonsterile venipuncture crosses the tricuspid valve first.
▪ **What other microorganisms are associated with the development of this condition?**	**Acute endocarditis** develops in previously normal valves; *S. aureus*, *Neisseria gonorrhoeae*, and *Streptococcus pneumoniae* are common culprits. **Subacute endocarditis** is diagnosed in previously abnormal or damaged valves, and is often secondary to previous rheumatic fever. *S. viridans*, *S. epidermidis*, enterococci, and *Candida* are common causes of subacute endocarditis.
▪ **What is this condition called when it occurs with systemic lupus erythematosus?**	**Libman-Sacks endocarditis,** or "sterile endocarditis," occurs with systemic lupus erythematosus. This condition is believed to result from autoimmune damage to cardiac valves.
▪ **What characteristic of the microbe shown in Figure 5-8 confers resistance to penicillin?**	*S. aureus* secretes penicillinase (a β-lactamase), which inactivates penicillin.

■ **How does vancomycin resistance develop?**	*S. aureus* may acquire a gene that changes the vancomycin binding site from a D-ala D-ala sequence to D-ala D-lac on bacterial cell wall precursors. Loss of the binding site results in resistance to vancomycin.
■ **Which of this microbe's virulence factors increase the risk of chordae tendineae rupture?**	*S. aureus* secretes hyaluronidase, an enzyme that digests connective tissue.

▶ Case 11

A 3-year-old boy is brought to his pediatrician by his mother because he has had a high fever for the past week. Physical examination reveals bilateral injected conjunctiva, palmar erythema, oral mucositis, cervical lymphadenopathy, and solar erythema.

What is the most likely diagnosis?	Kawasaki disease, or mucocutaneous lymph node syndrome.
What symptoms are common at presentation?	Kawasaki disease commonly presents with fever lasting >5 days; erythematous rash (usually truncal; see Figure 5-9 below); edema in the conjunctivae, lips, and mouth ("strawberry tongue"); palmar and solar erythema; cervical lymphadenitis; and mucositis.
Which patients are most commonly affected?	Kawasaki disease is most common in children 6 months to 4 years old. Individuals of Asian ancestry are more often affected.
What is the pathophysiology of this disease?	This acute disorder is characterized by necrotizing vasculitis of small and medium-sized vessels. It is believed to be of autoimmune or infectious origin.
What is the most appropriate treatment for this condition?	High-dose aspirin or intravenous immunoglobulin G is the preferred treatment. Steroids are contraindicated! Patients should be treated as promptly as possible to prevent acute complications, including coronary aneurysm, myocardial infarction, severe heart failure, and hydrops of the gallbladder.
Which other infectious diseases commonly present as palmar and solar erythema?	Syphilis, Rocky Mountain spotted fever, meningococcemia, and coxsackievirus A infection can also present as palmar and solar erythema.

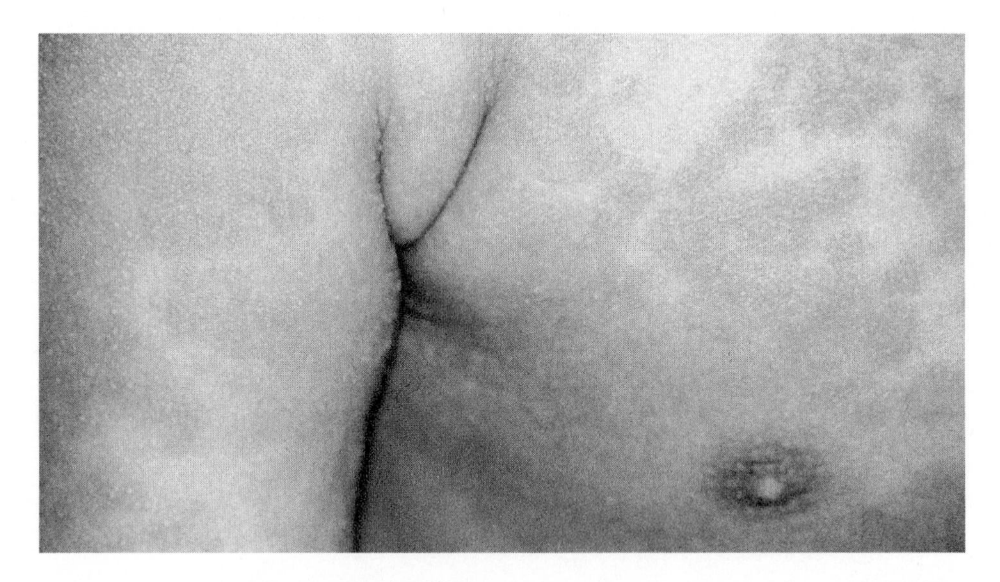

FIGURE 5-9. Erythema in Kawasaki disease. (Reproduced, with permission, from Wolff K, Johnson RA, Suurmond D. *Fitzpatrick's Color Atlas & Synopsis of Clinical Dermatology*, 5th ed. New York: McGraw-Hill, 2005: 423.)

▶ Case 12

A 56-year-old woman presents to the emergency department complaining of severe pain in her lower jaw and neck that has developed over the past hour. The pain is not sharp, and it is not relieved by rest or by changes in position. She took ibuprofen when the pain started, but the drug provided no relief. She also complains of nausea that began shortly before the onset of jaw and neck pain. On further questioning, she admits to a "heavy" feeling in her chest, which she describes as a squeezing or crushing sensation. She is profusely diaphoretic.

What is the most likely diagnosis?	Acute myocardial infarction (AMI).
How does this condition typically present?	Pain is the most common presenting symptom in patients with AMI. The pain is typically felt substernally or in the epigastrium, and is described by patients as "crushing" or "squeezing," and less commonly as "stabbing" or "burning" pain. An AMI may also present as pain in the left arm and/or jaw, sudden onset of shortness of breath, fatigue, or as adrenergic symptoms.
What serum markers are useful in making this diagnosis?	Serum cardiac markers such as creatinine kinase-MB fraction, cardiac-specific troponin I (cTnl), aspartate aminotransferase, and lactate dehydrogenase are released into the blood at varying times in response to cardiac tissue necrosis after AMI. **cTnl**, which is more specific than the other markers for AMI, is used within the first 4 hours, and cTnl levels may remain elevated for 7–10 days. **CK-MB** levels peak about 20 hours after the onset of coronary artery occlusion.
What test is the gold standard for diagnosing this condition in the first 6 hours after symptom onset?	Electrocardiogram. Figure 5-10 below shows ST segment elevation in leads V_2 and V_3. Total occlusion of an artery causing an AMI results in ST segment elevation. If there is subtotal occlusion, if the occlusion is transient, or if there is adequate collateral circulation, then ST segment elevation does not occur. Most patients who present with ST segment elevation eventually develop Q waves on ECG unless treated rapidly.
What complications are associated with this condition?	Complications of AMI include cardiac arrhythmia, left ventricular failure, thromboembolus as a result of a mural thrombus, cardiogenic shock (if the infarct involves a large area), and death. In addition, cardiac structures, including the ventricular wall, interventricular septum, or papillary muscles, may rupture. Fibrinous pericarditis and cardiac tamponade are additional possible complications.

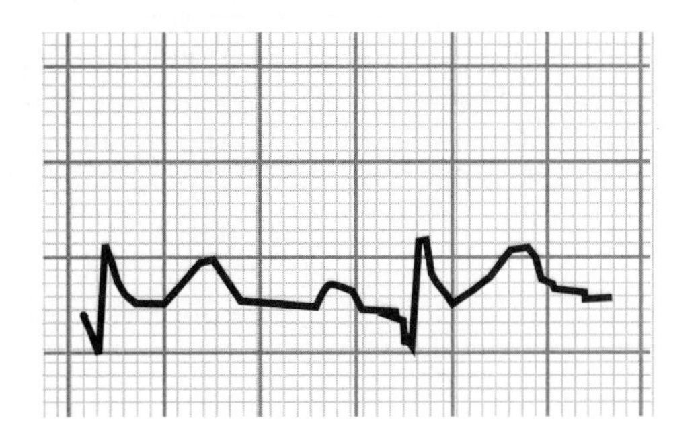

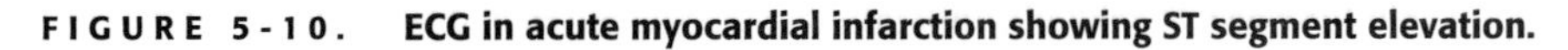

FIGURE 5-10. ECG in acute myocardial infarction showing ST segment elevation.

► **Case 13**

A 62-year-old woman comes to the emergency department with "excruciating" abdominal pain that began suddenly, waking her up from sleep early the same morning. She has no history of colitis or irritable bowel, and had an appendectomy as a teenager, but has had no surgeries since. On physical examination, she appears very uncomfortable, and her abdomen is slightly distended with hypoactive bowel sounds. She has only minimal pain on palpation, in the midepigastric area. She has no rebound or guarding. She denies changes in bowel habits, but her stool is heme positive.

- **What is the most likely diagnosis?**

This is a case of mesenteric ischemia, as suggested by the patient's severe gastrointestinal symptoms being out of proportion to the physical signs elicited. Given the sudden onset, this is most likely an embolic event. Ischemia affecting the small bowel will initially present with severe pain, with peritoneal signs developing later. Ischemia of the large bowel is less painful, and typically presents with hematochezia.

- **What organs are most likely affected by this condition?**

This case most likely represents ischemia of the midgut, which is supplied by the superior mesenteric artery (SMA) (see Figure 5-11 below). The SMA supplies part of the duodenum and part of the head of the pancreas (the territory of inferior pancreaticoduodenal artery), jejunum, ileum, ascending colon, and proximal two- thirds of the transverse colon.

- **What is the vascular supply of the hindgut?**

The inferior mesenteric artery (IMA). The hindgut includes the distal one-third of the transverse colon (splenic flexure), the descending colon, the sigmoid colon, and the rectum. The branches of the IMA are the left colic and sigmoid arteries. The IMA continues distally as the superior rectal artery. The left colic artery supplies the descending colon and the sigmoid arteries supply the sigmoid colon. The superior rectal artery supplies the proximal part of the rectum, piercing the muscular rectal wall to the submucous level as far as the mucocutaneous junction of the anal canal (anal columns). The muscle coat of the mid- and inferior rectum are supplied by branches of the internal iliac artery and internal pudendal artery, respectively. The anal canal below the mucocutaneous junction (pectinate line) is supplied by the inferior rectal artery branch of the internal pudendal artery.

- **What is the venous drainage of the midgut?**

The midgut is drained by the superior mesenteric vein, which lies anterior and to the right of the superior mesenteric artery. The superior mesenteric vein unites with the splenic vein behind the neck of the pancreas to form the portal vein.

- **After evaluating the patient, the surgeon decides to operate. Through what layers will the surgeon incise if he makes an incision 4 cm below the umbilicus?**

A midline incision through the anterior abdominal wall inferior to the umbilicus will cut through skin, superficial fascia and fat, the anterior layer of the rectus sheath (which is formed by the aponeuroses of the external oblique, internal oblique, and the transverses abdominis), then transversalis fascia, and finally peritoneum. Note that at the umbilicus and above, there is also a posterior layer of the rectus sheath.

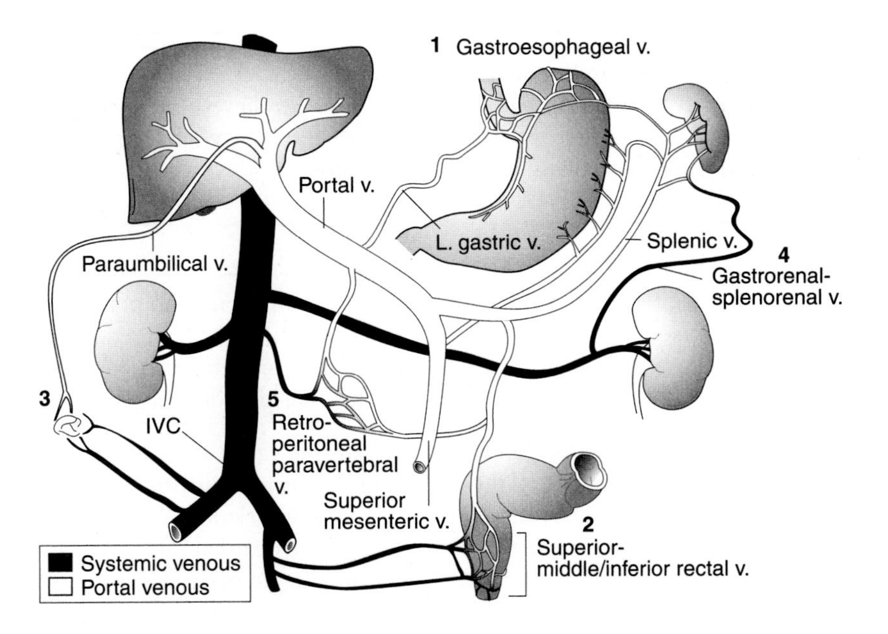

FIGURE 5-11. Portal-systemic anastomoses. Left gastric-azygos (1), superior-middle/inferior rectal (2), paraumbilical-inferior epigastric (3), retroperitoneal-renal (4), and retroperitoneal-paravertebral (5). (Reproduced, with permission, from Bhushan V, Le T, et al. *First Aid for the USMLE Step 1: 2006*. New York: McGraw-Hill, 2006: 264.)

▶ Case 14

A 47-year-old man presents to the emergency department after experiencing substernal chest pain. The pain is worsened with inspiration and is relieved only when he leans forward. He says he recently recovered from an upper respiratory infection. Cardiac examination reveals a friction rub and distant heart sounds.

■ **What is the most likely diagnosis?**	Pericarditis.
■ **What is an ECG likely to show?**	Diffuse ST segment elevations are consistent with pericarditis (see Figure 5-12 below). This is in contrast to ST segment elevations in some myocardial infarctions, in which the elevations are limited to ischemic regions. The classic finding is PR depression.
■ **How is this patient's condition classified?**	Preceding viral infection is a possible cause of serous pericarditis in this patient. Other causes of **serous pericarditis** include systemic lupus, rheumatoid arthritis, and uremia. Causes of **fibrinous pericarditis** include uremia, myocardial infarction, and rheumatic fever. Causes of **hemorrhagic pericarditis** include tuberculosis and malignancy.
■ **Which physical examination and ECG findings would be suspicious for cardiac tamponade in this patient?**	**Tamponade** is compression of the heart by fluid in the pericardium. This compression causes an equilibration of pressure in all four chambers of the heart and a reduction in blood pressure. **Pulsus paradoxus,** a decrease in arterial blood pressure >10 mm Hg during inspiration, is a sign of tamponade. Electrical **alternans,** or beat-to-beat variations in the amplitude of the QRS complex, may also be noted (see Figure 5-12 below).
■ **Why would an increase in jugular venous pressure on inspiration be of concern with this patient?**	This sign, known as the **Kussmaul sign,** indicates constrictive pericarditis, which can lead to compromise of cardiac output.
■ **What diagnosis would one consider if the patient had had a myocardial infarction 2 weeks earlier?**	**Dressler's syndrome,** or post-infarction pericarditis, describes the development of fibrinous pericarditis several weeks after myocardial infarction or cardiac surgery. It is likely an autoimmune response to myocardial antigens.

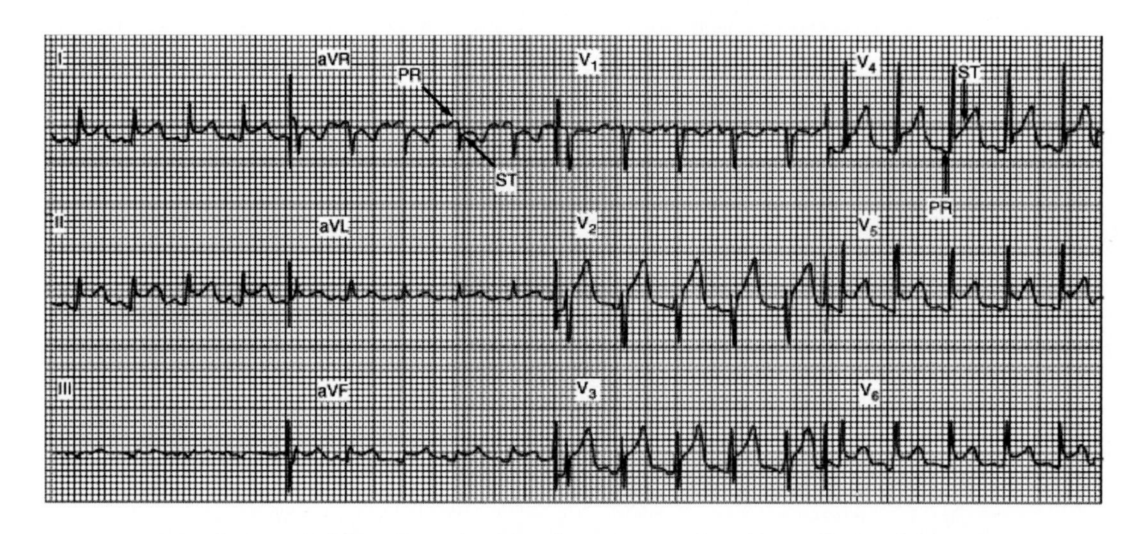

FIGURE 5-12. ECG strip in pericarditis. (Reproduced, with permission, from Kasper DL, et al. *Harrison's Principles of Internal Medicine,* 16th ed. New York: McGraw-Hill, 2005: 1318.)

▶ Case 15

A 35-year-old woman presents to her physician complaining of fatigue and fever. She also reports occasional abdominal pain, headaches, and muscle pain, and has lost 7 kg (15 lb) over the past 2 months. On physical examination, her blood pressure is 154/92 mm Hg. Retinal examination reveals cotton-wool spots, and skin examination is notable for palpable purpura. Her laboratory values are as follows:

Erythrocyte sedimentation rate: 121 mm/hr
Alanine aminotransferase (ALT) level: 1700 IU/L
Aspartate aminotransferase (AST) level: 1200 IU/L

▪ **What is the most likely diagnosis?**	Polyarteritis nodosa.
▪ **What is the pathophysiology of this disease?**	Polyarteritis nodosa is an autoimmune disorder characterized by segmental, transmural inflammation of small and medium-sized arteries due to necrotizing immune complexes. Vessels supplying the kidneys, heart, liver, and gastrointestinal tract are most often involved.
▪ **What laboratory test would be helpful in establishing a diagnosis?**	The presence of **P-ANCA** (perinuclear pattern of antineutrophil cytoplasmic antibodies) correlates with disease activity. P-ANCAs are more commonly seen in small artery disease.
▪ **What syndrome should be suspected if eosinophilia were also present?**	**Churg-Strauss syndrome;** this is a variant of polyarteritis nodosa characterized by eosinophilia and asthma.
▪ **What is the relevance of the ALT and AST levels?**	About 30% of cases of polyarteritis nodosa are associated with hepatitis B virus infection.

▶ **Case 16**

A 33-year-old woman who recently immigrated from India presents to her physician complaining of profound shortness of breath. Over the past few weeks, she has been progressively unable to walk up a flight of stairs without stopping to catch her breath. For the past few nights, she has been waking up suddenly, gasping for air. She also notes that she has recently been unable to fit into her dress shoes. The patient says she is generally healthy, leads an active lifestyle, and takes no medication except for vitamin supplements. Her past medical history is significant only for a 2-week hospitalization when she was a teenager for fever, sore throat, and joint pain. On physical examination her blood pressure is 110/80 mm Hg, heart rate is 100/min, and respiratory rate is 24/min. Jugular venous distention is noted, as are diffuse wheezes and rales at both lung bases. There is trace edema of her ankles bilaterally. Heart auscultation reveals a low-pitched, diastolic murmur with an opening snap, heard best at the apex.

▪ **What is the most likely diagnosis?**	Mitral stenosis (fish-mouth buttonhole deformity), resulting from a previous rheumatic fever infection. **Rheumatic heart disease** primarily affects the mitral and aortic valves; involvement of tricuspid and pulmonary valves is rare.
▪ **What histological changes are likely present in the myocardium in this condition?**	The histological hallmark of rheumatic heart disease is **Aschoff bodies,** which are areas of fibrinoid and collagen necrosis surrounded by multinucleated giant cells and other large cells **(Anitschkow myocytes)** (see Figure 5-13 below).
▪ **What hemodynamic changes occur in the heart in this condition?**	Left atrial diastolic pressure increases in cases of mitral stenosis because the left atrium must pump against a small, stiff valve. This can result in increased pulmonary hydrostatic pressure and, eventually, right heart failure.
▪ **What pathogen is responsible for the underlying infection in this condition?**	Rheumatic heart disease is a result of group A β-hemolytic streptococci infection. Valvular heart disease, as in this patient, often occurs many years after the acute infection. Antistreptolysin O antibodies are often seen in patients long after the acute infection resolves.
▪ **What is the most appropriate treatment for this condition?**	Cautious use of diuretics and sodium restriction to relieve pulmonary congestion is recommended. Surgery for valve replacement may be indicated for patients with severe symptoms. Prophylactic antibiotics for endocarditis may also be indicated.

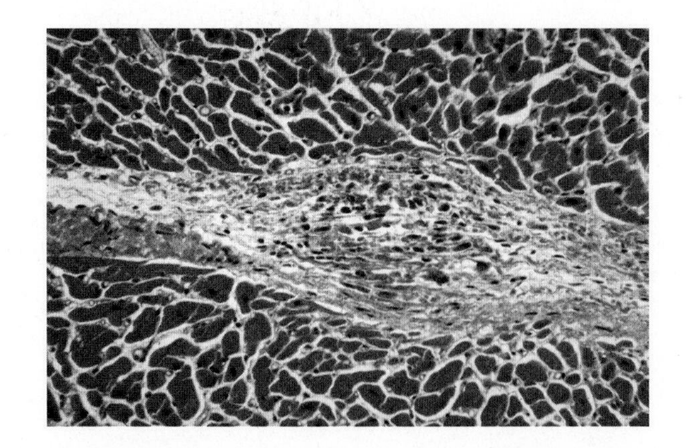

FIGURE 5-13. Aschoff bodies. (Reproduced with permission of the Pathology Education Instructional Resource Digital Library (http://pier.net) at the University of Alabama, Birmingham.)

► Case 17

A 59-year-old woman consults her physician because she has recently begun experiencing brief episodes of blurred vision in her right eye when reading the newspaper. On further questioning, she reports she has recently started to have headaches, which worsen at night.

What is the most likely diagnosis?	Temporal arteritis.
How is this condition diagnosed?	An elevated erythrocyte sedimentation rate and elevated C-reactive protein levels are nonspecific markers associated with temporal arteritis. Definitive diagnosis, however, requires biopsy of the temporal artery.
Which histopathologic features are associated with this condition?	Temporal arteritis is a systemic vasculitis of large and medium-sized vessels. One would expect to find mononuclear infiltrates in vessel walls and frequent giant cell formation (see Figure 5-14 below).
What is the most appropriate treatment for this condition?	Corticosteroids should be started as soon as possible. Nonsteroidal anti-inflammatory drugs can be given for pain.
What complications are associated with this condition?	Blindness in one or both eyes is the most common complication of untreated temporal arteritis, due to involvement of the ophthalmic artery or posterior ciliary arteries. Patients may also have fever, fatigue, new-onset headache, and jaw or arm claudication. More serious complications, such as thoracic aneurysm, occur less frequently. Additionally, temporal arteritis is often associated with **polymyalgia rheumatica.**

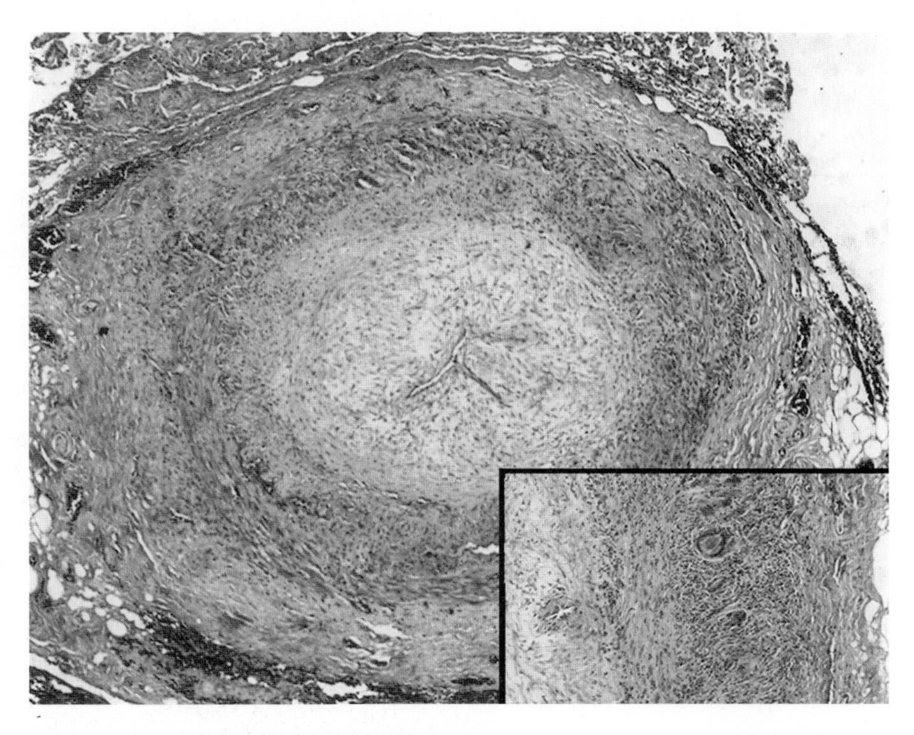

FIGURE 5-14. Histology of temporal arteritis. (Reproduced, with permission, from Hellmann DB. Vasculitis. In: Stobo J, et al. [eds]. *Principles and Practice of Medicine.* Norwalk, CT: Appleton & Lange, 1996.)

► Case 18

A 13-month-old boy is brought to the pediatrician by his mother, who reports he hyperventilates and becomes blue around his lips and in his fingertips after crying, eating, or any exertion. She has also noticed he tends to squat when he gets these symptoms.

What is the most likely diagnosis?	Tetralogy of Fallot (cyanotic congenital heart disease) presents as dyspnea on exertion, such as feeding or crying. Exertion results in systemic vasodilation, which lowers left-sided resistance, therefore increasing the right-to-left shunting of blood. This increasing bypass of the lungs causes cyanosis.
What anatomical findings are characteristic of this condition?	**PROVe** (refer to Figure 5-15 below): **P**ulmonary stenosis (1), **R**ight ventricular hypertrophy (2), **O**verriding aorta (deviation of the origin of the aorta to the right (3), and **V**entricular septal defect (VSD; 4).
Which congenital defect is responsible for this condition?	VSD. Specifically, the infundibular septum (portion of the septum adjacent to the outflow tracts) is anteriorly and superiorly displaced, leaving a hole in the ventricular septum. This displacement also causes pulmonary stenosis by blocking flow to the pulmonary artery. This results in increased pressure on the right side of the heart and right ventricular hypertrophy. Right-to-left shunting is increased when pressures on the left are decreased.
What is the characteristic radiologic finding in this condition?	Chest radiographs typically show a boot-shaped heart, due to right ventricular hypertrophy.
What additional physical finding is commonly associated with this condition?	Clubbing of the fingers in an adult (see Figure 5-16 below) also suggests chronic hypoxemia.

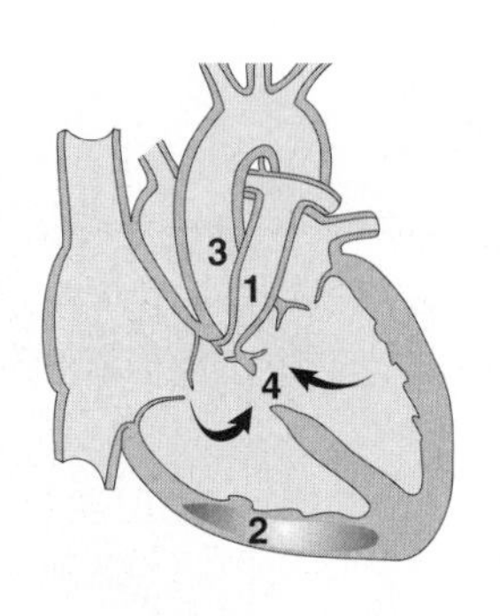

FIGURE 5-15. Drawing of heart in tetralogy of Fallot. (Adapted, with permission, from Chandrasoma P, Taylor CR. *Concise Pathology*, 3rd ed. Stamford, CT: Appleton & Lange, 1997: 345.)

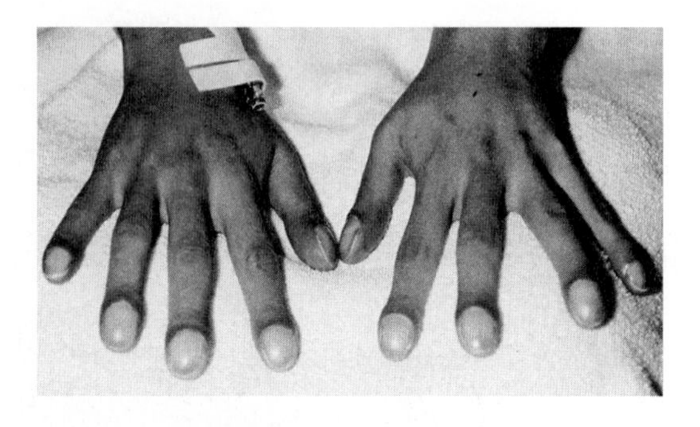

FIGURE 5-16. Clubbing of fingers. (Reproduced, with permission, from Knoop KJ, et al. *Atlas of Emergency Medicine*, 2nd ed. New York: McGraw-Hill, 2002: 369.)

▶ Case 19

A 61-year-old man with chronic sinusitis presents to his physician with cough and hemoptysis of 3 weeks' duration. He also complains of frequently becoming short of breath. Laboratory tests reveal his level of central pattern of antineutrophil cytoplasmic antibodies (C-ANCA) is elevated, and urinalysis reveals hematuria with RBC casts.

▪ **What is the most likely diagnosis?**	Wegener's granulomatosis.
▪ **What is the pathophysiology of this disease?**	Necrotizing granulomatous vasculitis of small and medium-sized vessels leads to manifestations in the kidney and lungs (see Figure 5-17 below).
▪ **What laboratory test would be helpful in establishing the diagnosis?**	The presence of C-ANCA is associated with Wegener's granulomatosis. In particular, Wegener's granulomatosis must be differentiated from **Goodpasture's syndrome,** an autoimmune disorder that also presents with hemoptysis and renal disease secondary to anti–glomerular basement membrane antibodies.
▪ **What are the likely findings on gross pathology?**	Renal involvement in Wegener's granulomatosis commonly manifests as a pauci-immune, or type III rapidly progressive glomerulonephritis. Immunofluorescence would reveal no antibodies or immune complex deposition.
▪ **If this patient also had severe renal dysfunction, which treatment should be avoided?**	Methotrexate can be nephrotoxic in patients with Wegener's granulomatosis. Preferred treatments include cyclophosphamide and corticosteroids.
▪ **What other findings are common in patients with this condition?**	Perforation of the nasal septum (the so-called "saddle nose" deformity, see Figure 5-18 below), chronic sinusitis, mastoiditis, cough, hemoptysis, hematuria, and RBC casts are common findings in patients with Wegener's granulomatosis.

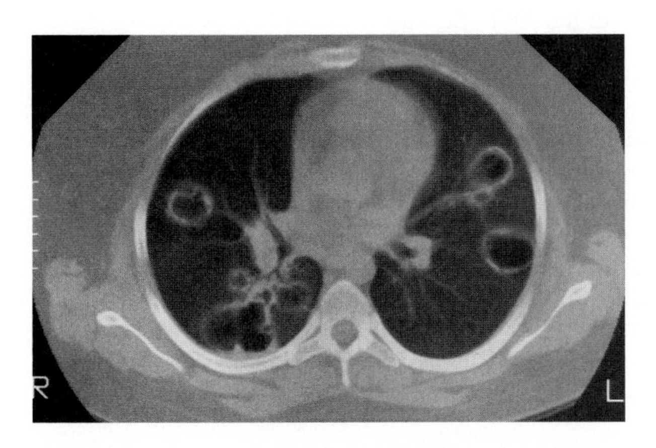

FIGURE 5-17. Lung findings in Wegener's granulomatosis. (Reproduced, with permission, from Kasper DL, et al. *Harrison's Principles of Internal Medicine,* 16th ed. New York: McGraw-Hill, 2005: 2004.)

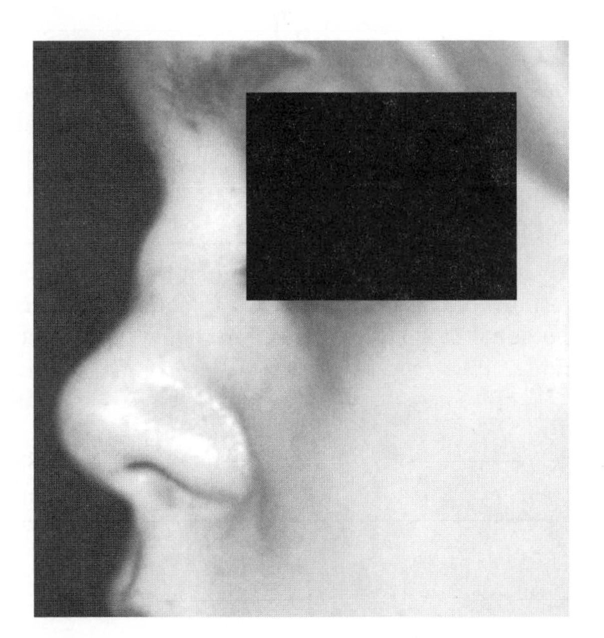

FIGURE 5-18. Nasal septum perforation in Wegener's granulomatosis. (Reproduced, with permission, from Imboden J, Hellmann DB, Stone JH. *Current Rheumatology Diagnosis & Treatment.* New York: McGraw-Hill, 2004.)

▶ Case 20

A 22-year-old man comes to his physician for a routine preemployment physical examination. Medical history reveals he is generally healthy, has no known medical conditions, and takes no medications. However, he admits he has recently experienced a few episodes of shortness of breath, dizziness, and palpitations. These episodes have no clear triggers. Results of physical examination are unremarkable. However, the patient's ECG is notable for the following: normal sinus rhythm at 65/min, a shortened PR interval (<0.12 sec), a prolonged QRS complex (>0.12 sec), and a slurred, slow-rising onset of the QRS complex (known as a **delta wave;** see Figure 5-19 below).

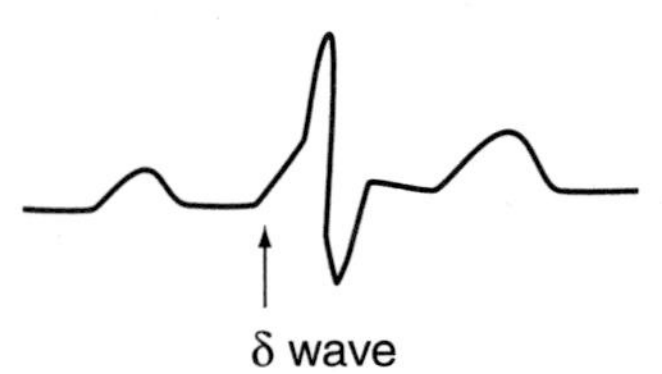

FIGURE 5-19. (Reproduced, with permission, from Bhushan V, Le T, et al. *First Aid for the USMLE Step 1: 2006*. New York: McGraw-Hill, 2006: 223.)

■ **What is the most likely diagnosis?**	Wolff-Parkinson-White (WPW) syndrome, or preexcitation syndrome.
■ **What is the pathophysiology of this condition?**	The presence of an abnormal band of myocytes creates an accessory conduction pathway, distinct from the atrioventricular (AV) node, between the atrial and ventricular systems. Because this accessory pathway is often faster than the AV node, the ventricles are excited more quickly than usual, causing the "preexcitation" syndrome. The presence of an accessory pathway, and the fact that accessory pathways have shorter refractory periods, predispose patients to reentrant tachycardias, atrial fibrillation, and atrial flutter.
■ **Why is the PR interval on ECG shortened in this condition?**	The PR interval is the interval between atrial contraction (the P wave) and ventricular contraction (the QRS complex). Thus, it is analogous to the conduction time through the AV node. It is shortened in WPW syndrome because AV conduction occurs via a faster, accessory pathway (frequently, the bundle of Kent), which bypasses the AV node.
■ **What ion channels are predominantly responsible for the upstroke in an action potential of a pacemaker cell in the AV node?**	Pacemaker cells depolarize due to the opening of voltage-gated calcium channels. These slow channels produce a slow conductance through the AV node, allowing for an interval between atrial and ventricular contraction. Without this interval, ventricles would not have time to fill. Atrial and ventricular myocytes (nonpacemaker cells), in contrast, depolarize via fast voltage-gated sodium channels; this produces the characteristic rapid upstroke of myocyte action potentials.

■ **Why are class II and class IV antiarrhythmic drugs not useful in this condition?**	Class II and IV antiarrhythmics, the β-blockers and calcium channel blockers, should not be used in patients with WPW syndrome because they act by increasing AV node refractoriness and decreasing AV node conduction velocity. They do **not** slow conduction over accessory pathways, and may even shorten the refractory period for accessory pathways. This may exacerbate atrial fibrillation or flutter, causing hemodynamic collapse. Rather, quinidine, disopyramide, and procainamide may be used to control arrhythmias in this syndrome.
■ **What is the most appropriate treatment for this condition?**	For most patients with WPW syndrome, electrophysiologic ablation is performed to ablate the accessory pathway. Cure is achieved in 90% of cases with no need for medication.

NOTES

Endocrine System

▶ Case 1

A 4-year-old girl is brought to her pediatrician for a routine checkup. The child is found to have high blood pressure. Upon reviewing the patient's chart, the physician finds the girl was born with ambiguous genitalia, namely, clitoral enlargement and labial fusion. The physician orders laboratory tests, which reveal the following:

Sodium: 142 mEq/L
Potassium: 3.1 mEq/L
Chloride: 102 mEq/L
Bicarbonate: 25 mEq/L

What enzyme deficiency is responsible for this condition?	11β-hydroxylase deficiency, as suggested by the constellation of **hyper**tension, masculinization, and **hypo**kalemia.
A similar enzyme deficiency also presents as masculinization of the external genitalia. How are these two enzyme deficiencies differentiated clinically?	21β-hydroxylase deficiency presents with **hypo**tension rather than hypertension, and **hyper**kalemia, rather than hypokalemia. Both deficiencies present with masculinization of the external genitalia. A review of adrenal steroid synthesis is shown in Figure 6-1 on the following page.
How does this enzyme deficiency result in hypertension?	11β-hydroxylase converts 11-deoxycorticosterone into corticosterone, and 11-deoxycortisol into cortisol. Deficiency of the enzyme results in a deficiency of cortisol and aldosterone. However, the precursor, 11-deoxycortisone, is a weak mineralocorticoid, and causes hypertension.
What treatment is most appropriate for this condition?	The goal of treatment is to replace the missing corticosteroid, which may be done by administering either dexamethasone or hydrocortisone. The patient should be treated with the lowest effective dose to avoid the cushingoid adverse effects of glucocorticoids, such as bone demineralization and growth retardation.
What is the mode of inheritance of this disorder?	11β-hydroxylase deficiency is inherited in an autosomal recessive manner, with mutations in the *CYP11B1* gene. All of the congenital adrenal hyperplasias are inherited in an autosomal recessive manner.

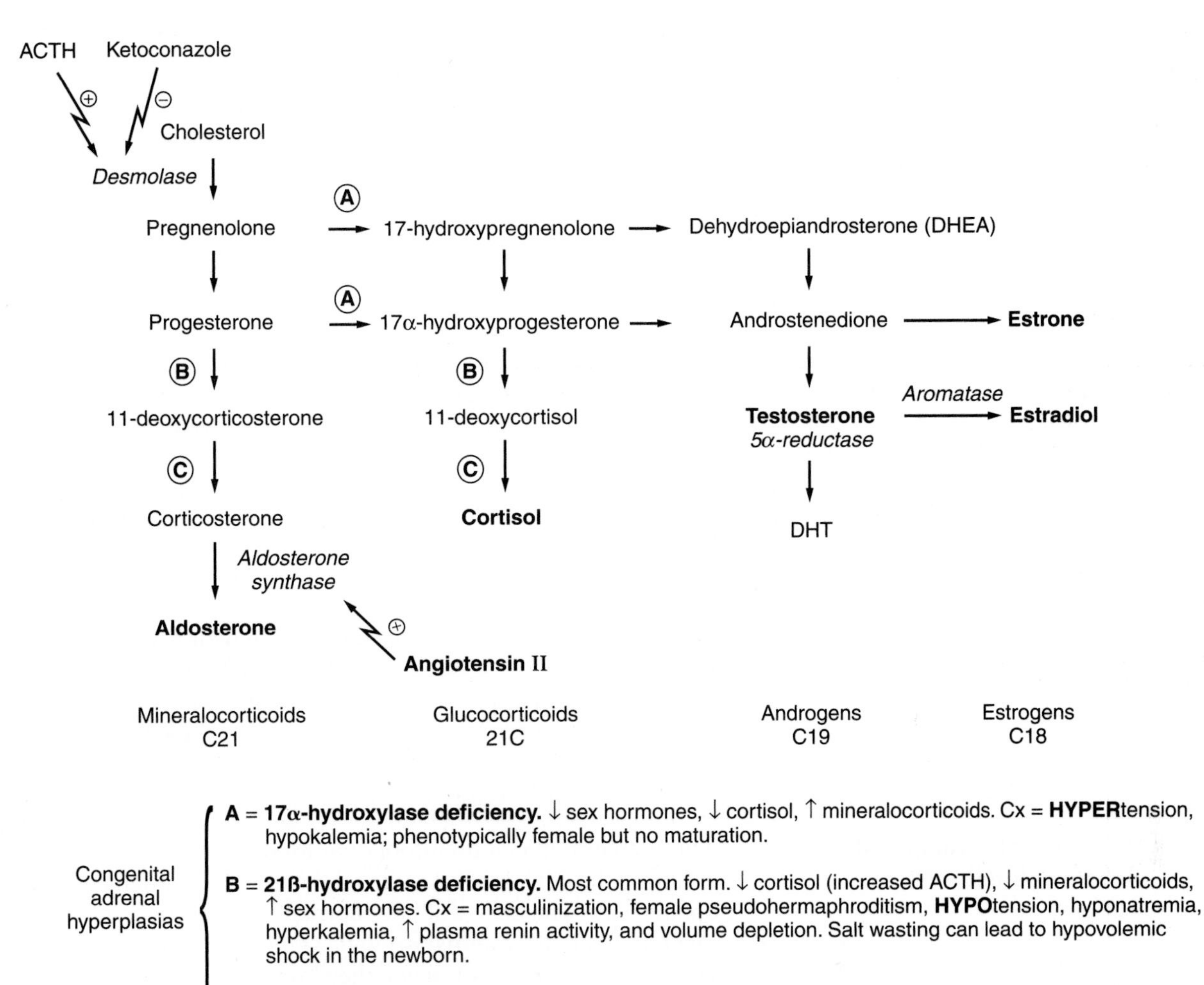

FIGURE 6-1. Adrenal steroid synthesis. (Reproduced, with permission, from Bhushan V, Le T, et al. *First Aid for the USMLE Step 1: 2006*. New York: McGraw-Hill, 2006: 249.)

▶ Case 2

A baby is born to a healthy mother, without complications. Physical examination reveals the neonate has ambiguous genitalia, with an enlarged clitoris that resembles a penis, and fused labia. The baby is also found to be dangerously hypotensive, and intravenous fluids are started.

▪ **What is the most likely diagnosis?**	The baby has congenital adrenal hyperplasia, as suggested by the ambiguous external genitalia (masculinization) and **hypo**tension. These signs are caused by lack of cortisol and aldosterone.
▪ **What enzyme deficiency is responsible for this condition?**	The defective enzyme is 21β-hydroxylase, which is an enzyme in the pathway that converts cholesterol into aldosterone and cortisol (see Figure 6-1 on page 125). This enzyme deficiency leads to buildup of its substrates, which get shunted into synthesis of sex hormones. Decreased cortisol leads to loss of feedback inhibition, and thus, increased adrenocorticotropic hormone, which further stimulates the conversion of cholesterol into sex hormone precursors.
▪ **What are the likely findings on laboratory testing?**	Patients with this enzyme deficiency will be **hyponatremic** and **hyperkalemic** because mineralocorticoids (which are low in these patients) are responsible for the retention of sodium and the excretion of potassium. The salt wasting causes hypotension, which leads to activation of the renin-angiotensin system, ultimately resulting in elevated serum renin levels.
▪ **Is this as example of hermaphroditism or pseudohermaphroditism?**	This is an example of **pseudohermaphroditism,** which is defined as having the gonads of one sex and the external genitalia of the opposite sex. The baby will have normal female gonads, but ambiguous, male-like external genitalia. **True hermaphroditism,** which is very rare, occurs when the child has both male and female gonadal tissue (ie, both testicular and ovarian tissues).
▪ **What is the most appropriate treatment for this condition?**	Congenital adrenal hyperplasia is treated with replacement of the deficient hormones.

▶ Case 3

A 40-year-old woman visits her physician because of fatigue, weakness, nausea, and constipation of several weeks' duration. She says she often feels lightheaded when she first gets out of bed in the morning. Review of symptoms is otherwise negative. Physical examination reveals several patches of hyperpigmentation on the skin (see Figure 6-2 below). Relevant laboratory findings are as follows:

Sodium: 126 mEq/L
Potassium: 5.2 mEq/L
Chloride: 97 mEq/L
Bicarbonate: 19 mEq/L
Cortisol: 4.3 mg/dL

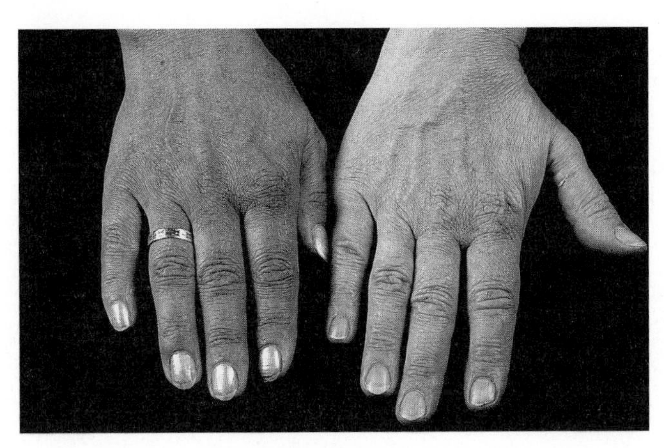

FIGURE 6-2. (Reproduced, with permission, from Wolff K, Johnson RA, Suurmond D. *Fitzpatrick's Color Atlas & Synopsis of Clinical Dermatology*, 5th ed. New York: McGraw-Hill, 2005: 445.)

- **What is the most likely diagnosis?**

Addison's disease, or primary adrenal insufficiency. This diagnosis is suggested by the clinical history of weakness and orthostatic hypotension, as well as hyperpigmentation, hyponatremia, hyperkalemia, and low serum cortisol level.

- **What are common etiologies of this disease?**

Most cases of Addison's disease are idiopathic/autoimmune-related. Other causes include:

- Disseminated intravascular coagulation
- **Waterhouse-Friderichsen syndrome** (hemorrhagic necrosis of the adrenal medulla secondary to meningococcemia)
- Granulomatous diseases such as tuberculosis
- Human immunodeficiency virus infection
- Neoplasm
- Trauma
- Vascular iatrogenic causes

- **What is the cause of this patient's metabolic abnormalities?**

Adrenal insufficiency causes a deficiency of cortisol. Hyponatremia, hyperkalemia, and a low bicarbonate level can result from low aldosterone levels associated with primary adrenal insufficiency.

- **How would this patient's cortisol level change if she were administered adrenocorticotropic hormone (ACTH)?**

The cortisol level should not change appreciably in response to ACTH, as the levels are low due to a **primary** adrenal insufficiency. This is suggested by the hyperpigmentation, reflecting the association between ACTH release and melanocyte-stimulating hormone, as well as low aldosterone levels, which would be normal in a secondary insufficiency.

- **Describe the secondary and tertiary forms of this condition.**

Secondary adrenal insufficiency is caused by decreased ACTH secretion by the pituitary gland. Administration of ACTH will result in a cortisol response. This syndrome does not cause hyperpigmentation. In contrast, **tertiary adrenal insufficiency** is caused by a decrease in corticotropin-releasing hormone production by the hypothalamus.

▶ Case 4

A 35-year-old woman presents to her internist complaining of recent episodes during which she feels weakness and tingling in her extremities. She has also been experiencing polyuria, nocturia, and polydipsia. Although her blood pressure was normal in the past, her blood pressure on the day of her visit is 160/100 mm Hg. Laboratory studies reveal a serum sodium level of 147 mEq/L, a potassium level of 2.8 mEq/L, and very low serum renin activity.

- **What is the most likely diagnosis?**

Primary hyperaldosteronism, also known as Conn's syndrome, as suggested by the patient's history, hypertension, hypernatremia, and hypokalemia. About 30%–60% of these cases are due to solitary adrenal adenomas in the zona glomerulosa, the layer of the adrenal cortex that secretes aldosterone. Bilateral hyperplasia of the zona glomerulosa can also cause Conn's syndrome.

- **How is aldosterone regulated?**

Renin, produced by the **juxtaglomerular cells** of the kidney, cleaves **angiotensinogen** (produced by the liver) to form **angiotensin I.** Angiotensin I, in turn, is cleaved by angiotensin-converting enzyme **(ACE)** to form **angiotensin II.** In response to volume contraction, **angiotensin II** is a potent stimulator of aldosterone synthase, a key enzyme in aldosterone synthesis.

- **Another patient presents with similar symptoms, but his laboratory tests show increased serum renin activity. What is his most likely diagnosis?**

Secondary hyperaldosteronism, resulting from an extra-adrenal source of renin hypersecretion. Causes include a renin-secreting tumor, renovascular disease (renal artery stenosis, malignant hypertension), and a decreased effective circulating volume (as in congestive heart failure, cirrhosis, nephrotic syndrome, hypovolemia, or the use of diuretics). Note that in primary hyperaldosteronism, renin is decreased, while it is increased in secondary hyperaldosteronism.

- **Given the patient's serum potassium level, what are the most likely findings on ECG?**

The typical ECG findings (see Figure 6-3 below) include:

- Prominent U waves
- Flattened T waves
- ST segment depression

- **What is the most appropriate treatment for this condition?**

Hypertension and hypokalemia in patients with Conn's syndrome are treated with spironolactone, which antagonizes aldosterone in the principal cells of the collecting tubule. Major adverse effects of spironolactone are due to its antiandrogen effects. These include gynecomastia, loss of libido, menstrual irregularities, and impotence.

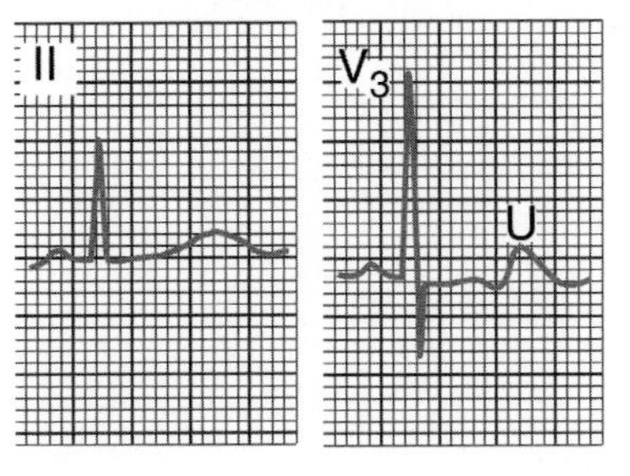

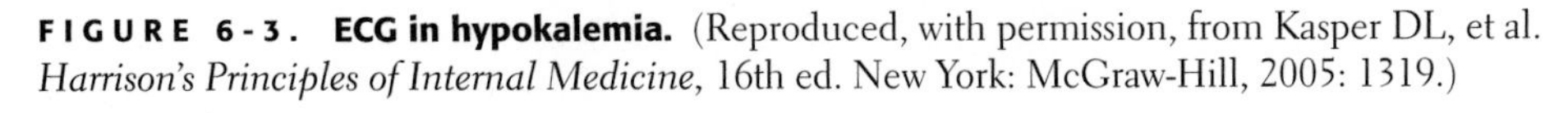

FIGURE 6-3. ECG in hypokalemia. (Reproduced, with permission, from Kasper DL, et al. *Harrison's Principles of Internal Medicine,* 16th ed. New York: McGraw-Hill, 2005: 1319.)

▶ Case 5

A 36-year-old woman with a history of hypertension, easy bruising, hirsutism, amenorrhea, and acne presents to her physician for a checkup. Physical examination reveals central obesity, proximal weakness, edema, and abdominal striae. Relevant laboratory findings are as follows:

Sodium: 140 mEq/L
Potassium: 3.4 mEq/L
Chloride: 92 mEq/L
Bicarbonate: 25 mEq/L
Glucose: 225 mg/dL

- **What is the most likely diagnosis?**

Cushing's syndrome. Common causes include:
- Adrenal hyperplasia/neoplasia
- Adrenocorticotropic hormone (ACTH)–producing tumor (most commonly secondary to small cell lung cancer)
- Iatrogenic (exogenous glucocorticoid administration is the most common cause)
- Pituitary adenoma (**Cushing's disease**)

- **What is the most likely etiology of the patient's syndrome?**

Cushing's syndrome is caused by excess glucocorticoids, either from increased cortisol production or from exogenous glucocorticoid therapy.

- **What laboratory tests can help confirm the diagnosis?**

- 24-hour urine test: demonstrates hypercortisolism
- Dexamethasone suppression test: oral administration of low-dose dexamethasone (a glucocorticoid) will not result in cortisol suppression

- **What diagnostic tests can elucidate the source of this patient's hormonal abnormalities?**

Serum ACTH levels can be an indicator of the source:
- High ACTH: pituitary adenoma or an ectopic ACTH-producing neoplasm
- Low ACTH: adrenal neoplasm/hyperplasia, or exogenous glucocorticoid administration

A pituitary adenoma may be differentiated from an ectopic ACTH-producing tumor by administering a high-dose **dexamethasone suppression test:** Pituitary adenomas respond to high-dose glucocorticoids by reducing their release of ACTH, whereas tumors that ectopically produce ACTH usually do not.

- **What are the most appropriate treatments for this condition?**

- Ketoconazole: inhibits glucocorticoid production
- Metyrapone: inhibits cortisol formation in adrenal pathway
- Aminoglutethimide: inhibits the synthesis of steroids

The most appropriate treatment for adrenal neoplasia is surgery.

▶ **Case 6**

A mother brings her 7-year-old child in to see the pediatrician. She says the boy has been less active, taking more naps, and wetting his bed, which he had stopped doing 2 years prior. Chart review reveals that, in the past year, his height has dropped from the 75th percentile curve to the 50th percentile. The mother is surprised by this and comments that he has been eating and drinking even more than usual. Relevant laboratory findings are as follows:

WBC count: 11,400/mm^3, with a normal differential
Sodium: 132 mEq/L
Potassium: 5.0 mEq/L
Chloride: 100 mEq/L
Blood urea nitrogen: 14 mg/dL
Creatinine: 1.2 mg/dL
Glucose: 350 mg/dL

- **What is the most likely diagnosis?**

Type 1 diabetes mellitus. Insulin deficiency is the result of autoimmune destruction of the islet cells of the pancreas (see Figure 6-4 below). Common presenting symptoms include polydipsia, polyphagia, weight loss, and polyuria (osmotic diuresis secondary to glucosuria).

- **What are the two types of this condition, and how do they differ?**

While **type 1 diabetes** is characterized by absolute insulin deficiency, **type 2 diabetes** is characterized by insulin resistance and increased insulin levels. Type 1 diabetes typically presents in thin individuals <30 years old, and is HLA-linked. Type 2 diabetes typically affects obese individuals >30 years old. Both types of diabetes can result in complications, including retinopathy, nephropathy, and neuropathy.

- **What are the major risks of rapid insulin therapy in this patient?**

- Cerebral edema from rapidly decreasing extracellular osmolality and subsequent influx of water into neurons
- Hypokalemia as insulin drives potassium into cells
- Hypoglycemia from too much insulin

- **What is DKA?**

DKA (**diabetic ketoacidosis**) results from a lack of insulin. Increased levels of fatty acids are delivered to the liver, where ketogenesis occurs. Presenting symptoms include **Kussmaul hyperpnea** (deep respirations), abdominal pain, dehydration, and nausea/vomiting.

- **What is the most appropriate treatment for this condition?**

Because these patients' insulin levels approach zero, they require lifelong insulin replacement. Oral hypoglycemic agents, which are effective for treating type 2 diabetes, will not work in patients with type 1 diabetes.

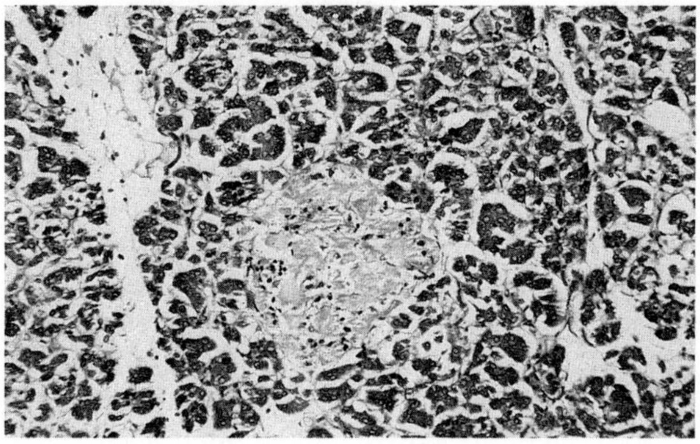

FIGURE 6-4. Pancreatic islet cells in type 1 diabetes mellitus. (Reproduced, with permission, from Bhushan V, Le T, et al. *First Aid for the USMLE Step 1: 2006*. New York: McGraw-Hill, 2006: Color Image 67B.)

▶ Case 7

A 40-year-old man presents to the clinic complaining of pain in his left big toe. He claims the pain is so severe that he is unable to walk normally. The pain began suddenly the same morning, waking him from sleep. He does not recall any trauma or bug bites to the area, and denies any accompanying symptoms. Upon questioning, the patient says the night before, he and his fiancée had a dinner of liver paté, cheese, and chianti wine. Physical examination reveals a warm and red metatarsophalangeal joint on his left foot, exquisitely sensitive to movement. Arthrocentesis of the affected toe is performed. Laboratory studies are significant for a serum uric acid level of 9 mg/dL.

- **What is the most likely diagnosis?**

Gout, secondary to hyperuricemia. Gout characteristically causes monoarticular arthritis, most commonly affecting the metatarsophalangeal joint **(podagra).**

- **What is the pathophysiology of this condition?**

Hyperuricemia secondary to overproduction (breakdown product of purine metabolism), or underexcretion of urate. Urate crystal deposition in the joints leads to acute and chronic inflammation.

- **What are some common causes of this condition?**

Uric acid overproduction resulting from:

- Excessive cell turnover (such as myelo- or lymphoproliferative disease, chronic hemolytic anemia, cytotoxic drugs, or severe muscle exertion)
- Excess dietary alcohol intake
- Excessive dietary purine intake
- Inherited enzyme defects
- Lesch-Nyhan syndrome

Uric acid underexcretion resulting from:

- Dehydration
- Impaired renal function
- Lactic acidosis
- Use of certain drugs (such as diuretics, salicylates, cyclosporine A)

- **What enzyme defects could result in this condition?**

Excess uric acid in the serum could result from enzyme defects in the purine salvage pathway, including hypoxanthine guanine phosphoribosyltransferase **(HGPRT)** deficiency, which causes Lesch-Nyhan syndrome, and phosphoribosylpyrophosphate **(PRPP)** synthetase overactivity.

- **What are the most likely findings on arthrocentesis of the big toe in this case?**

Needle-shaped negatively birefringent crystals are diagnostic for gout. Analysis of a sample from a patient with pseudogout, in contrast, would reveal basophilic rhomboid crystals of calcium pyrophosphate composition; deposition in pseudogout typically occurs in larger joints such as the knees.

- **What are the most appropriate treatments for this condition?**

- Nonsteroidal anti-inflammatory drugs (naproxen, sulindac, indomethacin): reduce inflammation.
- Colchicine: used to treat acute gout attacks. Depolymerizes microtubules, thus impairing leukocyte chemotaxis.
- Probenecid: used in chronic gout. Inhibits renal reabsorption of uric acid.
- Allopurinol: used in chronic gout. Inhibits conversion of xanthine to uric acid by xanthine oxidase. (Allopurinol is contraindicated in patients taking mercaptopurine and thiazide diuretics.)
- Nonpharmacologic therapy: reduced intake of purine-rich foods (eg, meat, beans, spinach) and alcohol, and avoidance of dehydration.

▶ Case 8

A 30-year-old woman visits her physicians because of her "heart racing" in her chest. She also reports she has been sweating much more than usual, to the point where she sometimes needs to change her clothes in the middle of the day. Physical examination reveals the woman has marked proptosis, and her hair is fine and sparse. She appears anxious, and on further questioning reports that her anxiety and feelings of restlessness have begun to cause problems at her workplace.

- **What is the most likely diagnosis?**

The signs and symptoms in this patient are typical of Graves' disease.

- **What demographic group does this condition typically affect?**

Graves' disease occurs eight times more frequently in women than men. The prevalence varies among populations, being more prevalent in populations with a high iodine intake. The disease rarely occurs before adolescence and typically affects those in the fourth to sixth decades of life.

- **What is the pathophysiology of this condition?**

Graves' disease is an autoimmune-induced hyperthyroidism. Thyroid-stimulating immunoglobulins are directed against, and stimulate, the thyroid-stimulating hormone receptor.

- **What are other common causes of hyperthyroidism?**

- Iatrogenic
- Silent thyroiditis
- Struma ovarii
- Subacute thyroiditis
- Thyroid adenoma
- Toxic multinodular goiter (Plummer's disease)

Note: Infiltrative ophthalmopathy and pretibial myxedema are seen only in hyperthyroidism caused by Graves' disease.

- **What are the most appropriate treatments for this condition?**

Propylthiouracil and methimazole inhibit iodine organification and coupling in the thyroid. Propylthiouracil also inhibits the peripheral conversion of thyroxine to triiodothyronine.

▶ Case 9

A 62-year-old woman presents with a month-long history of vague abdominal pain, constipation, and nausea/vomiting. Upon questioning, she says she also has experienced diffuse bone pain over the past month or so, but had attributed it to "just getting old." Physical examination reveals diffuse abdominal tenderness. Relevant laboratory findings are as follows:

Sodium: 140 mEq/L
Chloride: 110 mEq/L
Potassium: 4.0 mEq/L
Blood urea nitrogen/creatinine: 20:1.2 mg/dL
Calcium: 12.3 mg/dL
Bicarbonate: 26 mEq/L
Phosphate: 2.0 mg/dL

- **What is the most striking laboratory finding?**

Hypercalcemia. A useful mnemonic for common causes of hypercalcemia is **MISHAP: M**alignancy, **I**ntoxication with vitamin D, **S**arcoidosis, **H**yperparathyroidism, **A**lkali syndrome, and **P**aget's disease of the bone.

- **How is calcium regulated in the body?**

- **Parathyroid hormone (PTH)** stimulates increased calcium reabsorption from bone (by stimulating osteoclasts), increased calcium reabsorption in the distal convoluted tubules of the kidney, and increased production of 1,25-$(OH)_2$ vitamin D by the kidney (PTH also causes decreased reabsorption of phosphate by the kidney).
- **Vitamin D** promotes calcium reabsorption from bone as well as calcium absorption from the small intestine.
- **Calcitonin,** though probably not important in normal calcium homeostasis, inhibits the activity of osteoclasts, thereby decreasing reabsorption of calcium from bone.

- **The patient is found to have an elevated PTH level. How does this help explain the patient's overall clinical presentation?**

The patient has abdominal and bone pain in the context of an elevated calcium level and elevated PTH level. She has **hyperparathyroidism.** A useful mnemonic for the symptoms of hyperparathyroidism (and hypercalcemia, in general) is: "Painful bones, renal stones (nephrolithiasis), abdominal groans (abdominal pain, nausea, vomiting, anorexia), and psychic moans (changes in mental status)."

- **What are the most appropriate treatments for hypercalcemia?**

Hypercalcemia can often be corrected with hydration. If the electrolyte abnormality persists, a loop diuretic can be used (these cause increased calcium excretion). If needed, calcitonin and bisphosphonates can also be prescribed.

- **Describe the three forms of this condition.**

- **Primary hyperparathyroidism** occurs when the parathyroids produce PTH even in the face of elevated calcium—they are not responsive to the normal feedback regulation via an increased calcium concentration.
- **Secondary hyperparathyroidism** is the term given to a high production of PTH as a response to decreased calcium levels, as from renal failure.
- **Tertiary hyperparathyroidism** is refractory hyperparathyroidism in the setting of long-standing hyperparathyroidism, as seen in end-stage renal failure.

Because this patient has high levels of both PTH and calcium, she has primary hyperparathyroidism.

► Case 10

A 52-year-old woman presents to the clinic complaining of several months of generalized weakness, cold intolerance, and weight gain. Physical examination reveals alopecia, a thick and beefy tongue, myxedema, and delayed deep tendon reflexes. Her heart rate is 55/min and her blood pressure is 100/70 mm Hg. She is not taking any medications. Relevant laboratory findings are as follows:

Free thyroxine (T_4): 4.5 pmol/L (normal is 10.3–35 pmol/L)
Thyroid-stimulating hormone (TSH): 31 μU/mL (normal is 0.8–2 μU/mL)
Cholesterol: 230 mg/dL

▪ **What is the most likely diagnosis?**	Primary hypothyroidism. This is suggested by the history of cold intolerance, weight gain, myxedema, and fatigue and the prolonged relaxation phase of deep tendon reflexes.
▪ **What is the most common cause of this condition?**	**Hashimoto's thyroiditis,** resulting from autoimmune destruction of the thyroid gland. These patients are typically positive for **antithyroid peroxidase (antimicrosomal) antibodies.** Additional causes of hypothyroidism include Riedel's thyroiditis, subacute thyroiditis, and silent thyroiditis.
▪ **What endocrine disorder is associated with low free T_4 and low serum TSH levels?**	Low T_4 levels in the setting of low or normal TSH levels implies **secondary hypothyroidism,** the most common cause of which is **hypopituitarism.** Other manifestations of hypopituitarism include sexual dysfunction and diabetes insipidus.
▪ **What is thyroid storm?**	**Thyroid storm** is an acute, life-threatening surge of thyroid hormone in the blood, usually precipitated by surgery, trauma, infection, an acute iodine load, or long-standing hyperthyroidism. Manifestations include tachycardia (>140/min), heart failure, fever, agitation, delirium, psychosis, stupor, or coma. Gastrointestinal symptoms can also be present. This condition is treated with the β-blocker methimazole (to prevent hormone synthesis) and agents to reduce peripheral T_4 to triiodothyronine conversion.
▪ **What is the most appropriate treatment for this condition?**	Levothyroxine (synthetic T_4 hormone). Levels of T_4 typically take 4–6 weeks to reach steady state after initiating therapy.

▶ Case 11

A 58-year-old woman presents to her physician with a 2-month history of hoarseness and occasional palpitations and headaches. Her blood pressure is 170/90 mm Hg. Physical examination reveals a lump at the base of her neck. Results of biopsy of the mass are shown in Figure 6-5 below. Laboratory values are significant for hypercalcemia.

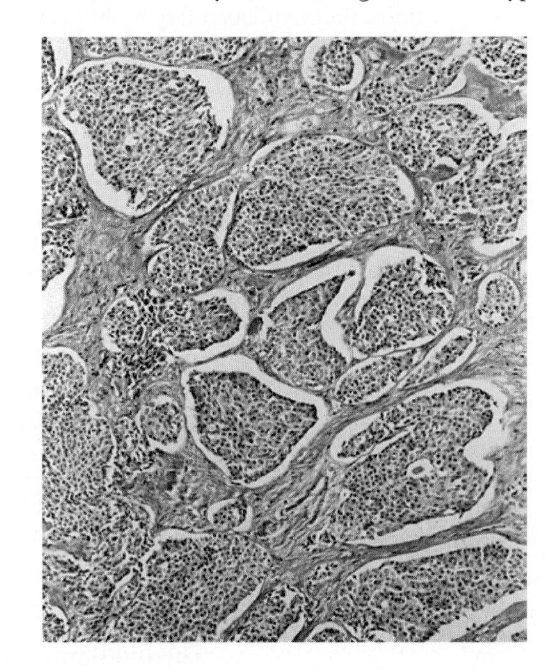

FIGURE 6-5. (Reproduced with permission of the Pathology Education Instructional Resource Digital Library (http://peir.net) at the University of Alabama, Birmingham.)

■ **What is the most likely diagnosis?**	Multiple endocrine neoplasia (MEN) type IIA, or Sipple syndrome. This syndrome is characterized by medullary carcinoma of the thyroid, pheochromocytoma, and hyperparathyroidism (due to either hyperplasia or tumor). Figure 6-5 shows the lobular pattern of growth of this tumor, which is accentuated to some degree by shrinkage artifact.
■ **What are the likely findings on gross pathologic examination of the neck mass?**	Medullary carcinoma of the thyroid is characterized by nests of cells in amyloid stroma.
■ **What genetic screening tests would be useful in confirming the diagnosis?**	The presence of the *RET* oncogene mutation in the setting of medullary carcinoma would be highly suspicious for MEN IIA. A variant of the *RET* mutation is also seen in MEN IIB, characterized by pheochromocytoma, medullary carcinoma, and mucocutaneous neuromas. However, parathyroid hyperplasia (hyperparathyroidism) is not a feature of MEN IIB.
■ **What additional laboratory tests would be useful in confirming the diagnosis?**	■ Elevated calcitonin levels due to medullary carcinoma ■ Elevated parathyroid hormone and calcium levels from parathyroid hyperplasia or adenoma ■ Elevated urinary or plasma levels of catecholamines and catecholamine metabolites (vanillylmandelic acid, metanephrine, and normetanephrines) in pheochromocytoma
■ **If this patient and her father have the *RET* mutation, what is the probability of her sibling's developing this condition?**	MEN IIA is an autosomal dominant disease. Thus, the probability of her sibling's having the mutation is 50%.

▶ Case 12

A 50-year-old woman presents to the emergency department complaining of a 2-hour history of vertigo, headache, palpitations, blurry vision, and diaphoresis. She has a history of occasional tension headaches, but no significant cardiac history. She does not smoke, and has no history of hypertension. At presentation her blood pressure is 200/140 mm Hg, heart rate is 120/min, and she is afebrile. Physical examination reveals her skin is sweaty and flushed. Imaging of the brain is negative for blood or other mass lesions. Her blood pressure is stabilized pharmacologically. Laboratory testing reveals increased plasma metanephrine and catecholamine levels. Results of a thyroid-stimulating hormone test and urinalysis of a 24-hour specimen are within normal limits.

What is the most likely diagnosis?	Pheochromocytoma, which is a catecholamine-secreting tumor of chromaffin cells of the adrenal medulla.
Describe the key steps in epinephrine catabolism.	As shown in Figure 6-6 below, catecholamines are substrates for monoamine oxidase (MAO) and catechol-O-methyltransferase (COMT). Epinephrine can undergo two paths of catabolism. In the first path, COMT converts epinephrine into metanephrine, which MAO then converts into 3-methoxy-4-hydroxymandelic acid. In the second path, MAO converts epinephrine into dihydroxymandelic acid, which COMT then converts into 3-methoxy-4-hydroxymandelic acid (the same product as the first pathway).
What receptors do catecholamines act on to produce hypertension?	α_1 and β_1 receptors. Activation of α_1 receptors leads to vascular smooth muscle contraction, and activation of β_1 receptors in the heart increases heart rate, conduction velocity, and contractility.
During removal of an adrenal gland, the surgeon must identify the superior, middle, and inferior suprarenal (adrenal) arteries. Where does each of these arteries originate?	The blood supply is symmetric for the right and left adrenal glands. The superior suprarenal arteries originate from the inferior phrenic artery. The middle suprarenal artery originates from the aorta. The inferior suprarenal artery originates from the renal artery.
What is the probability that this patient's condition is malignant?	There is approximately a 10% chance of malignancy. The "**rule of 10's**" for pheochromocytomas is: 10% malignant, 10% bilateral, 10% extra-adrenal, 10% calcify, 10% pediatric, 10% familial, and 10 times more likely to show up on the boards than in real life.

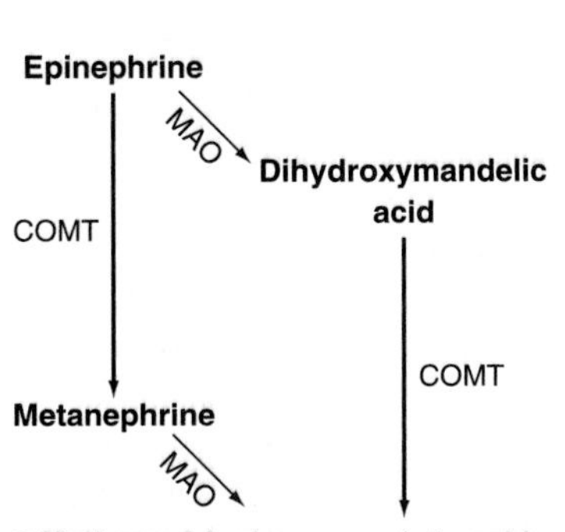

FIGURE 6-6. Epinephrine catabolism.

ORGAN SYSTEMS

ENDOCRINE SYSTEM

▶ Case 13

A 10-year-old girl is brought to her pediatrician for a workup of new-onset seizure. The patient had been in her usual state of health until 3 months previously, when she developed numbness and tingling in her fingertips and frequent muscle cramps. Last week, she suddenly had a grand mal seizure. CT of the head at that time revealed no intracranial lesions. Her parents deny a family history of seizures. Physical examination is notable for short stature, shortened fourth and fifth metacarpals, and positive Chvostek's and Trousseau's signs. Relevant laboratory findings are as follows:

Calcium: 7 mg/dL
Phosphate: 6 mg/dL
Parathyroid hormone (PTH): 100 pg/dL (normal 10–60 pg/dL)

■ **What is the most likely diagnosis?**	Pseudohypoparathyroidism (Type 1a), characterized by renal unresponsiveness to PTH. A genetic cause of this disorder results from a mutation in the G_s-α_1 protein of adenylyl cyclase. **Albright's hereditary osteodystrophy** is also present in type 1a pseudohypoparathyroidism, and some patients have growth hormone–releasing hormone resistance.
■ **What would hypocalcemia with a low serum PTH level suggest?**	**Primary hypoparathyroidism,** usually caused by accidental removal/injury of the parathyroid glands during thyroid surgery, causes decreased PTH levels, which results in decreased serum calcium levels.
■ **What are Chvostek's and Trousseau's signs?**	**Chvostek's sign** (twitching of ipsilateral facial muscles upon tapping of facial nerve just anterior to ear) and **Trousseau's sign** (carpal contractions provoked by inflating a blood pressure cuff above systolic blood pressure for over 3 minutes) are signs of hypocalcemia.
■ **How is the serum calcium level regulated?**	Serum calcium levels are regulated by both PTH and vitamin D. **PTH** has two major sites of action: in bone, it increases bone turnover, liberating calcium; in the kidney, PTH increases enzymatic formation of 1,25-$(OH)_2$-cholecalciferol from vitamin D, increases phosphate excretion, and increases calcium reabsorption. The active form of **vitamin D,** a steroid hormone, stimulates calcium and phosphate absorption in the gut and stimulates bone resorption.
■ **Where is PTH synthesized?**	PTH is made in the **chief cells** of the four parathyroid glands.

▶ Case 14

A 55-year-old woman with a history of external neck radiation therapy as a child presents to her physician for her yearly checkup. Physical examination reveals a nodule in the neck. Biopsy and imaging confirm the presence of a papillary carcinoma 1.2 cm in diameter in the left lobe of the thyroid and small metastases in the contralateral lobe. Two weeks later, the patient undergoes a near-total thyroidectomy.

- **How many parathyroid glands are there?**

Most people (83%) have four parathyroid glands. However, 13% have more than four glands, and 3% have fewer than four glands.

- **Describe the embryological origin of the parathyroid glands.**

The superior parathyroid glands are derived from the fourth pharyngeal pouch. The inferior parathyroids are derived from the third pharyngeal pouch. Most ectopic sites are derived from the carotid sheath and mediastinum.

- **What layers of muscle are incised during a thyroidectomy?**

- Platysma (facial nerve innervation)
- Cervical fascia
- The muscles listed below are flat and are referred to as "strap" muscles:
  - Sternohyoid
  - Omnohyoid
  - Sternothyroid
  - Thyrohyoid
- Lobes of thyroid, isthmus, and pyramidal lobe

- **What nerves in this region are particularly at risk during thyroidectomy?**

Damage to the recurrent laryngeal nerve in the tracheoesophageal groove results in a hoarse voice. The external laryngeal artery branch of the superior laryngeal nerve accompanies the superior thyroid artery and therefore can be ligated with the artery in thyroid surgery (see Figure 6-7 below). It is spared by ligating the artery close to the gland. Damage results in changes in pitch.

- **What are common causes of hypothyroidism?**

- Alcohol
- Autoimmune (Hashimoto's thyroiditis)
- Drugs (amiodarone and lithium)
- Infection

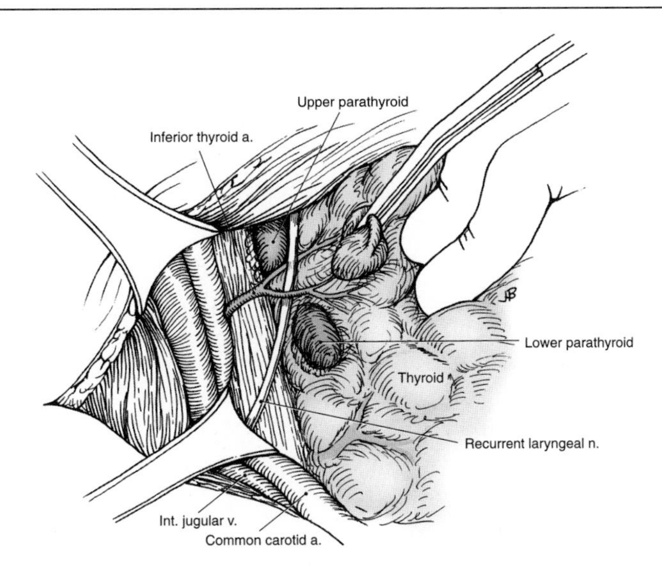

FIGURE 6-7. Relationship of the parathyroids to the recurrent laryngeal nerve. (Reproduced, with permission, from Brunicardi FC, et al. *Schwartz's Principles of Surgery*, 8th ed. New York: McGraw-Hill, 2005.)

NOTES

ORGAN SYSTEMS

ENDOCRINE SYSTEM

Gastrointestinal System

▶ Case 1

A 50-year-old man comes to his physician because of problems swallowing over the past several months. He says he encounters the greatest difficulty swallowing solid foods, although recently liquids have become problematic as well. Occasionally he also regurgitates bits of undigested food and often has a feeling of discomfort in his chest after eating. His physical examination is unremarkable.

What is the most likely diagnosis?	Achalasia.
What type of imaging or testing could help confirm this diagnosis?	A barium esophogram in a patient with achalasia will demonstrate a "bird's beak" appearance of the esophagus (as shown in Figure 7-1 below). Esophageal manometry confirms the diagnosis with a complete absence of peristalsis and failure of the lower esophageal sphincter (LES) to relax with swallowing.
What other conditions should be considered in the differential diagnosis?	Chagas' disease is indistinguishable from idiopathic forms of achalasia and should be considered in a patient from Central or South America, where the disease is endemic. Certain malignancies affect the gastroesophageal junction and give a picture known as "pseudoachalasia." Diffuse esophageal spasm and esophageal scleroderma must also be ruled out.
What is the pathophysiology of this condition?	Achalasia is an idiopathic motility disorder caused by impaired relaxation of the LES and loss of peristalsis in the smooth muscle that composes the lower two-thirds of the esophagus. The myenteric plexus of the esophagus contains nitric oxide–producing inhibitory neurons that are lost in achalasia, resulting in the clinical picture described above.
What is the most appropriate treatment for this condition?	Pneumatic dilation of the LES provides effective relief in most patients. Surgical myotomy and an antireflux procedure, typically performed laparoscopically, are also effective. In patients who are not surgical candidates, treatment includes multiple injections of botulinum toxin in the LES.

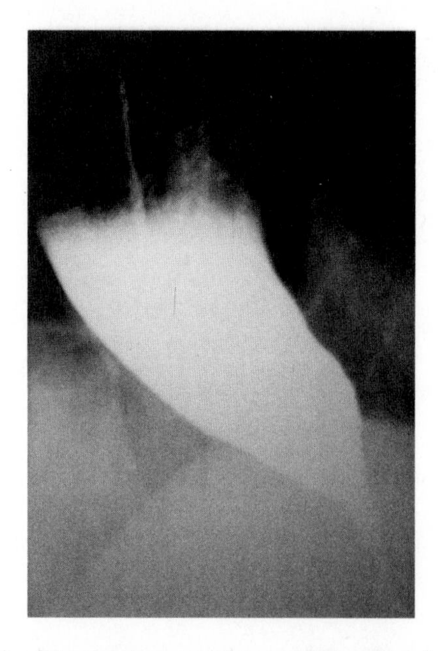

FIGURE 7-1. "Bird's beak" appearance of the esophagus in achalasia. (Reproduced, with permission, from Lalwani AK. *Current Diagnosis & Treatment in Otolaryngology—Head & Neck Surgery*. New York: McGraw-Hill, 2004.)

► Case 2

A 48-year-old man with human immunodeficiency virus (HIV) infection presents to his primary care physician with a 1-day history of nausea and vomiting. The man also complains of severe epigastric pain, which radiates to his back and is worse when he is lying down. Review of the patient's medical history reveals he is taking the reverse transcriptase inhibitor didanosine. Laboratory testing reveals his amylase level is five times higher than normal, and his lipase level is six times higher than normal.

▪ **What is the most likely diagnosis?**	Acute pancreatitis.
▪ **What are the most common causes of this condition?**	Acute pancreatitis is caused when pancreatic enzymes (trypsinogen, chymotrypsinogen, phospholipase A) are activated in pancreatic tissue rather than in the lumen of the intestine, resulting in the autodigestion of pancreatic tissue. The most common causes are **G**allstones, **E**tOH, **T**rauma, **S**teroids, **M**umps, **A**utoimmune diseases, **S**corpion stings, **H**yperlipidemia, and certain **D**rugs, including didanosine (mnemonic: **GET SMASHeD**).
▪ **What other conditions should be considered in the differential diagnosis?**	▪ Cholelithiasis ▪ Diabetic ketoacidosis ▪ Dissecting aortic aneurysm ▪ Intestinal obstruction ▪ Mesenteric ischemia ▪ Myocardial infarction ▪ Nephrolithiasis ▪ Perforated ulcer In this patient, the elevated amylase and lipase levels are sensitive and specific for acute pancreatitis.
▪ **Why is there an increased incidence of this condition in patients with HIV infection?**	Patients with HIV or acquired immunodeficiency syndrome (AIDS) are often infected with organisms such as cytomegalovirus, the *Mycobacterium avium* complex, and *Cryptosporidium*, all of which can cause pancreatitis. Patients with HIV/AIDS also take medications such as didanosine, pentamidine, and trimethoprim-sulfamethoxazole, which predispose to acute pancreatitis.
▪ **What is the most appropriate treatment for this condition?**	Most cases (85%–90%) are self-limited and spontaneously resolve within 4–7 days of the start of treatment. Typical treatment for acute pancreatitis include morphine for pain relief, intravenous fluid resuscitation, avoiding all oral intake (NPO), and possibly nasogastric tube placement to decrease the amount of gastrin in the stomach. Antibiotics do not affect outcome in mild or moderate acute pancreatitis, but they continue to be used prophylactically in cases of severe acute pancreatitis.

▶ **Case 3**

A 42-year-old man presents to his doctor for a regular checkup. He has an extensive past medical history of smoking, alcohol use, and remote intravenous drug use and has not seen a doctor for several years. During the review of systems, the patient says he has noticed increased bleeding from his gums recently as well as increased bruising. Physical examination reveals an overweight white man who appears older than his stated age. He also has mild gynecomastia and palmar erythema, with mild pitting edema in his lower extremities. Abdominal examination reveals shifting dullness. Relevant laboratory findings are as follows:

WBC count: 3200/mm^3	Potassium: 4.0 mEq/L
Platelets: 90,000/mm^3	Chloride: 98 mEq/L
Hemoglobin: 9 g/dL	Bicarbonate: 24 mEq/L
Hematocrit: 28%	Creatinine (Cr): 1.5 mg/dL
Prothrombin time (PT): 14 sec	Albumin: 3.3 g/dL
Partial thromboplastin time (PTT): 40 sec	Aspartate aminotransferase (AST): 100 U/L
Sodium: 138 mEq/L	Alanine aminotransferase (ALT): 60 U/L
	Blood urea nitrogen (BUN): 36 mg/dL

- **What is the most likely diagnosis?**

Alcoholic cirrhosis of the liver. The ascites, palmar erythema, and gynecomastia all suggest liver failure. The moderately elevated transaminase levels suggest a chronic process (too many hepatocytes have already died off to cause the dramatic rise that would be seen in an acute process). Further indicators of a chronic process include the decreased albumin level, elevated PT and PTT, thrombocytopenia from splenic sequestration, and decreased hematocrit (suggesting a bleed from some undetermined source or hemolytic anemia, promoted by a coagulopathy). An AST level higher than the ALT level suggests an alcoholic etiology rather than a viral one.

- **What are the causes of this patient's gynecomastia and bleeding gums?**

The liver normally degrades estrogen. Because this patient has liver injury, he likely has elevated estrogen levels in his serum, which explains the gynecomastia. The bleeding from his gums is likely due to thrombocytopenia from splenic sequestration.

- **How do ascites form?**

Ascites (an abnormal accumulation of serous fluid in the abdominal cavity) form as a result of increased intrahepatic sinusoidal pressure (which develops because of the intrahepatic obstruction that occurs in a cirrhotic liver), decreased degradation of aldosterone by the liver (leading to sodium and water retention), and decreased plasma osmotic pressure (resulting from decreased hepatic production of albumin). Signs of ascites on physical examination include shifting dullness, bulging flanks, and a fluid wave.

■ **What findings would be likely on urinalysis?**	BUN and Cr levels are elevated, and the BUN:Cr ratio is >20, suggesting prerenal failure. The kidneys are likely not being perfused appropriately because of decreased intravascular volume (as a result of the patient's ascites).
■ **Describe the findings in Figure 7-2 below.**	One can see a micronodular liver architecture that is characteristic of alcoholic liver damage. Fibrous bands are also observed in Figure 7-2 and are characteristic of alcoholic liver damage.

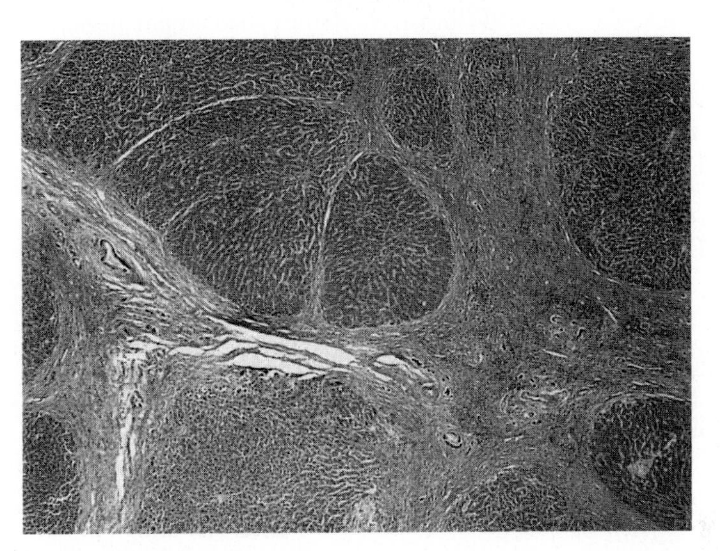

FIGURE 7-2. Cirrhosis, microscopic. Regenerative lesions are surrounded by fibrotic bands of collagen ("bridging fibrosis"), forming the characteristic nodularity. (Reproduced with permission of the Pathology Education Instructional Resource Digital Library (http://peir.net) at the University of Alabama, Birmingham.)

▶ Case 4

A 25-year-old woman presents to her physician complaining of a 3-day history of crampy abdominal pain that started in the epigastric region. She also reports nausea, a low-grade fever, and complete loss of appetite. Her last menstrual period was 2 weeks prior to presentation, and she denies any possibility that she could be pregnant. She denies changes in frequency or burning with urination or recent contact with a sick person. Relevant laboratory findings are as follows:

WBC count: 13,000/mm^3
β-Human chorionic gonadotropin: negative
Urinalysis: negative for blood, WBCs, leukocyte esterase, and protein

---

- **What is the most likely diagnosis?**

Appendicitis.

- **Which conditions should be considered in the differential diagnosis?**

- Genitourinary: ruptured Graafian follicle, ectopic pregnancy, pelvic inflammatory disease, ovarian torsion
- Gastrointestinal: Crohn's disease, Meckel's diverticulitis, perforated bowel, *Yersinia enterocolitica* infection, intussusception
- Renal: urinary tract infection, renal colic
- Lymphatics: mesenteric lymphadenitis

- **What is the pathophysiology of this condition?**

Two causes are possible: **obstruction** or **infection.** The appendiceal lumen may be obstructed by mucosal secretions, which distends the appendix. Alternatively, bacteria may attack the wall of the appendix, blocking the venous system and creating increased intraluminal pressure, which can then lead to arterial insufficiency.

- **What is McBurney's point?**

McBurney's point is the area to which right lower quadrant pain typically localizes in appendicitis. Specifically, it is one-third the distance from the anterior superior iliac spine to the umbilicus.

- **Which antibiotics are used to cover against enteric organisms?**

Ampicillin and sulbactam are commonly used empirically to treat *Escherichia coli* and *Bacteroides fragilis* infections. Gentamicin, clindamycin, imipenem, second-generation cephalosporins, and piperacillin/tazobactim are also effective.

- **What is the most appropriate treatment for this condition?**

Because appendicitis in this patient results from obstruction, surgery is still the preferred treatment, with supportive intravenous fluids and empiric antibiotics in case of rupture. The gold standard for diagnosis is CT of the abdomen; Figure 7-3 below is a contrast-enhanced CT showing a calcified appendolith.

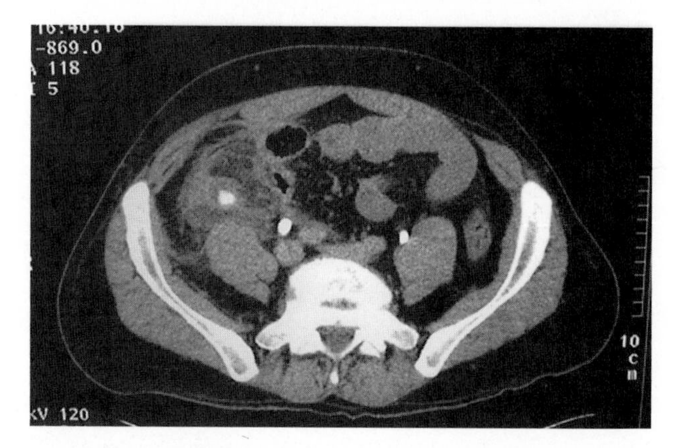

FIGURE 7-3. Contrast-enhanced CT showing a calcified appendolith. (Reproduced, with permission, from Stone CK, Humphries RL. *Current Emergency Diagnosis & Treatment*, 5th ed. New York: McGraw-Hill, 2004: 269.)

▶ Case 5

A 55-year-old man comes to his physician with a complaint of a burning pain in his chest. The pain often radiates to his neck and typically occurs after eating, although it also awakens him from sleep on occasion. The patient also complains of difficulty swallowing, which is most noticeable with solid foods. He reports he has had these symptoms for several years, but now seeks medical attention because they seem to be worsening. Endoscopy reveals gastric columnar epithelium in the distal esophagus.

▪ **What is the most likely diagnosis?**	Barrett's esophagus.
▪ **In the absence of positive findings on endoscopy, what other conditions should be considered in the differential diagnosis?**	▪ Angina pectoris ▪ Erosive esophagitis ▪ Esophageal stricture ▪ Gastroesophageal reflux disease (GERD) ▪ Peptic ulcer disease ▪ Pill esophagitis ▪ Malignancy ▪ Schatzki's ring
▪ **What type of epithelium is normally found in the distal esophagus?**	Nonkeratinized squamous epithelium. In Barrett's esophagus, this is replaced by gastric (columnar) epithelium in response to chronic injury from gastroesophageal reflux (see Figure 7-4 below). The border between the squamous epithelium of the esophagus and the columnar epithelium of the stomach is known as the squamocolumnar junction, or **"Z line."**
▪ **Patients with this condition are at greatly increased risk for what other condition?**	Adenocarcinoma of the esophagus. Compared to the general population, patients with Barrett's esophagus are 30 times more likely to develop esophageal adenocarcinoma, with a mean annual incidence of about 1%. However, Barrett's esophagus does not increase the risk of developing squamous cell carcinoma.
▪ **What factors increases the risk of developing esophageal cancer?**	Barrett's esophagus is the major risk factor for adenocarcinoma. Squamous cell cancer is strongly associated with alcohol and cigarette smoking. The risk factors for esophageal cancer may be remembered with the mnemonic **ABCDEF: A**chalasia/**A**frican-American male, **B**arrett's esophagus, **C**orrosive esophagitis/**C**igarettes, **D**iverticuli (ie, Zenker's diverticulum), **E**sophageal web/**E**tOH, and **F**amilial/**F**ood low in fruits and vegetables.

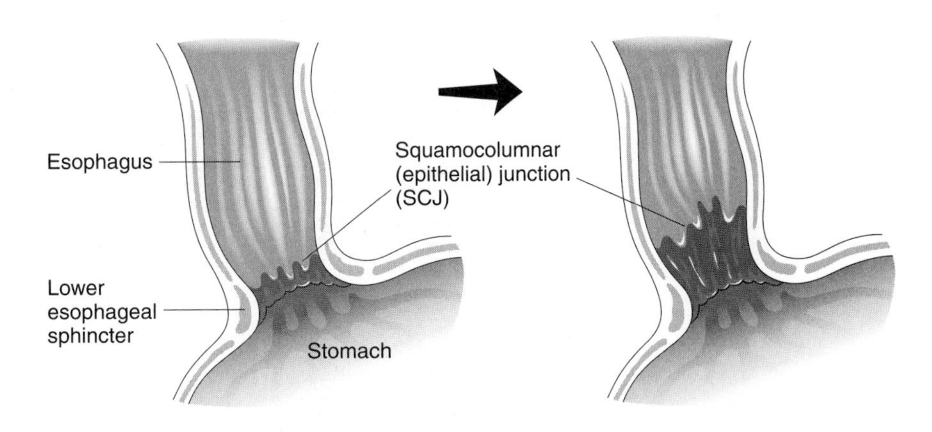

FIGURE 7-4. Barrett's esophagus. Note how the columnar epithelium of the stomach has migrated superior to the LES. (Reproduced, with permission, from Bhushan V, Le T, et al. *First Aid for the USMLE Step 1: 2006*. New York: McGraw-Hill, 2006: 274.)

ORGAN SYSTEMS

GASTROINTESTINAL SYSTEM

▶ Case 6

A 42-year-old obese woman presents to the urgent care facility with a sudden onset of right upper quadrant and epigastric pain that began after she dropped off her youngest child at school 8 hours earlier. She describes the pain as steady in nature, and notes some pain behind her right shoulder. After eating dinner, she found the pain increased significantly. Physical examination reveals inspiratory arrest with deep palpation of the right upper quadrant (Murphy's sign). Relevant laboratory findings are as follows:

Total bilirubin: 2 mg/dL
Aspartate aminotransferase: 44 U/L
Alanine aminotransferase: 49 U/L
Blood urea nitrogen: 16 mg/dL
Creatinine: 1.05 mg/dL

- **What is the most likely diagnosis?**

A gallbladder obstructed by gallstones (cholelithiasis).

- **Which bacteria are commonly associated with this condition?**

Escherichia coli, Enterobacter cloacae, Enterococcus, and *Klebsiella* infections secondary to obstruction from cholelithiasis are commonly associated with infection in an obstructed gallbladder.

- **How does the obstruction in this patient form?**

Cholesterol gallstones are most common in the United States and occur when cholesterol is more predominant than bile acid, allowing cholesterol crystals to form. Risk factors for gallstones can be remembered as the **Four F's: Fat, Fertile, Female,** and **Forty.** Patients with decreased gallbladder emptying secondary to oral contraceptive use, spinal cord injury, or diabetes mellitus are predisposed to gallstones. Intestinal and liver disease are also risk factors. Worldwide, **pigmented gallstones** are the most common form. These form secondary to bile duct/gallbladder infection or hemolysis (causing excess bilirubin to be excreted from the liver) or impaired hepatic synthesis of bilirubin.

- **What is the pathophysiology of the patient's pain?**

Gallstones produce pain by obstructing the ampulla of Vater or the cystic duct, which creates distention of the gallbladder. The pericholecystic fluid and thickened gallbladder wall make visualization of gallstones difficult on CT.

- **What is the most appropriate treatment for managing this patient's pain?**

Gallstone pain is relieved when the gallstone moves back into the gallbladder, moves into the common bile duct, or passes through the ampulla of Vater. Pain of biliary colic accompanies spasms of the sphincter of Oddi. Therefore, **meperidine** should be given for pain, as morphine causes spasms of the sphincter of Oddi.

- **The hepatoduodenal ligament includes which three structures?**

Three structures run through the hepatoduodenal ligament (see Figure 7-5 on the following page):

- **Portal vein:** brings blood from the digestive tract to the liver
- **Hepatic artery:** brings oxygen and nutrients to the liver
- **Common bile duct:** connects liver and gallbladder to the small intestine

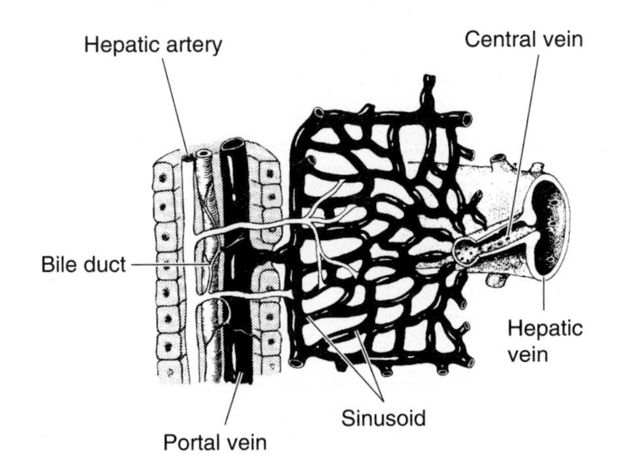

FIGURE 7-5. Vascular anatomy of the liver lobule. (Reproduced, with permission, from Doherty GM. *Current Surgical Diagnosis and Treatment,* 12th ed. New York: McGraw-Hill, 2006: 542.)

▶ Case 7

A 6-day-old girl born to a Jewish couple is brought to her pediatrician because her skin and eyes have become progressively more yellow since birth. The parents also report the baby has been sleeping through the night and napping throughout most of the day. They are concerned because the baby seems weak and floppy. Physical examination reveals a jaundiced infant with scleral icterus, without other obvious abnormalities. Relevant laboratory findings are as follows:

Total bilirubin: 34 mg/dL
Direct bilirubin: undetectable
Aspartate aminotransferase: 10 U/L
Alanine aminotransferase: 12 U/L
Coombs' test: negative

■ **What is the most likely diagnosis?**	Crigler-Najjar syndrome.
■ **What is the pathophysiology of this condition?**	This disease is an inherited disorder of bilirubin metabolism. It is the result of a mutation in glucuronyl transferase, the enzyme responsible for conjugating bilirubin with glucuronic acid. Unconjugated bilirubin is less water soluble than conjugated bilirubin and is less easily excreted in urine and bile.
■ **What are the two subtypes of this condition, and how do they differ in severity?**	■ **Crigler-Najjar type I:** Glucuronyl transferase activity is completely absent and there is a high likelihood of death in the first year of life. ■ **Crigler-Najjar type II:** Glucuronyl transferase activity is low but still present. This portends a much better prognosis. Table 7-1 on the following page compares these two subtypes.
■ **This patient is at risk for what life-threatening complication?**	The mental status change that the baby has presented with suggests the onset of **kernicterus,** an abnormal accumulation of bile pigment in the brain and other nervous tissues. Unconjugated bilirubin that is not bound to albumin can penetrate the blood-brain barrier and cause neuronal death. Kernicterus can be fatal.
■ **What is the most appropriate treatment for this condition?**	In Crigler-Najjar type I, phototherapy is used to prevent kernicterus. Liver transplantation is the only cure. In the less severe Crigler-Najjar type II, the hyperbilirubinemia often responds to phenobarbital treatment.

TABLE 7-1. Principal Differential Characteristics of Crigler-Najjar Syndromes

Feature	Crigler-Najjar Syndrome	
	Type I	Type II
Total serum bilirubin, mg/dL	18–45 (usually >20)	6–25 (usually ≤20)
Routine liver tests	Normal	Normal
Response to phenobarbital	None	Decreases bilirubin by >25%
Kernicterus	Usual	Rare
Hepatic histology	Normal	Normal
Bile characteristics		
Color	Pale or colorless	Pigmented
Bilirubin fractions	>90% unconjugated	Largest fraction (mean: 57%) monoconjugates
Bilirubin UDP-glucuronosyltransferase activity	Typically absent; traces in some patients	Markedly reduced: 0%–10% of normal
Inheritance (both autosomal)	Recessive	Predominantly recessive

Modified, with permission, from Kasper DL, et al. *Harrison's Principles of Internal Medicine,* 16th ed. New York: McGraw-Hill, 2005: 1819.

▶ **Case 8**

A 64-year-old woman presents to her physician complaining of gas, constipation, and abdominal discomfort, which is worse on her left side. She reports the pain increases after meals but persists throughout the day. She has also felt lightheaded and fatigued for roughly a week. The patient has a history of chronic constipation, but the current symptoms are worse than is typical for her. She has not noticed any bloody stools, but reports having had massive gastrointestinal bleeding last year. After that episode was controlled, she received a barium enema; her roentgenogram is shown in Figure 7-6. She is currently taking aspirin once a day for her heart, but is taking no other medication. Physical examination reveals a fever of 38.6° C (101.5° F), blood pressure of 110/70 mm Hg, heart rate of 105/min, and respiratory rate of 18/min. Relevant laboratory findings are as follows:

WBC count: 13,400/mm^3
Platelets: 250,000/mm^3
Hemoglobin: 13 g/dL
Hematocrit: 38%
Sodium: 136 mEq/L
Potassium: 4.3 mEq/L
Chloride: 100 mEq/L
Bicarbonate: 24 mEq/L
Creatinine: 1.2 mg/dL
Stool guaiac test: negative

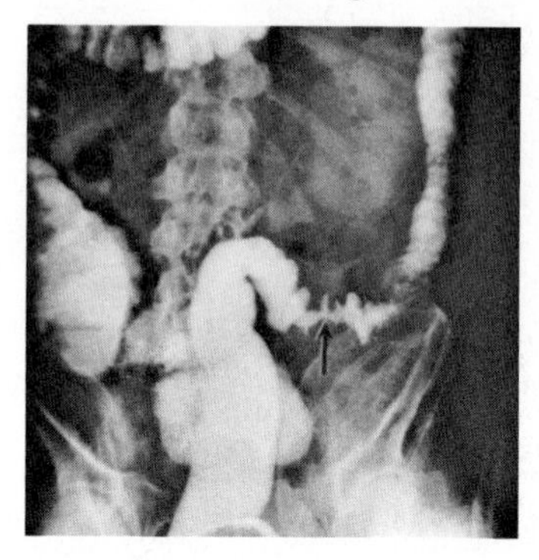

FIGURE 7-6. (Reproduced, with permission, from Doherty GM, Way LW. *Current Surgical Diagnosis & Treatment*, 12th ed. New York: McGraw-Hill, 2006: 715.)

- **What is the most likely diagnosis?**

The patient has diverticular disease, which is seen on imaging as contrast-filled diverticula in the distal colon. This suggests that the cause of the patient's previous history of gastrointestinal bleeding was likely the result of diverticulosis.

- **Which of the clinical signs and symptoms help confirm the diagnosis?**

The patient's constipation, flatus, left-sided abdominal pain, tenderness, fever, tachycardia, and elevated WBC count are all abnormal and characteristic of diverticulitis.

- **What tests could help confirm the diagnosis?**

The patient should undergo x-ray of the abdomen to check for intraperitoneal air (resulting from diverticular rupture) or distention. CT of the abdomen should also be ordered. In cases of diverticulitis, one might typically see bowel wall thickening, fistulas, or abscesses on CT. A colonoscopy is contraindicated in the acute setting, as it might induce perforation; however, it should be completed on follow-up.

- **What factors increase the risk of this condition, and what steps can prevent recurrence?**

The patient's age, chronic constipation, previous diverticulosis, and aspirin use all heighten her risk for diverticulitis. A high-fiber diet and good hydration reduce the risk of progression to diverticulitis.

- **What is the most appropriate treatment for this condition?**

Broad-spectrum antibiotics such as metronidazole and ciprofloxacin should be started. She should also stay on a clear liquid diet for a week and take analgesics for pain. A follow-up colonoscopy should be completed after her acute symptoms resolve.

► Case 9

The mother of a newborn girl complains to the pediatrician that the infant is coughing, drooling excessively, and vomiting immediately after every feeding. The infant was treated for gestational polyhydramnios. X-ray of the chest reveals the nasogastric tube is unable to reach the stomach, which is full of air.

▪ **What is the most likely diagnosis?**	Esophageal atresia with tracheoesophageal fistula. As depicted in Figure 7-7 below, this variant accounts for 85% of these malformations.
▪ **How did the patient's polyhydramnios develop?**	Normally, fetuses swallow amniotic fluid in utero. The fluid is absorbed in the gastrointestinal tract into the infant's circulation and returned to the mother via the placenta, or eliminated through the urinary system. When the fetus does not have the ability to swallow, amniotic fluid builds up, resulting in **polyhydramnios** (an increased amount of amniotic fluid).
▪ **The lung buds are derived from which embryonic structure?**	The lung buds, which will become the bronchial tree, begin as evaginations from the primitive foregut. The foregut also gives rise to the esophagus. Thus, abnormalities in this process can result in a variety of tracheoesophageal fistulae.
▪ **Which pathogens are most likely to cause pneumonia in this patient?**	**Anaerobes,** given the increased risk of aspiration with frequent vomiting and pooling of fluids in the esophageal pouch.
▪ **What other congenital condition is associated with polyhydramnios and bilious vomiting?**	**Duodenal atresia.** Bilious vomiting is indicative of gastrointestinal obstruction distal to the opening of the bile duct. There is an increased incidence of duodenal atresia in infants with trisomy 21 (Down's syndrome).

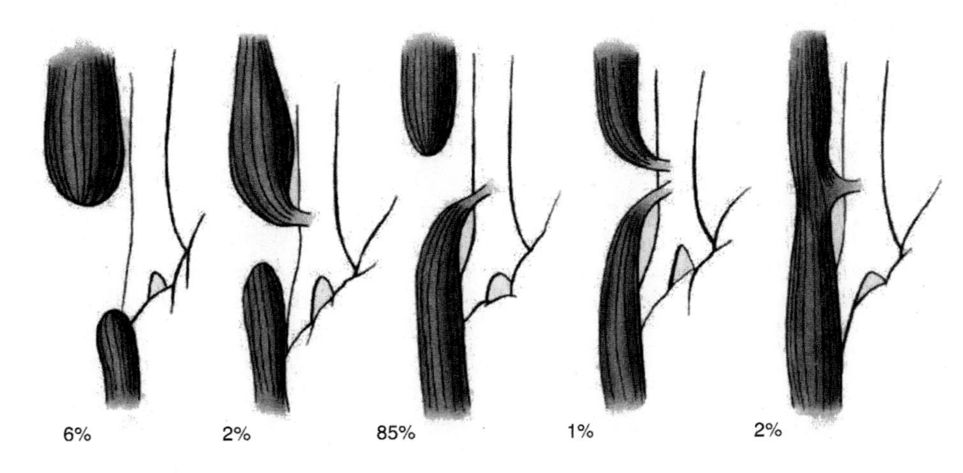

FIGURE 7-7. Variants of esophageal atresia and their prevalence. (Reproduced, with permission, from Brunicardi FC, et al. *Schwartz's Principles of Surgery*, 8th ed. New York: McGraw-Hill, 2005.)

► **Case 10**

A 65-year-old woman presents to her physician with left lower quadrant pain, a 3-week history of nausea and vomiting, diarrhea, and an unintentional 15.9-kg (35-lb) weight loss over the past month. She has a complicated medical history including type 2 diabetes mellitus, hypertension, breast cancer, erosive esophagitis, and chronic peptic ulcer disease. The patient is taking several medications, including a β-blocker. CT of the abdomen reveals a 5 × 5 mass involving the head of the pancreas. Relevant laboratory findings are as follows:

Gastric pH: <2.0
Gastrin: 97 pg/mL (normal: <90 pg/mL)
Hematocrit: 26%
Basal gastric acid output: >15 mEq/hr (normal: <15 mEq/hr)

- **What is the most likely diagnosis?**

Gastrinoma. Gastrinoma is a non–β islet cell tumor of the pancreas or duodenal wall that produces gastrin. Gastrinomas cause gastric hypersecretion of hydrochloric acid, which may result in the development of disseminated gastrointestinal ulcers.

- **What are the two most common neuroendocrine tumors?**

Gastrinoma (two-thirds are malignant) and **insulinoma** (usually benign) are the two most common neuroendocrine tumors.

- **What signs and symptoms are diagnostic of these tumors?**

- Diarrhea
- Epigastric pain
- Gastroesophageal reflux disease
- Hematemesis
- Hematochezia
- Increased resting gastrin level
- Melena
- Nausea/vomiting
- Peptic ulcer disease
- Ulcers in unusual locations such as the proximal jejunum
- Weight loss

- **With what syndrome are these tumors commonly associated?**

Zollinger-Ellison syndrome, which is the triad of increased gastric acid secretion, peptic ulcer disease, and diarrhea. About 20%–30% of gastrinomas are associated with multiple endocrine neoplasia type I (Wermer's syndrome).

- **What is the most appropriate treatment for this tumor?**

- Surgical: Whipple procedure, duodenotomy.
- Medical: proton pump inhibitors, somatostatin. Octreotide is a somatostatin analogue with a longer half-life. Both somatostatin and octreotide act by inhibiting release of somatotropin, insulin, gastrin, glucagons, and vasoactive intestinal peptide.

▶ Case 11

A 34-year-old man with a history of alcohol and drug abuse comes to the emergency department complaining of nausea and vomiting. He notes no recent change in diet or lifestyle and has been in a monogamous relationship for the past year. Workup is negative for gonorrhea and chlamydia. Physical examination reveals a fever of 38.3° C (101° F), a heart rate of 80/min, and a respiratory rate of 18/min. Icterus is present and there is tenderness in the right upper quadrant and midepigastric region. Relevant laboratory findings are as follows:

Alanine aminotransferase (ALT): 1310 U/L
Aspartate aminotransferase (AST): 1200 U/L
Alkaline phosphatase: 98 U/L

- **What is the most likely diagnosis?**

Hepatitis.

- **What is the etiology of this condition?**

Hepatitis can be caused by alcohol, viral infection, ischemia, congestive heart failure, or toxins such as acetaminophen or aflatoxin. The history, in addition to roughly equivalent increases of serum transaminases (by >1000 U/L), suggests an acute viral etiology. If this were an alcoholic hepatitis, AST would be increased out of proportion to ALT, and generally would not rise above 1000 U/L.

- **A workup for hepatitis B virus (HBV) is conducted, with the following results:**
  HBsAg: negative
  HBeAg: negative
  Anti-HBeAg antibody: positive
  Anti-HBcAg antibody: positive
  Anti-HBsAg antibody: negative
  Does the patient have HBV infection?

The patient is in the so-called "window phase" of HBV infection, which occurs after HBsAg has disappeared but before anti-HBsAg antibody is detectable (see Table 7-2 below). This is indicated by the presence of anti-HBeAg and anti-HBcAg antibodies. The patient is not a carrier because he is negative for HBsAg. The patient is not highly infective because he is negative for HBeAg. Finally, the patient is not immune because he does not yet have anti-HBsAg.

- **What percentage of patients with this acute condition develop it chronically?**

Ten percent of adults with acute HBV infection develop chronic hepatitis, while 90% of affected neonates develop the chronic disease.

- **What are the most appropriate treatments for this condition?**

- Adefovir
- α-Interferon
- Lamivudine

TABLE 7-2. Hepatitis B Virus Infection

Test	Acute Disease	Window Phase	Complete Recovery	Chronic Carrier
HBsAg	+	–	–	+
HBsAb	–	–	+	–[b]
HBcAb	+[a]	+	+	+

[a] IgM in acute stage; IgG in chronic or recovered stage.
[b] Patient has surface antibody but available antibody is bound to HBsAg.
Reprinted, with permission, from Bhushan V, Le T, et al. *First Aid for the USMLE Step 1: 2006.* New York: McGraw-Hill, 2006: 158.

► Case 12

A nursing student gives a patient an intramuscular injection and, while attempting to recap the needle, accidentally sticks himself. The patient is known to have chronic, active hepatitis C virus (HCV) infection, so the student immediately goes to Occupational Health to report the needle stick. At Occupational Health, the student has blood drawn for antibody testing, which is found to be negative for anti-HCV antibody. Four weeks later, the nursing student is still negative for anti-HCV antibody, but at 12 weeks, results of antibody testing are positive.

Was the third antibody test a false-positive? Why or why not?	No, this patient has acute HCV infection. It takes weeks to months for the body to develop an antibody response to HCV (see Figure 7-8 on the following page). However, because the student had two negative tests before a positive test, it does establish that he did not have a preexisting infection with HCV, nor had he been exposed in the past.
What other laboratory findings are typically found in patients with this infection?	In acute HCV infection, damage to the liver cells will result in release of intracellular enzymes, causing increased serum aspartate aminotransferase and alanine aminotransferase levels. HCV RNA would also be detectable in the serum by polymerase chain reaction.
What is the course of acute HCV infection?	The majority of patients with acute HCV infection are asymptomatic. About 25% of patients will become jaundiced. The patient will likely have flulike symptoms lasting between 2 and 12 weeks. While only a small percentage of those exposed to HCV by needle stick will develop acute hepatitis, 60%–80% of those who develop acute hepatitis will develop a chronic infection. **Chronic infection** has a variable but slowly progressive course, and about 20% of patients with chronic infection develop cirrhosis. Excessive alcohol consumption is a major risk factor for developing cirrhosis.
What are the most appropriate treatments for this infection?	Treatment with a combination of ribavirin and pegylated α-interferon is about 40% effective for inducing remission of chronic, active HCV infection. Ribavirin is a guanosine analog that inhibits viral mRNA synthesis. Pegylated α-interferon is an endogenous cytokine that induces antiviral host enzymes. It causes significant flulike adverse effects.
If the patient develops cirrhosis, he will be at increased risk for what neoplasm?	The risk of developing **primary hepatocellular cancer** is increased in patients infected with HCV-associated cirrhosis. This is in contrast to patients who are infected with hepatitis B virus, who may develop hepatocellular cancer without cirrhosis.

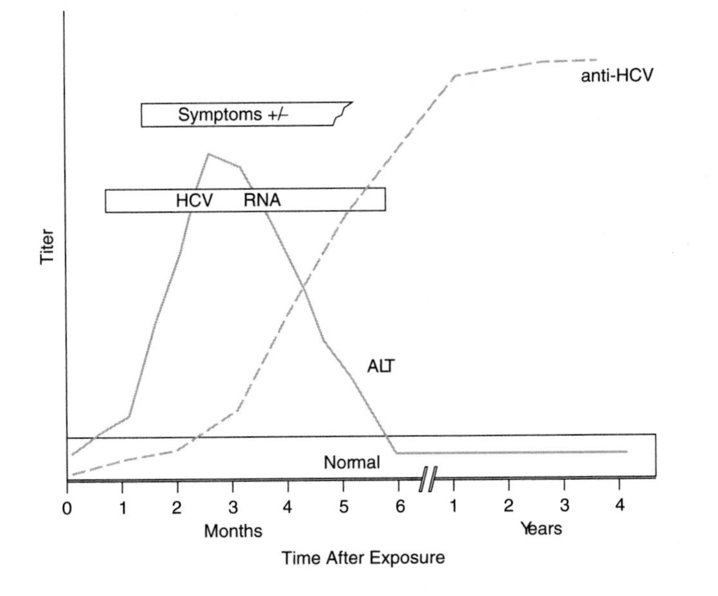

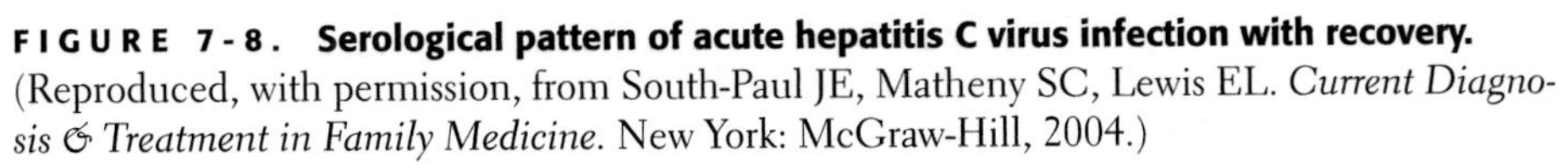

FIGURE 7-8. Serological pattern of acute hepatitis C virus infection with recovery. (Reproduced, with permission, from South-Paul JE, Matheny SC, Lewis EL. *Current Diagnosis & Treatment in Family Medicine.* New York: McGraw-Hill, 2004.)

▶ **Case 13**

An otherwise healthy 36-hour-old male infant born at 37 weeks' gestation to a G3P2 mother is noted to have yellowed skin over his entire body. A blood sample shows the baby is slightly anemic, but has normal WBC and platelet counts. Other relevant laboratory findings are as follows:

Direct bilirubin: 0 mg/dL
Serum total bilirubin (STB): 19 mg/dL (95th percentile of normal at this age is 11 mg/dL)
Direct Coomb's test: weakly positive
Mother's blood type: O+
Infant's blood type: B+

■ **What is the most likely diagnosis?**	Hyperbilirubinemia.
■ **Is this neonate's condition likely due to cholestatic jaundice?**	No, cholestatic jaundice is unlikely because the direct bilirubin level is 0 mg/dL, indicating conjugated bilirubin is being excreted properly.
■ **The infant is given phototherapy, in which his skin is exposed to light. One mechanism of phototherapy is the irreversible conversion of unconjugated bilirubin into lumirubin, which is more similar to conjugated bilirubin. Why is this therapeutic?**	**Lumirubin,** like conjugated bilirubin, is more soluble than unconjugated bilirubin and can be excreted in bile and urine, thus reducing STB levels.
■ **The infant is given a blood transfusion for his anemia. What ABO blood types of the packed RBC donor and of the plasma donor should be chosen in order to minimize hemolysis upon transfusion?**	The RBC donor should be type O to avoid hemolysis of donor cells by maternal anti-B antibodies in the infant's blood. The plasma donor should be type B or AB, so that the plasma will not contain anti-B antibodies to make it incompatible with the infant's blood.
■ **Which drugs, when ingested by the mother, increase the baby's risk of kernicterus?**	Drugs that are highly bound to albumin, including aspirin, ceftriaxone, and sulfa-based drugs, may displace bilirubin from albumin, thus increasing the level of neurotoxic free bilirubin in the blood.
■ **Despite phototherapy, the infant's STB climbs to 26 mg/dL, and an infusion of albumin followed by an exchange transfusion is ordered. In an exchange transfusion, several aliquots of the infant's blood are removed and replaced with an equal volume of fresh or reconstituted whole blood. Why is the infusion of albumin helpful?**	Infused albumin binds free bilirubin, helping to draw extravascular bilirubin from tissues into the blood to be removed by exchange transfusion.

▶ Case 14

A 75-year-old woman comes to the emergency department (ED) after passing two bright red, plum-sized clots of blood into the toilet. There was no stool passed with the clots. The patient denies any abdominal discomfort or cramping, but states she becomes lightheaded upon standing. She also reports she has been very constipated over the past few months. She takes one 81-mg aspirin per day. In the ED, her hematocrit is 28% and her blood pressure is 110/70 mm Hg supine, 80/50 mm Hg standing.

▪ Where is the likely origin of the blood?

The blood is most likely from the lower gastrointestinal (GI) tract, specifically distal to the ligament of Treitz. The presentation of **hematochezia** (maroon or bright red blood/clots per rectum) is a hallmark of a lower GI bleed. In contrast, **hematemesis** (vomiting of blood or coffee ground-like material) and/or **melena** (black, tarry stools) is characteristic of an upper GI bleed. While this distinction is not absolute, it is a good rule of thumb.

▪ What conditions should be considered in the differential diagnosis?

- Anatomical (diverticulosis)
- Hemorrhoids
- Inflammatory (infectious, ischemic, idiopathic inflammatory bowel disease, and radiation
- Neoplastic (polyp, carcinoma)
- Post-biopsy bleeding
- Ulcers
- Vascular (angiodysplasia, radiation-induced telangiectasia)

▪ What is the most likely cause of this patient's bleeding?

Diverticulosis. The most common causes of acute lower GI bleeding are diverticulosis (33%), cancers/polyps (19%), colitis/ulcers (18%), angiodysplasia (8%), and anorectal/hemorrhoids (4%). The cause is unknown approximately 16% of the time. Additionally, 30%–50% of massive rectal bleeding is caused by diverticulosis.

▪ What is the pathophysiology of this condition?

Diverticulosis occurs when **diverticula** (saclike protrusions of the colonic wall) form, exposing the surrounding arterial vasculature to injury and causing thinning of the media. This predisposes to rupture, which in turn leads to arterial bleeding and potentially rapid loss of blood per rectum. This is in contrast to **angiodysplasia,** which can cause venous bleeding into the large intestine. Although most diverticula form on the left colon, the wider necks of right-sided diverticula predispose them to more frequent bleeds. Risk factors for diverticula formation include nonsteroidal anti-inflammatory drugs, lack of fiber, advancing age, and constipation. By age 85, about 65% of the population has diverticula.

▪ What is the initial diagnostic test for this condition?

Colonoscopy is the initial choice for diagnosis and treatment. Additional tests include radionuclide imaging and mesenteric angiography.

▶ Case 15

A 53-year-old man with a history of hepatitis C virus infection and cirrhosis presents to his physician with increasing jaundice, increased abdominal girth, weight loss, and early satiety. He says he is often fatigued and feels lightheaded when he stands. A complete blood count reveals he is anemic, and additional blood work demonstrates hyperbilirubinemia and an increased serum α-fetoprotein level.

▪ **Describe the blood supply to the liver.**

The liver is supplied by the portal vein (75% of blood flow) and hepatic artery. Efferent blood is carried from the hepatic vein to the inferior vena cava. The porta hepatis or hilum is a central area where the hepatic ducts and the lymphatic vessels leave the liver, and the hepatic artery and portal vein enter the liver. Branches of these vessels divide the liver into the left and right lobes.

▪ **What are hepatocytes?**

Hepatocytes are parenchymal cells that constitute the majority of the liver and are important in bile formation, carbohydrate regulation, and metabolism. They lie next to the sinusoids in sheets that radiate from the portal triad to central veins. Blood flowing into the liver passes between plates of hepatocytes, and nutrients are exchanged across the spaces of Disse.

▪ **Which structures are adjacent to the liver?**

The **gallbladder** lies beneath and the **right kidney** is immediately below the liver. The **cystic duct** from the gallbladder joins the common hepatic duct so that bile can drain directly into the duodenum or be stored in the gallbladder. The **ampulla of Vater** is the site where the common bile duct and pancreatic duct enter the duodenum.

▪ **Describe the fetal blood supply to the liver.**

The umbilical vein supplies nutrients to the developing fetus and is the major blood supply to the fetal liver. On entering the abdomen at the umbilicus, the umbilical vein joins the left portal vein. A small amount of placental blood perfuses the liver. The major portion of placental blood, however, bypasses the liver and is shunted by the ductus venosus to the left hepatic vein and continuing to the inferior vena cava and ultimately to the right atrium. The umbilical vein and ductus venosus disappear 2–5 days after birth, becoming the ligamentum teres and ligamentum venosum, respectively.

▪ **Where is the falciform ligament?**

During development, the **falciform ligament** connects that portion of the primitive foregut that will form the liver, to the anterior abdomen at the umbilicus. This connection enables the umbilical vein from the placenta to enter its free border at the umbilicus and reach the portal vein at the porta hepatis. The falciform ligament on the anterior surface of the liver divides the liver into the left and right anatomical lobes.

▶ Case 16

A 47-year-old white man is brought to the emergency department by the police. He was found wandering the streets and is incoherent. He is incontinent with diarrhea. Physical examination reveals a pigmented, scaling rash on his neck, arms, and hands (see Figure 7-9 below) as well as glossitis.

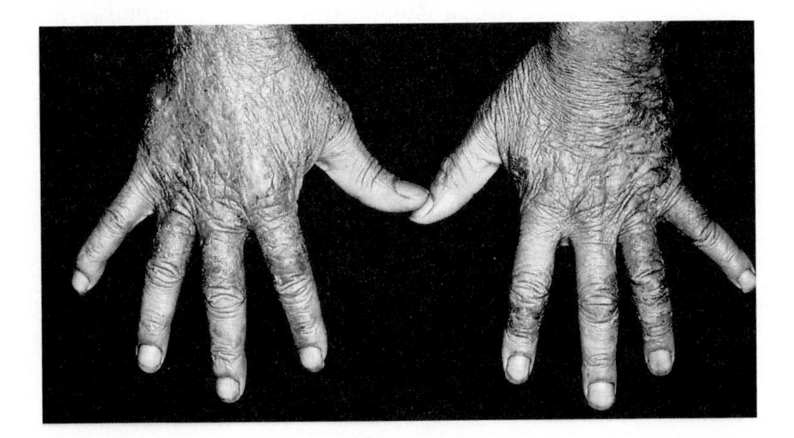

FIGURE 7-9. (Reproduced, with permission, from Wolff K, Johnson RA, Suurmond D. *Fitzpatrick's Color Atlas & Synopsis of Clinical Dermatology*, 5th ed. New York: McGraw-Hill, 2005: 457.)

■ **What is the most likely diagnosis?**	Vitamin B_3 (niacin) deficiency. This is also known as pellagra.
■ **What is the function of vitamin B_3?**	Niacin serves as a precursor for two coenzymes, NAD+ and NADPH. **NAD** is involved in carrying reducing equivalents away from catabolic processes. The most important example is the reactions involved in oxidative phosphorylation. **NADPH** is used as a supply of reducing equivalents in anabolic reactions, including the biosynthesis of steroids and fatty acids, in addition to the maintenance of reduced glutathione and in the oxygen-dependent respiratory burst of macrophages.
■ **From what amino acid is vitamin B_3 derived?**	Niacin is derived from tryptophan.
■ **What are the most likely causes of this presentation?**	In well-developed nations, pellagra is seen most commonly in alcoholics (due to malnutrition). However, it can also be seen in patients with Hartnup's disease (due to malabsorption of tryptophan) and in patients with carcinoid syndrome (due to increased conversion of tryptophan to serotonin). Isoniazid is an inhibitor of the conversion of tryptophan to niacin; thus, patients receiving isoniazid therapy are often prescribed niacin replacement.
■ **What are the symptoms of overdose of vitamin B_3?**	Niacin is often used as a treatment for hypertriglyceridemia. A common adverse effect is prostaglandin-mediated flushing. Prophylaxis with aspirin often prevents this reaction.

▶ Case 17

An 84-year-old man is hospitalized for a course of intravenous clindamycin to treat an abscess. A week later, the patient begins to develop profuse diarrhea; no blood is visible in the stool, but the stool is heme positive. The patient also complains of nausea and malaise. He is febrile, with a temperature of 38.8° C (101.9° F). Physical examination reveals substantial abdominal tenderness and distention. The WBC count is 19,000/mm^3 with a differential of 91% neutrophils, 7% monocytes, and 2% lymphocytes. Sigmoidoscopy reveals 0.2- to 2-cm raised, adherent, yellow plaques.

▪ **What is the most likely diagnosis?**	This is a typical presentation of pseudomembranous colitis: the patient is taking clindamycin, is hospitalized, and developed profuse watery diarrhea during the course of antibiotic therapy. Confirmatory findings would include the presence of fecal leukocytes, anorexia, and dehydration.
▪ **What is the causative organism of this condition?**	*Clostridium difficile*. This anaerobic gram-positive rod often colonizes the bowel after normal flora have been altered by the use of broad-spectrum antibiotics, such as clindamycin, penicillins (especially ampicillin), and cephalosporins.
▪ **What is the underlying pathophysiology of this condition?**	*C. difficile* releases two exotoxins (**proteins A** and **B**) that bind to receptors on intestinal epithelial cells. These toxins cause cell shedding into the lumen, which in turn results in ulceration of the mucosal surface. This **pseudomembrane** is composed of inflammatory cells, proteins, and mucus, as seen in the autopsy specimen shown in Figure 7-10 below.
▪ **What are other manifestations of infections with this organism?**	Infection with *C. difficile* can result in a broad spectrum of symptoms, ranging from asymptomatic carriage to fulminant colitis. Antibiotic-associated diarrhea can be mild or profuse and can occur with or without colitis. The colitis itself can appear pathologically nonspecific, or demonstrate pseudomembranes. Fulminant colitis can result in toxic megacolon or even perforation.
▪ **What are the most appropriate treatments for this condition?**	First-line therapy for pseudomembranous colitis is oral metronidazole. Intravenous metronidazole can be used in serious cases. Oral vancomycin can be used to treat *C. difficile* enterocolitis as it is poorly absorbed and will predominantly remain in, and pass through, the gut. Interestingly, both vancomycin and metronidazole have been implicated as causes of pseudomembranous colitis.

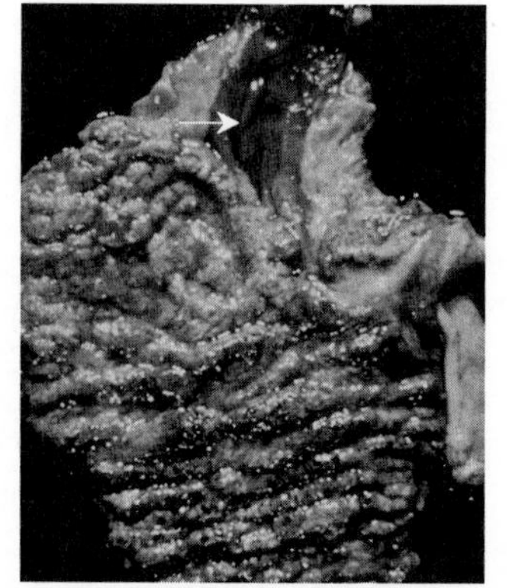

FIGURE 7-10. Autopsy specimen showing confluent pseudomembranes covering the cecum of a patient with pseudomembranous colitis. (Reproduced, with permission, from Kasper DL, et al. *Harrison's Principles of Internal Medicine*, 16th ed. New York: McGraw-Hill, 2005: 760.)

▶ Case 18

A 3-month-old female infant has been maintained on parenteral nutrition since a length of her bowel was resected secondary to the development of necrotizing enterocolitis at 2 weeks of age. The length of bowel removed included her ascending colon, ileum, and distal portion of the jejunum. She is unable to thrive on enteral feeding alone.

▪ **What is the name for this condition?**	Short bowel syndrome.
▪ **After resection of the ileum, which specific molecules will be malabsorbed?**	**Vitamin B_{12}** and bile salts are absorbed exclusively in the ileum, and thus are deficient in short bowel syndrome.
▪ **The remainder of the patient's jejunum has adapted by increasing the number of cells in the villi, thereby lengthening the villi. What term describes this type of adaptation?**	**Hyperplasia.** Hyperplasia refers to increasing the number of cells within a tissue. This is in contrast to **hypertrophy,** in which the cells increase in size.
▪ **During bowel transplantation, which branch(es) of the aorta must be identified and anastomosed to supply blood to the jejunum, ileum, and ascending colon?**	▪ The **superior mesenteric artery** (SMA). The SMA supplies blood to intestine from the proximal jejunum to the proximal transverse colon. ▪ The **celiac trunk** supplies the stomach, liver, spleen, and duodenum. ▪ The **inferior mesenteric artery** supplies the distal transverse colon, descending colon, and sigmoid colon.
▪ **How might octreotide be used in this patient?**	As a **somatostatin analog,** octreotide inhibits the release of gastrin, thus reducing gastric secretions and subsequent losses due to malabsorption resulting from lack of adequate intestinal length.
▪ **How will malabsorption of bile salts affect this patient's prothrombin time (PT) and partial thromboplastin time (PTT)?**	PT and PTT should both increase secondary to depletion of vitamin K as a result of malabsorption of fat and fat-soluble vitamins.

▶ Case 19

A 37-year-old woman with a 20-year history of Crohn's disease presents to her primary care physician complaining of fatigue. Physical examination reveals tachycardia (heart rate 106/min), pale conjunctivae, angular cheilosis, and a beefy tongue. Relevant laboratory findings include a hematocrit of 21% and a mean corpuscular volume of 105 fl.

▪ **What is the most likely diagnosis?**	Vitamin B_{12} deficiency.
▪ **What are the functions of this vitamin, and how does its deficiency result in this presentation?**	Vitamin B_{12} serves as a cofactor for methionine synthase. This enzyme catalyzes the transfer of a methyl group from N-methyltetrahydrofolate to homocysteine, producing tetrahydrofolate (TH4) and methionine. Decreased production of TH4 interferes with DNA synthesis required for hematopoiesis (see Figure 7-11A on the following page), resulting in megaloblastic anemia. Vitamin B_{12} is also a cofactor for methylmalonyl CoA mutase (see Figure 7-11B on the following page), an enzyme involved in the catabolism of odd-numbered fatty acid chains.
▪ **What are the possible causes of this patient's condition?**	The most common etiology of vitamin B_{12} deficiency is pernicious anemia, an autoimmune destruction of the gastric parietal cells that produce **intrinsic factor,** a protein necessary for vitamin B_{12} absorption. Other causes include malabsorption (celiac sprue, enteritis, *Diphyllobothrium latum* infection) and absence of the terminal ileum (due to Crohn's disease or surgical resection) where vitamin B_{12} is absorbed. Vitamin B_{12} deficiency is rarely due to insufficient dietary intake of the vitamin. However, since vitamin B_{12} is found only in animal products, strict vegetarians may present with deficiency.
▪ **For what other condition is this patient at risk?**	Neurologic problems often manifest as paresthesias and ataxia. Over time, symptoms such as spasticity and paraplegia can develop. The exact role vitamin B_{12} deficiency plays in this pathology is unclear, though we do know its deficiency causes a defect in myelin formation. These symptoms are unfortunately irreversible.
▪ **What other vitamin deficiency can also cause megaloblastic anemia?**	**Folic acid deficiency.** However, this deficiency does not cause neurologic symptoms.

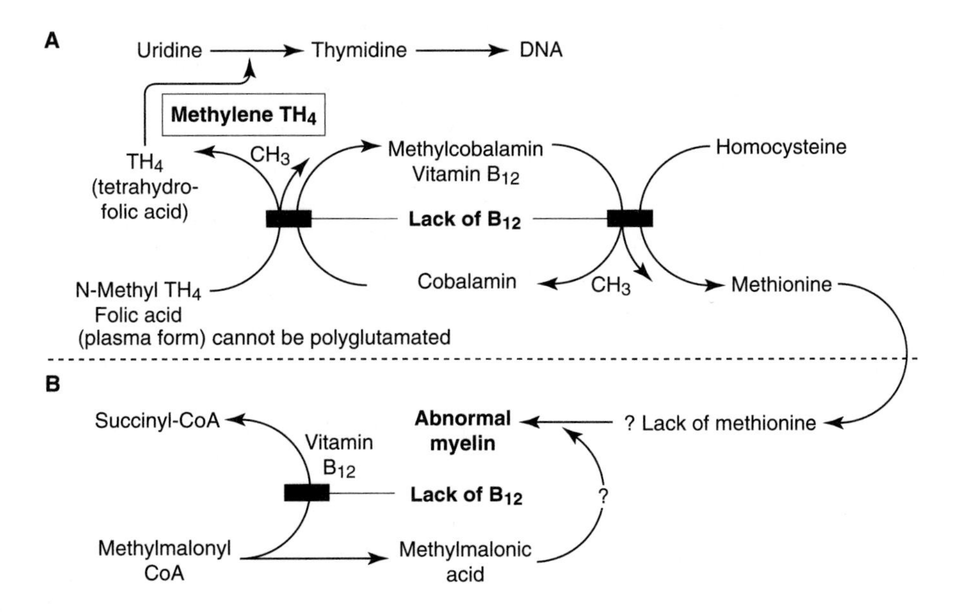

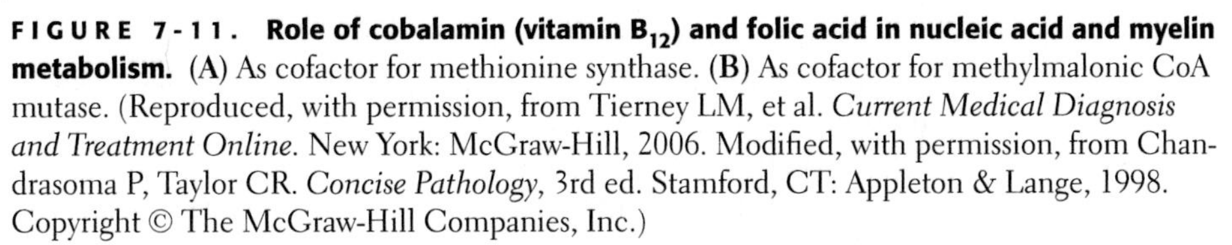

FIGURE 7-11. Role of cobalamin (vitamin B_{12}) and folic acid in nucleic acid and myelin metabolism. (**A**) As cofactor for methionine synthase. (**B**) As cofactor for methylmalonic CoA mutase. (Reproduced, with permission, from Tierney LM, et al. *Current Medical Diagnosis and Treatment Online*. New York: McGraw-Hill, 2006. Modified, with permission, from Chandrasoma P, Taylor CR. *Concise Pathology*, 3rd ed. Stamford, CT: Appleton & Lange, 1998. Copyright © The McGraw-Hill Companies, Inc.)

▶ Case 20

A 45-year-old man presents to the emergency department after vomiting approximately half a cup of blood. Two days prior to admission, the patient began having colicky, nonradiating abdominal pain and nausea. He has an extensive history of alcohol abuse, and admits to currently drinking 8–10 beers a day. He has been treated for pancreatitis, and is known to have bouts of vomiting after alcohol intake. Digital rectal examination reveals his stool is dark and heme positive. He denies any use of nonsteroidal anti-inflammatory drugs.

■ **What anatomical structure distinguishes an upper gastrointestinal (GI) bleed from a lower GI bleed?**	The **ligament of Treitz,** which marks the junction between the duodenum and the jejunum. Bleeding proximal to the ligament of Treitz is defined as an upper GI bleed.
■ **How is upper GI bleeding and lower GI bleeding distinguished clinically?**	**Hematemesis** (bloody or coffee ground–appearing vomit) and/or **melena** (black, tarry stools from digested hemoglobin) indicate an upper GI source. **Hematochezia** (bloody stools) usually indicates a lower GI source, but can also result from a brisk, upper GI bleed in cases in which transit time does not allow for heme breakdown.
■ **What is the most likely diagnosis, and what are its major causes?**	This patient most likely has an upper GI bleed. Common causes include: ■ Acute hemorrhagic gastritis ■ Arteriovenous malformations ■ Esophagitis ■ Esophagogastric varices ■ Mallory-Weiss tears ■ Peptic ulcer disease (55%) ■ Tumors Patients with chronic alcohol abuse are particularly prone to developing esophageal varices and **Mallory-Weiss tears.** A history of vomiting in an alcoholic is strongly suggestive of a Mallory-Weiss tear.
■ **What factors increase the risk of developing peptic ulcer disease?**	■ Chronic obstructive pulmonary disease ■ Cirrhosis ■ *Helicobacter pylori* infection ■ Nonsteroidal anti-inflammatory drugs ■ Smoking ■ Uremia ■ Zollinger-Ellison syndrome (gastrinoma causing increased gastrin secretion)
■ **When is nasogastric tube lavage indicated?**	In cases of massive hematemesis, **nasogastric tube lavage** is indicated to prevent aspiration. It is also used to distinguish between upper and lower sources of GI bleeding, and to identify high-risk lesions as sources of bleeding.

► Case 21

A 35-year-old woman presents to her physician complaining of severe, gnawing epigastric pain of several days' duration. The pain is worse between meals and is somewhat relieved with milk, food, and antacids. She has had three peptic ulcers in the past 2 years. Additionally, she sometimes has diarrhea associated with the gnawing pain. She denies seeing blood in her stools or urine, and also denies alcohol or tobacco use. Upper endoscopy reveals prominent gastric folds and an erosion in the first portion of the duodenum. The patient's fasting gastrin level is 700 pg/dL.

■ **What is the most likely diagnosis?**	A history of recurrent peptic ulcers suggests Zollinger-Ellison syndrome, in which there is hypersecretion of gastrin from a gastrinoma, resulting in high gastric acid output.
■ **With what endocrine disorder is this condition associated?**	Twenty percent of patients with Zollinger-Ellison syndrome have the disease in association with multiple endocrine neoplasia type I (**MEN I,** also known as Wermer's syndrome). Such patients will also have parathyroid adenomas, resulting in hyperparathyroidism, and/or anterior pituitary tumors.
■ **How is secretion of gastric acid regulated?**	Gastric acid is secreted by **parietal cells** of the stomach in response to gastrin, acetylcholine (vagal input), and histamine (paracrine regulation by enterochromaffin-like cells) (see Figure 7-12 below). Acid secretion is inhibited by somatostatin.
■ **What is the pathophysiology of diarrhea in patients with this condition?**	Many patients with this syndrome present with diarrhea because the excessive, voluminous acid secretion overwhelms the buffering capacity of pancreatic bicarbonate. Therefore, pancreatic enzymes are inactivated in this acidic environment, resulting in maldigestion; as well, the excess acid interferes with the emulsification of fats, leading to steatorrhea.
■ **What are the most appropriate treatments for this condition?**	■ Surgical: Resection of the gastrinoma (typically at the head of pancreas) ■ Medical: Proton-pump inhibitors to suppress gastric acid secretion

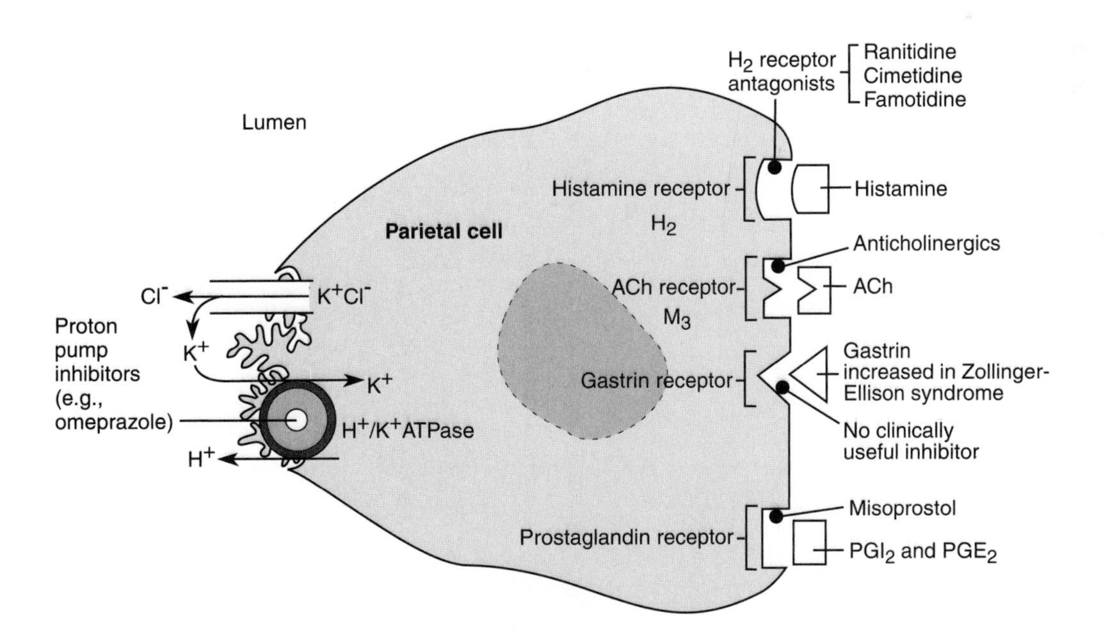

FIGURE 7-12. Regulation of gastric acid secretion. (Reproduced, with permission, from Bhushan V, Le T, et al. *First Aid for the USMLE Step 1: 2006*. New York: McGraw-Hill, 2006: 270.)

NOTES

Hematology and Oncology

► Case 1

A 27-year-old woman comes to the physician complaining of severe abdominal pain of 3 days' duration. She says she has had similar attacks in the past, starting in early adolescence. However, she thought the pain was due to menstruation, and did not seek medical attention. Review of systems reveals a history of depression and insomnia. On physical examination, the patient is hyporeflexic in the lower extremities and has generalized weakness, which is worse in the lower extremities than in the upper extremities. Urinalysis reveals the urine color is initially light but darkens on exposure to air and light, and the porphobilinogen level is 110 mg/24 hr.

What is the most likely diagnosis?	Acute intermittent porphyria (AIP).
Which biochemical defect is responsible for this condition?	AIP is caused by a deficiency in **porphobilinogen deaminase**, an enzyme required for hemoglobin production. Virtually all of the porphyrias are autosomal dominant disorders. Typically patients have accumulation of porphobilinogen and present with neuropathy and attacks of abdominal pain. Unlike other porphyrias, cutaneous disease is rarely present in AIP.
What are the most likely precipitants of this patient's attacks?	Endogenous and exogenous gonadal steroids, certain drugs (sulfonamides, many antiepileptic agents), alcohol, low-calorie diets, and sunlight can increase α-aminolevulinic (ALA) synthase activity, and can precipitate attacks.
What is the most appropriate treatment for this condition?	Avoiding common precipitants of attacks (as listed above). IV infusion of dextrose solution can also help abate acute attacks. Heme is a repressor of ALA synthase. The absence of heme causes an increase in the synthesis of ALA synthase. Intravenous injection of hemin (intravenous heme) leads to decreased synthesis of ALA synthase, which, in turn, often reduces the severity of symptoms. Hemin is used for refractory cases after failure of carbohydrate loading. Treatment of pain and monitoring for neurologic and respiratory compromise are essential.
What other condition should one consider if the patient had neurological manifestations but no abdominal pain?	Ascending muscle weakness and hyperreflexia is the classic presentation of **Guillain-Barré syndrome.** However, the high level of porphobilinogen in the urine is essentially pathognomonic of AIP. If the diagnosis were unclear, a lumbar puncture could be performed, as albumino-cytologic dissociation is seen in the cerebrospinal fluid in patients with Guillain-Barré syndrome.

▶ Case 2

A 67-year-old man presents to his physician with a 10-day history of fatigue, bleeding gums, and cellulitis, and a recent weight loss of 9 kg (20 lb). On physical examination, the patient is pale, but has no evidence of lymphadenopathy or hepatosplenomegaly. Results of a blood smear are as follows:

WBC count: 18,300/mm^3 (75% blastocytes, 20% lymphocytes)
Hemoglobin: 9.1 g/dL
Hematocrit: 29%
Platelet count: 98,000/mm^3

■ **What is the most likely diagnosis?**	Acute myelogenous leukemia (AML).
■ **What other symptoms are common at presentation?**	Epistaxis, skin rash, petechiae, bone pain, and shortness of breath can be seen with AML. Gingival hyperplasia can occur due to leukemic infiltration. Leukemia cutis in skin infiltrates can also be seen. Monocytic leukemia may be associated with central nervous system involvement. Disseminated intravascular coagulation is often seen with **acute promyelocytic leukemia** (a variant of AML).
■ **What are the likely findings on histology?**	The proliferation of myeloblasts with characteristic eosinophilic needle-like cytoplasmic inclusions, or **Auer rods,** is pathognomonic for AML (see Figure 8-1 below).
■ **How can genetic testing influence treatment?**	A t(15:17) chromosomal translocation indicates acute promyelocytic leukemia (M3 variant) as the specific diagnosis. This can be treated with all-*trans* retinoic acid (ATRA). This agent causes differentiation of promyelocytes into mature neutrophils, thereby inducing apoptosis of the leukemic promyelocytes.
■ **Cellulitis is commonly associated with this condition; how does this occur?**	Neutropenia caused by replacement of mature WBCs with leukemic cells leads to an increased susceptibility to infection.

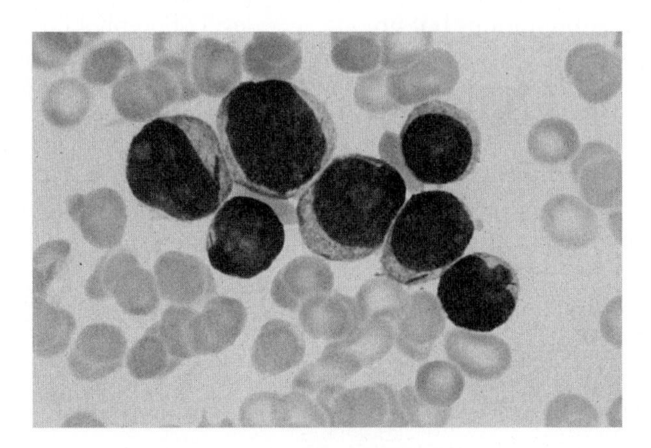

FIGURE 8-1. Auer rods in acute myelogenous leukemia. (Reproduced with permission of the Pathology Education Instructional Resource Digital Library (http://peir.net) at the University of Alabama, Birmingham.)

▶ Case 3

A 14-year-old boy presents to his physician with a laceration on his hand that has become badly infected. Upon questioning, the boy mentions he has felt fatigued for some time. Physical examination reveals pallor of the mucous membranes in addition to bleeding on the inside of his cheeks. He has petechiae covering his body, and patches of purpura on his thighs, trunk, and arms. Relevant laboratory findings are as follows:

WBC count: 27,000/mm^3
Hematocrit: 22%
Platelet count: 48,000/mm^3

■ **What is the most likely diagnosis?**	Aplastic anemia. This condition results from failure or autoimmune destruction of myeloid stem cells, which leads to pancytopenia. It is characterized by neutropenia (infection), anemia (pallor and fatigue), and thrombocytopenia (petechiae and purpura).
■ **What is the most likely cause of this patient's condition?**	Most cases of aplastic anemia are **idiopathic** (autoimmune). Other possible causes include **viral** agents (hepatitis C virus, Epstein-Barr virus, herpes zoster), and **drugs** such as alkylating agents, antimetabolite agents, and chloramphenicol. Some hereditary cases have been linked to mutations in the telomerase gene (dyskeratosis congenital aplastic anemia).
■ **What are the most likely findings on a peripheral blood smear?**	Hypocellularity and pancytopenia. The visualized cells are morphologically normal. Macrocytosis and dysplastic forms can be seen.
■ **What other test would be useful in confirming the diagnosis?**	Bone marrow biopsy would reveal hypocellular bone marrow with a fatty infiltrate. Figure 8-2A below shows a normal bone marrow biopsy, while Figure 8-2B below shows a biopsy sample from a patient with aplastic anemia.
■ **What type of treatment is most appropriate for this condition?**	Treatment includes RBC and platelet transfusions, allogeneic bone marrow transplant (sibling), granulocyte colony–stimulating factor or granulocyte macrophage colony–stimulating factor, and withdrawal of any toxic agent that may be a cause. If possible, transfusion should be avoided before bone marrow transplantation due to the risks of alloimmunization and graft rejection. Cyclosporin, antithymocyte globulin, and cyclophosphamide are used if no donor can be found.

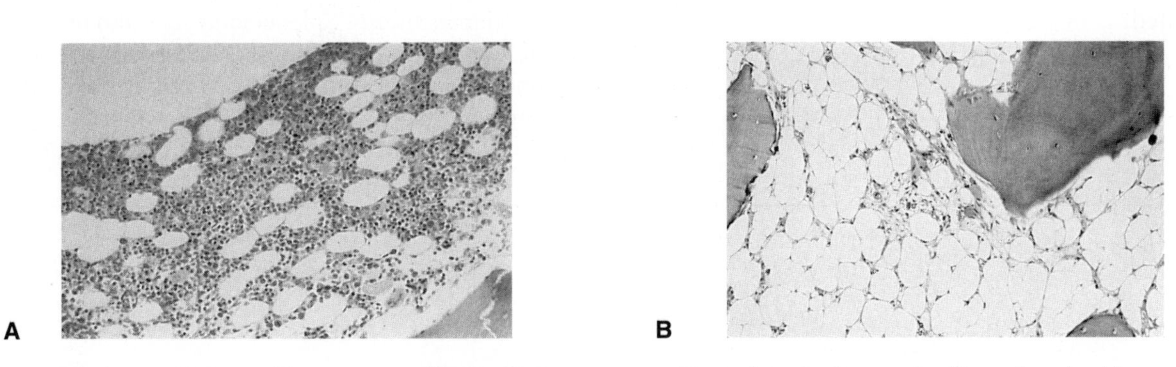

FIGURE 8-2. (A) Normal bone marrow biopsy. (B) Bone marrow biopsy in aplastic anemia. (Reproduced, with permission, from Kasper DL, et al. *Harrison's Principles of Internal Medicine*, 16th ed. New York: McGraw-Hill, 2005: 620.)

▶ Case 4

A 7-month-old Greek boy is brought to his pediatrician by his parents, who have noticed the baby has been jaundiced and dyspneic for about 2 weeks. The mother claims her son has been healthy up until now, and there were no complications during the pregnancy or delivery. Physical examination reveals tachycardia. Laboratory tests reveal a mean corpuscular volume of 75 fl and a reticulocyte count of 0.3%. The serum iron concentration is within normal limits.

▪ **What is the most likely diagnosis?**	β-Thalassemia major, a form of microcytic, hypochromic anemia, is the homozygous form of the genetically transmitted disease, thalassemia. This disease is prevalent in Mediterranean populations. Symptoms emerge after about 6 months of life due to the decline in normal hemoglobin F (α_2/γ_2) and rise in hemoglobin A (α_2/β_2).
▪ **What is the pathophysiology of this condition?**	In β-thalassemia, the β chain of hemoglobin is either underproduced (**thalassemia minor**) or absent (**thalassemia major**). As a result, the normal α hemoglobin chains build up and form insoluble aggregates that precipitate out into the RBCs. This results in either hemolysis of or damage to the RBCs, making them more susceptible to macrophage destruction and splenic sequestration. The result is a hemolytic anemia, in which the microcytic and hypochromic RBCs resemble those seen in severe iron deficiency (see Figure 8-3 on the following page). The reticulocyte count is low in these patients due to ineffective hematopoiesis. Target cells, nucleated RBCs, and microcytes are commonly seen. **Heinz body** precipitates are the oxidatively destructive α-globin chains in RBCs.
▪ **How is this condition diagnosed?**	Gel electrophoresis is used for diagnosis, as it can distinguish mutated and normal forms of hemoglobin. An increased concentration of hemoglobin F (fetal hemoglobin) may also be seen on electrophoresis.
▪ **What complications are associated with this condition?**	Complications include pulmonary hypertension, cardiac failure, leg ulcers, folate deficiency, and skeletal abnormalities.
▪ **What are the two common forms of this condition?**	The major form of the disease results in severe hemolytic anemia, whereas the minor form of the disease may be completely asymptomatic. Extramedullary hematopoiesis is common in **Cooley's anemia** (thalassemia major).
▪ **How is each form of this condition treated?**	Thalassemia major causes severe anemia, requiring treatment with repeated blood transfusions. Splenectomy may also be necessary to treat the resultant hypersplenism. Thalassemia minor is usually asymptomatic and its treatment merely requires avoidance of oxidative stressors of RBCs. Iron chelation for overload (ferritin level >2247 pmol/L) is important. But beware of *Yersinia enterocolitica* infection, which eats up the free iron!

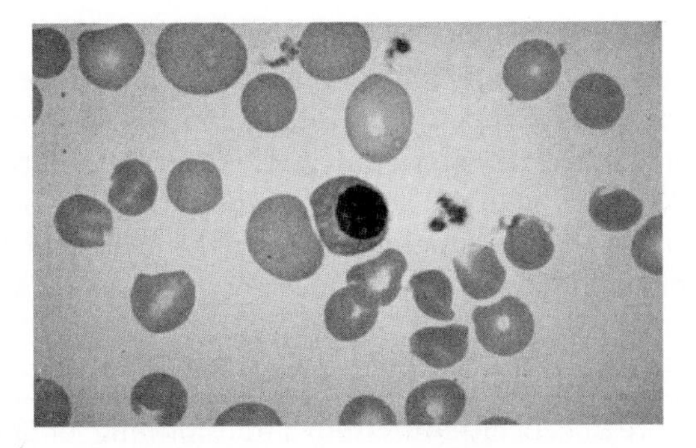

FIGURE 8-3. Peripheral blood smear in β-thalassemia. (Reproduced, with permission, from Kasper DL, et al. *Harrison's Principles of Internal Medicine,* 16th ed. New York: McGraw-Hill, 2005: 598.)

▶ Case 5

A 57-year-old nulliparous woman presents to her general practitioner concerned about a painless lump she has found in the right upper quadrant of her right breast. Her mother died of breast cancer at the age of 60. Her medical history is significant for mild obesity, an early onset of menarche, and late onset of menopause 3 years previously. She has noted some unilateral pain and dimpling of her right breast but has been scared to make an appointment with her physician. Laboratory tests show a serum calcium level of 9.7 mg/dL.

- **What is the pathophysiology of this condition?**

Breast cancer results from a transforming, or oncogenic, event that leads to clonal proliferation and survival of breast cancer cells. The events that trigger sporadic breast cancer are often unknown, but abnormalities in cell-cycle pathways, including Her-2, cyclin D1, c-myc, estrogen, and progesterone signaling, have been implicated. *BRCA1* and *BRCA2* genes have been linked to hereditary breast and ovarian cancer and are linked to defects in DNA mismatch repair.

- **What risk factors increase a person's likelihood of developing this condition?**

- Age
- Alcohol intake
- Breast density
- Early menarche
- Family history (50%–70% of women carrying the *BRCA1* or *BRCA2* genes will develop breast cancer)
- Female gender
- Hormone replacement therapy
- Nulliparity, late first pregnancy, or menopause
- Obesity (in postmenopausal women)
- Prior breast biopsy, particularly for lesions with atypia
- Radiation exposure

- **What are the common forms of this condition?**

Breast cancer is the leading cause of cancer death in women and the most common form of cancer in this group. Most tumors develop in upper/outer quadrants. Types of breast cancer include:

- Ductal carcinoma in situ (premalignant)
- Inflammatory carcinoma
- Invasive ductal carcinoma (most common form)
- Invasive lobular carcinoma
- Medullary, mucinous, tubular forms (less common)
- Paget's disease of the breast
- Phylloides tumors, lymphoma, sarcoma (very rare)

- **What are the patterns of metastasis in this condition?**

Bone, axillary lymph nodes, lungs, liver, and brain are common sites of metastasis. Metastases to bone are often blastic rather than lytic. Chest wall recurrences are common as well.

- **What are the most appropriate treatments for this condition?**

The most common treatment is modified mastectomy or lumpectomy with postoperative radiation. Adjuvant tamoxifen or aromatase inhibition (such as anastrazole or letrozole) is often added to reduce the risk of recurrence; these drugs are given for 5 years, and often longer. Recently, herceptin has been used in the adjuvant setting to reduce the risk of recurrence in Her-2-overexpressing tumors. Adjuvant chemotherapy (doxorubicin, cyclophosphamide, sometimes with a taxane) is often used for higher-risk patients to reduce the risk of recurrence. Chemotherapy is typically given prior to radiation therapy or hormone therapy.

▶ Case 6

A 35-year-old man presents to his primary care physician complaining of watery diarrhea over the past several months. He reports the diarrhea is often "greasy looking," but never bloody. On physical examination, the man's face is flushed, and his neck is covered by a blotchy, violaceous erythema. When asked about this flushing, the man says it has happened several times a day over the past few years, often while he is feeling stressed at work.

- **What is the most likely diagnosis?**

Carcinoid syndrome (secretory).

- **What symptoms are most commonly associated with this condition?**

Flushing and diarrhea are the two most common presenting symptoms (see Table 8-1 below). These symptoms occur in up to 73% of patients initially and up to 89% of patients during the course of disease. Flushing is typically sudden in onset and lasts 2–5 minutes, although it may persist as long as 1 hour later in the disease course. Diarrhea typically occurs with flushing, with steatorrhea present in up to 67% of cases.

- **Which laboratory test would be useful in confirming the diagnosis?**

Other conditions such as menopause and chronic myelogenous leukemia, as well as reactions to alcohol, glutamate, and calcium channel blockers, may cause flushing. However, flushing in conjunction with an increase in **5-hydroxyindoleacetic acid** on urinalysis occurs only in carcinoid syndrome (see Table 8-1 below).

- **What is the pathophysiology of this condition?**

Carcinoid syndrome occurs only when sufficient concentrations of substances secreted by carcinoid tumors (neuroendocrine cells) reach the circulation. Carcinoid tumors secrete a variety of gastrointestinal peptides, including gastrin, somatostatin, substance P, vasoactive intestinal polypeptide, pancreatic polypeptide, and chromogranin A, as well as serotonin. Diarrhea occurs when the liver can no longer metabolize serotonin due to the presence of metastases. Flushing is thought to be caused by excess histamine release.

TABLE 8-1. Clinical Characteristics in Patients with Carcinoid Syndrome

SYMPTOMS/SIGNS	AT PRESENTATION	DURING COURSE OF DISEASE
Diarrhea	32%–73%	68%–84%
Flushing	23%–65%	63%–74%
Pain	10%	34%
Asthma/wheezing	4%–8%	3%–18%
Pellagra	2%	5%
None	12%	22%
Carcinoid heart disease	11%	14%–41%

Modified, with permission, from Kasper DL, et al. *Harrison's Principles of Internal Medicine,* 16th ed. New York: McGraw-Hill, 2005: 2224.

- **What type of cardiac involvement is typically seen in patients with this condition?**

Right-sided valvular involvement occurs in 11% of patients initially and up to 41% during the course of the disease. Cardiac disease results from serotonin-mediated fibrosis in the endocardium, most commonly in the tricuspid valve. Up to 80% of patients with cardiac involvement develop heart failure. Cardiac involvement can also occur with certain diet drugs that affect serotonin (such as "Phen-Fen").

▶ Case 7

A 52-year-old man visits his primary care physician complaining of constant vague abdominal pain that has been increasing over the past month. He has noted recent weakness and weight loss, which he attributes to recently decreased appetite. His father was diagnosed with colorectal cancer in his late fifties. The patient admits he has never had a colonoscopy and eats a diet high in fat and low in fiber. Rectal examination reveals a palpable mass and occult blood. The patient's carcinoembryonic antigen level is elevated, and his hematocrit is 28%.

▪ What is the most likely diagnosis?

Colorectal cancer is the second leading cause of cancer deaths. These malignant polypoid, ulcerating, annular lesions are found in colonic or rectal mucosa. About 15% are mucinous adenocarcinoma, as staged by the Dukes' classification. Spread is via lymphatics and hematogenously to the liver and peritoneal cavity.

▪ What factors are associated with an increased risk of this neoplasm?

- Age >50 years old
- Genetics:
  - Lynch syndrome I and II
  - Hereditary nonpolyposis colorectal cancer
  - Long-standing chronic ulcerative pancolitis
  - Tumor suppressor gene and proto-oncogene changes
- Low-fiber and high-fat diets
- Male gender

▪ What signs and symptoms are commonly associated with this neoplasm?

- Abdominal pain
- Anemia
- Bleeding/mucus per rectum
- Change in bowel habit
- Rectal lesions
- Tenesmus

▪ What are the four major types of this neoplasm?

- Left colon (10% of cases):
  - Altered bowel habits
  - Bright red blood per rectum
  - One-third large bowel obstruction
- Sigmoid colon (20% of cases):
  - Altered bowel habits
  - Bright red blood per rectum
  - Mucus per rectum
- Right colon (20% of cases):
  - Anemia
  - Weight loss
  - Right iliac fossa mass
- Rectal (50% of cases):
  - Polyps (confined to wall)
  - Ulcer (through bowel wall)
  - Mass with nodal involvement

▪ What are the most appropriate treatments for this condition?

Surgical treatment is indicated. Radiotherapy may be used to shrink tumors preoperatively or for palliative care in inoperable cases. There is a 25% survival rate after resections with <5 liver metastases.

▶ Case 8

A 33-year-old African-American woman has been in the intensive care unit of the hospital for 2 days after being admitted for treatment of a severe bacteremia. Her prior medical history is noncontributory. Physical examination now reveals mucosal bleeding, oozing from intravenous access sites, and petechiae on her trunk and extremities. Laboratory tests reveal a prolonged bleeding time, prothrombin time (PT), and activated partial thromboplastin time (aPTT).

▪ **What is the most likely diagnosis?**	Disseminated intravascular coagulation (DIC).
▪ **What is the pathophysiology of this condition?**	Clotting throughout the body, rather than in a localized area, results in a depletion of coagulation factors. This causes both bleeding and thrombosis (see Figure 8-4 below). Causes of DIC include sepsis, trauma, acute leukemia (especially acute myelogenous leukemia), cavernous hemangiomas (Kassabach-Merritt syndrome), cancer (often found in patients with chronic DIC), amniotic fluid embolism, and snake envenomation.
▪ **Which clotting factors are involved in the intrinsic and extrinsic pathways?**	The **intrinsic pathway** involves all of the clotting factors except VII and XIII. The **extrinsic pathway** involves factors II, V, VIII, and X.
▪ **Which laboratory tests help differentiate this condition from thrombocytopenia?**	A prolonged bleeding time corresponds to a functional platelet abnormality. An elevated aPTT suggests a problem with the intrinsic pathway, while an elevated PT reveals a defect in the extrinsic pathway. **Thrombocytopenia** and DIC both have prolonged bleeding times, but in DIC, there is also a prolonged PT and aPTT because of the consumption of coagulation factors in addition to platelets.
▪ **Which laboratory tests help differentiate this condition from classic hemophilia and Christmas disease?**	Classic hemophilia and Christmas disease both have normal bleeding times along with prolonged aPTTs and normal PTs. They are distinguished from DIC by a positive factor VIII assay for **classic hemophilia,** and by a positive factor IX assay for **Christmas disease.**
▪ **Which laboratory tests help differentiate this condition from von Willebrand's disease and vitamin K deficiency?**	**von Willebrand's disease** results in ineffective platelet adhesion and functional factor VIII deficiency. Therefore, the bleeding time is prolonged, as is the aPTT. In **vitamin K deficiency,** the activities of factors II, VII, IX, and X are decreased, resulting in a prolonged PTT and aPTT and a normal bleeding time.

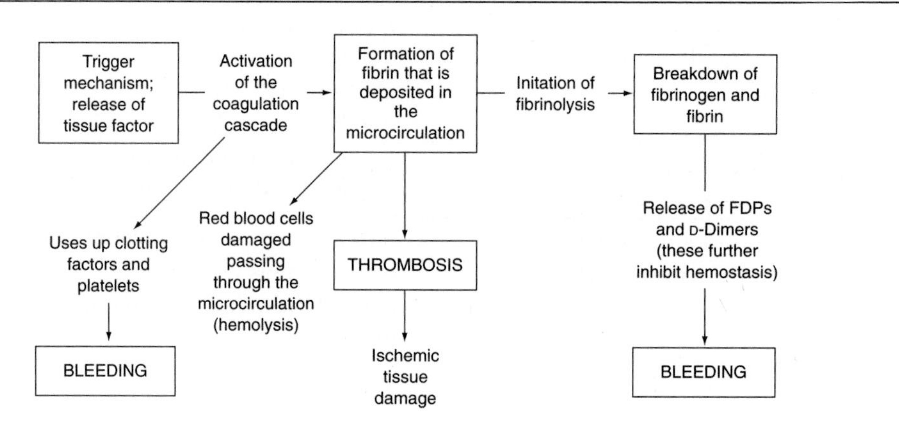

FIGURE 8-4. Pathophysiology of DIC. (Reproduced, with permission, from Tintinalli JE, et al. *Tintinalli's Emergency Medicine: A Comprehensive Study Guide*, 6th ed. New York: McGraw-Hill, 2004: 1328.)

▶ Case 9

A 56-year-old man presents to the emergency department complaining of 1 day of nausea and vomiting in the context of significant weight loss over the past few months. Careful questioning reveals he has noticed black specks in his emesis, resembling "coffee grounds." On review of systems, he notes early satiety with a decreased appetite, specifically for meat. He attributes his anorexia to a general feeling of fullness after eating. He has no diarrhea, constipation, known sick contacts, or recent travel history, but notes occasional fevers and chills with recent night sweats. Physical examination reveals the patient is afebrile with a nontender, nondistended, soft abdomen remarkable for a firm epigastric mass. Relevant laboratory findings are as follows:

Hematocrit: 28%
Hemoglobin: 9 g/dL
WBC count: 9000/mm^3
Stool test:
  Guaiac positive
  Negative for ova and parasites

- **What is the most likely diagnosis? What population is most at risk for this condition?**

The incidence of gastric cancer is decreasing in the United States, but it is still high in Japan. Men have twice the risk of women. People who consume a diet low in fruits and vegetables and high in starch are at increased risk, as are patients with previous gastric operations.

- **How is this condition classified?**

Adenocarcinoma is the most common type of gastric cancer.
- **Advanced carcinoma** develops partly inside the stomach.
- **Ulcerating carcinoma** penetrates all layers of the stomach and may involve neighboring organs.
- **Polypoid carcinoma** involves intraluminal growths that metastasize late in the disease.

- **What signs and symptoms are commonly associated with this condition?**

- Anorexia (especially for meat)
- Dysphagia (caused by lesions at cardia of stomach)
- Coffee ground emesis (if bleeding tumor)
- Palpable epigastric mass
- Postprandial heaviness
- Vomiting (in cases of pyloric obstruction)
- Weight loss

If disease has metastasized:
- Intra-abdominal masses
- Virchow's node (left supraclavicular node)

- **What findings are likely on laboratory testing?**

Anemia is present in 50% of patients. The stool is guaiac positive. Carcinoembryonic antigen levels are elevated in two-thirds of patients.

- **What is the most appropriate treatment for this condition?**

Diagnosis is via esophagogastroduodenoscopy and biopsy. However, only 50% of patients have resectable lesions, and there has been no proven efficacy of adjuvant chemotherapy.

▶ Case 10

A 56-year-old man who was previously in excellent health is brought to the emergency department after a rapid decline in mental status that began 3 days earlier. His wife notes he has been acting differently and was unable to understand her 2 days earlier. This morning, his wife found him unresponsive and extremely agitated. Currently, the patient is flailing his limbs and is unresponsive to stimuli or to verbal commands. His pupils are equal and reactive. The patient is subsequently sedated, and CT of the head demonstrates a large lesion in the right frontal lobe. MRI establishes the likely diagnosis.

What is the differential diagnosis of a brain lesion?	The most common brain tumor is a metastatic lesion. Primary brain tumors include gliomas, meningiomas, pituitary adenomas, vestibular schwannomas, and primary central nervous system lymphomas. Brain lesions can be infections (arising from abscesses, viral processes, progressive multifocal leukoencephalopathy, toxoplasmosis, or cysticercosis), vascular (resulting from cerebral hemorrhage or infarct), or inflammatory (associated with multiple sclerosis or postinfectious encephalopathy).
What is the most likely diagnosis?	Glioblastoma multiforme (GBM). MRI is the definitive test for a brain mass. Gliomas appear hypointense on T1-weighted imaging and hyperintense on T2-weighted imaging. They also heterogeneously enhance with contrast and can be distinguished from the surrounding edema. The rapidity of onset of this patient's symptoms without signs of infarct also suggests that his symptoms are the result of a highly malignant process.
Where are these tumors typically found?	GBM is the most commonly diagnosed primary brain tumor. GBM is a grade IV astrocytoma that is most commonly found in adults, in contrast to the peak childhood prevalence of low-grade (pilocytic) astrocytoma. GBM is typically found in the cerebral hemispheres and can cross the corpus callosum to form the characteristic "butterfly glioma."
What are the most common signs and symptoms associated with this tumor?	The most common symptoms associated with adult GBM are headache (found in 73%–86% of cases) and seizures (found in 26%–32% of cases). The most common neurologic signs are hyperparesis, papilledema, confusion, and aphasia. Symptoms can progress over the course of days to months, but the prognosis of GBM is quite grave, with the majority of patients surviving less than 1 year.
What is the most appropriate treatment for this condition?	Dexamethasone is used to alleviate the vasogenic edema resulting from blood-brain barrier disruption that occurs in the region surrounding many brain tumors. The mechanism of action of dexamethasone is unknown, but it is preferred to other steroids because its relative lack of mineralocorticoid activity decreases the risk of fluid retention.

▶ Case 11

A 42-year-old African-American man presents to the emergency department with sudden onset of shortness of breath. He complains of feeling fatigued and weak, and notes he saw blood in his urine for the first time this morning. He has no chest pain or palpitations and has no prior history of hypertension, coronary artery disease, or ischemic heart disease. He is being treated with trimethoprim-sulfamethoxazole for a urinary tract infection, but has no other significant medical history. He denies a history of alcohol or drug abuse. Physical examination reveals hepatosplenomegaly, mild scleral icterus, and tachycardia.

■ **What is the most likely diagnosis?**	Glucose-6-phospate dehydrogenase (G6PD) deficiency.
■ **What are the likely findings on a peripheral blood smear (PBS)?**	PBS will likely reveal bite cells and ghost cells, implying intravascular hemolytic anemia.
■ **What is the pathophysiology of this condition?**	G6PD protects cells from oxidative damage by converting nicotinamide adenine dinucleotide phosphate (NADP+) to its reduced form (NADPH). Patients with a deficiency in this enzyme are less able to deal with oxidative stresses, such as those that might result from ingestion of a sulfa drug such as sulfamethoxazole.
■ **How is this condition acquired?**	G6PD deficiency is an X-linked recessive trait and affects males predominantly. Heterozygous females are usually normal. Patients with G6PD deficiency are normal in the absence of oxidative stress. However, exposure to oxidative stress triggers the disease. G6PD in Mediterranean pedigrees results in **favism,** or hemolysis induced by the ingestion of fava beans.
■ **How are anemias classified in terms of cell volume?**	■ **Microcytic anemia** (mean corpuscular volume [MCV] <80 fl): Caused by iron deficiency, thalassemia, or lead poisoning. ■ **Normocytic anemia** (MCV 80–100 fl): Caused by enzyme deficiency (such as G6PD or pyruvate kinase), blood loss (as from trauma), anemia of chronic disease, or hemolysis (autoimmune or mechanical). ■ **Macrocytic anemia** (MCV >100 fl): Causes include vitamin B_{12}/folate deficiency, liver disease, drugs that inhibit DNA synthesis, and alcohol.
■ **What is the most appropriate treatment for this condition?**	Treatment is generally supportive with removal of offending agent.

▶ Case 12

A 55-year-old white man is brought to the emergency department after collapsing in a restaurant. He is conscious on arrival and claims he has not seen a doctor for many years. On physical examination, the patient appears jaundiced. An ECG demonstrates he is in atrial fibrillation. Laboratory studies reveal an elevated serum glucose level and the following iron parameters:

Serum iron: 400 μg/dL
Transferrin: 150 μg/dL
Iron saturation: 85%
Ferritin: 1100 ng/mL

What is the most likely diagnosis?	Hereditary hemochromatosis, which is an autosomal dominant disease resulting in excessive iron absorption. Excess iron gradually accumulates at a rate of approximately 0.5–1.0 g/yr. Normal body iron content is approximately 3–4 g, and symptoms are noticeable at a body iron content exceeding 20 g. As a result, most men are not diagnosed until after age 40, and women are not diagnosed until after cessation of their menstrual periods. Normal iron loss is 1 mg/day in men and 1.5 mg/day in menstruating women.
What is the pathophysiology of this condition?	Normally, iron homeostasis is achieved by regulating iron intake to compensate for losses through the skin, menses, pregnancy, and other processes. However, in hereditary hemochromatosis, an autosomal dominant mutation in chromosome 6 (***HFE* gene**) causes excessive iron to be absorbed through the intestine. This iron gradually deposits as hemosiderin throughout the body, particularly in the liver (see Figure 8-5 on the following page), skin, pancreas, joints, gonads, heart, and pituitary, which eventually leads to oxidative damage to these organs.
What signs and symptoms are commonly associated with this condition?	Clinical manifestations correspond to the organs with excessive iron deposits. Patients may present with the classic triad of cirrhosis, diabetes mellitus, and skin pigmentation (hence the moniker "bronze diabetes"), as well as arthropathy (pseudogout, often the second and third digits), impotence in men, cardiac enlargement, cardiac conduction defects, and weakness or lethargy (due to pituitary involvement).
What laboratory findings are common in this condition?	Iron saturation of >60% in men and >50% in women suggests hemochromatosis 90% of the time. A cutoff of 45% for both men and women is typically used, however, for simplicity. Other typical laboratory findings include hyperglycemia, elevated liver enzyme levels, elevated serum iron levels, decreased total iron binding capacity, and elevated ferritin levels.
What is the most appropriate treatment for this condition?	Serial phlebotomy with the possible use of deferoxamine, an iron-binding agent, especially for those with homozygous *HFE* mutations (C282Y) and iron overload. Compound heterozygotes with iron overload should also be treated.

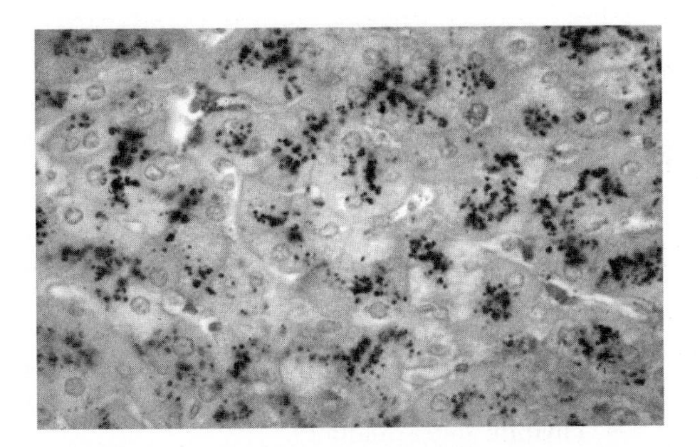

FIGURE 8-5. Iron deposits in the liver in hemochromatosis. (Reproduced with permission of the Pathology Education Instructional Resource Digital Library (http://peir.net) at the University of Alabama, Birmingham.)

▶ Case 13

A 67-year-old man presents to his physician with pain on swallowing and hoarseness. He has noted some swelling of the right side of his neck. The patient has smoked one pack of cigarettes per day since he was 15 years old and drinks two beers every night before dinner. Physical examination reveals a palpable neck mass and white plaques in his mouth.

▪ **What is the differential diagnosis of a neck mass?**	▪ **Congenital:** torticollis, thyroglossal duct cyst, brachial cleft cyst, cystic hygroma, dermoid cyst, carotid body tumor ▪ **Acquired:** lymphoma, mononucleosis (Epstein-Barr virus), other causes of lymphadenopathy, cervical lymphadenitis ▪ **Thyroid:** goiter (midline) ▪ **Malignancy (thyroid):** papillary, medullary, follicular, anaplastic, lymphoma ▪ Head and neck cancer (squamous)
▪ **What is the most likely diagnosis?**	Squamous cell tumor or adenocarcinoma of the head and neck.
▪ **Which risk factors increase this person's likelihood of disease?**	Tobacco and alcohol (for squamous cell carcinomas of the head and neck only).
▪ **Which procedures are useful in confirming this diagnosis?**	Diagnostic procedures include biopsy via fine needle aspiration of the mass and CT and/or MRI to determine the stage and possible vascular involvement and resectability. If lymphoma is suspected, excisional biopsy should be performed.
▪ **Where are these lesions commonly located?**	Head and neck cancers are typically found in the oral cavity, nasopharynx, larynx, oropharynx, and salivary glands.
▪ **What are the most appropriate treatments for this condition?**	Localized lesions are removed surgically or via radiotherapy. Palliative radiation is used for larger, more complex lesions. Combined chemotherapy and radiotherapy is the standard of care for advanced lesions.

▶ Case 14

An 11-year-old girl is brought to her physician because of frequent epistaxis and "purple spots" on her body. She reports no recent history of trauma. Physical examination reveals petechiae and purpura on her arms, outer thighs, and legs (see Figure 8-6 below). A peripheral blood smear (PBS) shows large platelets, but no helmet cells or schistocytes. Results of a Coombs' test are positive. Relevant laboratory findings are as follows:

Hemoglobin: 12.5 g/dL
Hematocrit: 36%
WBC count: 5000/mm^3
Platelet count: 11,000/mm^3

Bleeding time: 12 min
Prothrombin time (PT): 13 sec
Partial thromboplastin time (PTT): 25 sec

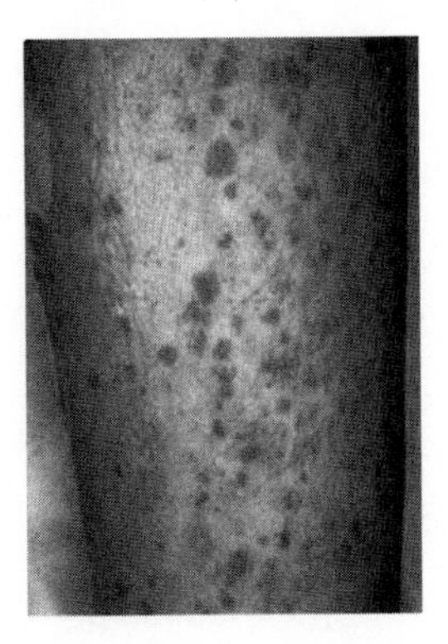

FIGURE 8-6. (Reproduced, with permission, from Bondi EE, Jegasothy BV, Lazarus GS [eds]. *Dermatology: Diagnosis & Treatment.* Norwalk, CT: Appleton & Lange, 1991. Copyright © by The McGraw-Hill Companies, Inc.)

■ **What is the most likely diagnosis?**	Idiopathic thrombocytopenic purpura (ITP), a disease in which the body makes antiplatelet antibodies.
■ **What would be the most likely diagnosis if schistocytes were evident on PBS and results of Coombs' test were negative?**	In this case, the likely diagnosis would be thrombotic thrombocytopenic purpura (TTP)/hemolytic-uremic syndrome. This idiopathic disease causes microthrombi to develop in small vessels.
■ **What are the three main causes of this condition?**	■ Splenic sequestration ■ Decreased production (due to stem-cell failure, leukemia, aplastic anemia, alcohol, aspirin, clopidogrel) ■ Increased destruction (due to ITP, TTP, heparin, quinidine)
■ **What clinical findings are commonly associated with this condition?**	ITP presents with mucous membrane bleeding, petechiae, and purpura (see Figure 8-6 above). Epistaxis (nosebleed) and easy bruisability are characteristic of bleeding disorders in general. The childhood form of ITP usually develops after a viral urinary tract infection or immunization. It is a self-limited disease. Adult ITP, in contrast, is a chronic disease.
■ **What additional tests are useful for confirming the diagnosis?**	Bleeding time is increased in ITP, with normal PT and PTT. A PBS reveals large (young) platelets. Antiplatelet antibodies can be present or absent, and thus are not helpful in the diagnosis. Bone marrow biopsy, if done, demonstrates increased megakaryocytes.

- **What are the most appropriate treatments for this condition?**

- ITP: First-line treatment is high-dose steroids. Second-line treatment includes intravenous immunoglobulin G (IVIG), anti-Rh (such as WinRho®), splenectomy, or rituximab (anti-CD20). Acute bleeding in ITP is treated with IVIG followed by platelets and pulse methylprednisolone.
- TTP: Plasma exchange until disease abates. This disease is fatal without treatment. Antibodies to von Willebrand cleaving enzyme are often found in patients with TTP; thus, this disease may involve immune aspects as well.

► Case 15

A 60-year-old woman presents to her primary care physician for her annual physical examination. She says she has been feeling "down" and tired lately. Upon questioning, she also admits to some constipation, abdominal pain, joint pain, and muscle aches. Physical examination reveals blue pigmentation in her gum-tooth line. A peripheral blood smear reveals basophilic stippling. Relevant laboratory findings are as follows:

Hemoglobin: 9.0 g/dL
Hematocrit: 26%
Mean corpuscular volume: 76 fl
WBC count: 5000/mm^3

- **What is the most likely diagnosis?**

Lead poisoning. This is suggested by the blue pigmentation of the gums **(Bruton's lines)**, the patient's microcytic anemia, and the characteristic basophilic stippling. Additional presenting symptoms include colicky abdominal pain, constipation, irritability, difficulty concentrating, depression/psychosis, decreased short-term memory, arthralgias and myalgias, headache, decreased libido, and anemia. Lead poisoning can also cause peripheral neuropathy, often presenting as extensor weakness (eg, wrist drop) due to segmental demyelination and degeneration of motor axons.

- **What is the most likely cause of the anemia?**

Lead poisoning is an environmental cause of porphyria through inhibition of porphobilinogen synthetase, which converts 5-aminolevulinic acid to porphobilinogen in one of the first steps of heme synthesis. This impairment results in decreased hemoglobin production, and therefore a microcytic, hypochromic anemia.

- **What are the common causes of microcytic, hypochromic anemia?**

Lead poisoning, **I**ron deficiency, and **T**halassemia are three causes of decreased hemoglobin synthesis. These can be remembered using the mnemonic "**LIT**tle RBCs."

- **Where does lead distribute in the body?**

Lead distributes in the blood, soft tissues, and skeleton, particularly bone and teeth. The vast majority (95%) of the body's lead burden is deposited in the skeleton, where its half-life is approximately 25 years. Therefore, events associated with bone turnover, such as hyperthyroidism, menopause, pregnancy, and breast-feeding, can cause lead to be released into the blood. This can cause acute lead intoxication in the absence of an acute exposure. Lead can also cross the placenta. In children, especially those 1–3 years old, lead can easily enter and harm their developing nervous system because the blood-brain barrier is not completely formed.

- **What do increased serum lead levels and increased free erythrocyte protoporphyrin (FEP) levels indicate about the duration of this condition?**

Increased serum lead levels indicate lead exposure within the past 3 weeks. FEP levels are a measure of intoxication in the past 120 days (the average lifetime of an RBC). Chelation therapy can be useful in addition to removing the source of the lead. Also, for patients with iron deficiency anemia, any iron supplementation should be suspended.

▶ Case 16

A 65-year-old woman presents to her physician with cough, hemoptysis, wheezing, and pleuritic pain. She has noted increased hoarseness of her voice and weight loss over the past few months. She also has noted progressively worsening shortness of breath when ascending or descending one flight of stairs. She has been hospitalized for pneumonia twice during the past 12 months. Sputum analysis reveals atypical cells. A complete blood count reveals her hematocrit is 25% and her WBC count is 12,000/mm^3.

- **What is the most likely diagnosis?**

Lung cancer **(Pancoast's syndrome).** This disease is caused by a tumor of the upper lobe of the lung, which causes pain in the ipsilateral arm and Horner's syndrome (ptosis, miosis, and ipsilateral anhydrosis). The tumor is often accompanied by ipsilateral pain or weakness/numbness in the ulnar distribution.

- **What are the major clinical features of this condition?**

Hoarseness is caused by recurrent laryngeal nerve involvement. Neck or facial swelling is due to superior vena cava obstruction. Diaphragmatic paralysis is due to phrenic nerve involvement. Dyspnea is secondary to obstruction and increased ventilation requirements. Metastasis to the liver, adrenal glands, brain and bone, and mediastinal lymph nodes is common. Extrathoracic signs include paraneoplastic syndromes such as Cushing's syndrome, hypercalcemia, syndrome of inappropriate secretion of ADH (SIADH), clubbing (hypertrophic osteoarthropathy), and Eaton-Lambert syndrome.

- **What laboratory findings are common in this condition?**

- Sputum analysis typically reveals atypical cells (not sensitive). Anemia of chronic disease is also common.
- Chest radiographs and CT typically reveals squamous cell carcinomas at the hilum and/or adenocarcinoma at the periphery.
- Ventilation-perfusion scanning can assess the pulmonary reserve.
- Positron emission tomography may be useful to evaluate mediastinal adenopathy and for staging.

- **What are the primary pathologic types of this condition?**

- **Non–small cell lung cancer** (which is the most common type) includes the following:
  - **Squamous cell carcinoma** accounts for 30% of lung cancers. It occurs centrally near the hilum; slower growth and cavitation are frequently seen.
  - **Adenocarcinoma** accounts for 30% of lung cancers. These tumors may be mucus secreting, as in acinar adenocarcinoma. They may also be bronchoalveolar in scar like carcinoma (more common among nonsmokers).
  - **Bronchoalveolar carcinoma** occurs more often in nonsmokers, and is associated with epidermal growth factor receptor (EGFR) mutations.
- **Large cell carcinoma,** which is rare.
- **Small cell carcinoma** accounts for 25% of lung cancers. These tumors occur centrally and are early to metastasize. They are very sensitive to chemotherapy but frequently relapse.

- **What are the most appropriate treatments for this condition?**

Surgery is considered for lesions without distant metastasis, if the patient has sufficient cardiopulmonary reserve. Radiotherapy is used to treat unresectable tumors. Adjuvant chemotherapy is also used with some patients undergoing surgery; patients with stage Ib disease or higher require chemotherapy. For patients with metastatic disease, chemotherapy is often used palliatively, often with biological agents (such as antiangiogenic agents and EGFR inhibitors).

▶ Case 17

A 45-year-old man presents to his physician for a regular checkup. He has no previous medical or surgical history. As part of the checkup, the physician orders routine laboratory tests; relevant findings are as follows:

Hemoglobin: 11 g/dL
Hematocrit: 33%
Reticulocyte count: 0.2%
Mean corpuscular volume: 120 fl

- **What is the most likely diagnosis?**

The tests are indicative of a macrocytic anemia. However, one must remember that macrocytic anemia is not a diagnosis in itself, and a cause for the anemia must always be pursued.

- **Which other test would be useful in confirming the diagnosis?**

A peripheral blood smear would reveal the presence of polymorphonuclear cells (PMNs). In megaloblastic anemias, PMNs are characterized by multilobed (>5) nuclei (see Figure 8-7 below).

- **What are some possible etiologies for this condition?**

- Alcoholism
- Folate deficiency
- Hypothyroidism
- Mild aplastic anemia
- Myelodysplastic syndrome
- Pharmaceutical agents (especially antimetabolites such as methotrexate or chemotherapeutic agents)
- Vitamin B_{12} deficiency

- **What diagnosis should be considered if the patient also had decreased vibration sensation in his feet?**

This neuropathy would indicate a vitamin B_{12} deficiency (subacute combined degeneration). A **Schilling test** would be helpful in excluding other possible causes, such as pellagra or celiac sprue. The Schilling test involves administering radiolabeled vitamin B_{12} and measuring urinary excretion of radioisotope before and after the administration of intrinsic factor. Beware, however, that bacterial overgrowth can cause false-positive results.

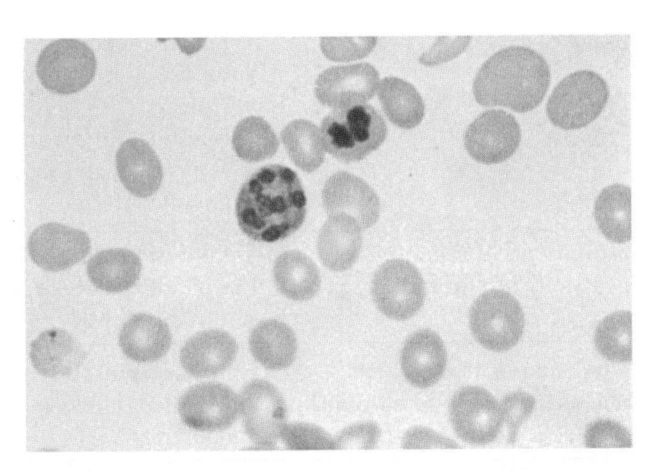

FIGURE 8-7. Multilobed PMNs characteristic of megaloblastic anemias. (Reproduced, with permission, from Kasper DL, et al. *Harrison's Principles of Internal Medicine*, 16th ed. New York: McGraw-Hill, 2005: 605.)

▶ Case 18

A 66-year-old postmenopausal woman presents to her physician with complaints of fatigue, dyspnea, dizziness, and tachycardia. She also says she craves chewing on ice cubes. Physical examination reveals pallor of the mucous membranes of her mouth. The cells on a peripheral blood smear are microcytic and hypochromic (see Figure 8-8 below). Relevant laboratory findings are as follows:

Hemoglobin: 11 g/dL
Hematocrit: 30%
Reticulocyte count: 0.2%
Mean corpuscular volume: 74 fl

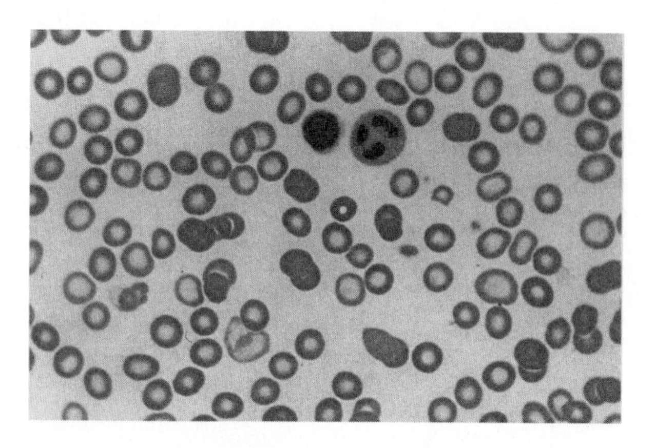

FIGURE 8-8. (Reproduced, with permission, from Bhushan V, Le T, et al. *First Aid for the USMLE Step 1: 2006*. New York: McGraw-Hill, 2006: Color Image 20.)

■ **What is the most likely diagnosis?**	Iron deficiency anemia. This diagnosis would be further supported by laboratory studies demonstrating a decreased iron concentration, *increased* total iron binding capacity, and *decreased* ferritin levels. However, iron deficiency anemia is not a diagnosis, as the physician must always search for the underlying reason for a patient's iron deficiency.
■ **What factors can lead to this disease?**	■ Chronic blood loss (especially gastrointestinal blood loss secondary to colon cancer) ■ Dietary deficiency (increased demand or decreased absorption) ■ Increased iron requirement (as in pregnancy or childhood growth) ■ Intestinal hookworm infection (this is the most common cause worldwide, and should be considered in patients who have immigrated from developing countries)
■ **Why are measurements of the total iron binding capacity important?**	Total iron binding capacity is high in iron deficiency anemia and low in anemia of chronic disease. Both illnesses have decreased serum iron levels.
■ **What other conditions is this patient at a greatly increased risk for developing?**	**Plummer-Vinson syndrome,** due to an extreme lack of iron. This syndrome is characterized by atrophic glossitis, esophageal webs, and anemia.
■ **What are the common causes of microcytic, hypochromic anemia?**	Microcytic anemia results from either decreased hemoglobin production or faulty hemoglobin function. Thalassemia, lead poisoning, sideroblastic anemia, and iron deficiency are the four possible etiologies of microcytic, hypochromic anemia.

▶ Case 19

A 62-year-old African-American man comes to his physician complaining of lower back pain of recent onset. His past medical history is unremarkable except for two recent attacks of pneumonia that were successfully treated. Relevant laboratory values are as follows:

Sodium: 140 mEq/L
Bicarbonate: 25 mEq/L
Magnesium: 1.8 mg/dL
Potassium: 4.0 mEq/L
Calcium: 14 mEq/L
Phosphate: 3.6 mg/dL
Chloride: 106 mEq/L
Blood urea nitrogen: 15 mg/dL
Creatine: 2.0 mg/dL

- **What is the most likely diagnosis?**

Back pain, increased recent susceptibility to infection, and elevated serum calcium and creatinine levels strongly suggest multiple myeloma.

- **What is the pathophysiology of this condition?**

Multiple myeloma is a clonal proliferation of B cells that have then differentiated into plasma cells. These mature B cells cause lytic lesions in the bones, called **punched-out lesions.** These cells produce massive quantities of identical immunoglobulin molecules, usually IgG or IgA, that are either κ or λ light chain (κ more common than λ). Rarely, IgD or nonsecretory myeloma can be diagnosed.

- **What aspects of the condition are responsible for this patient's symptoms?**

The abnormal lymphocytes are incapable of mounting a normal immunologic response, which explains the patient's recent susceptibility to infection. The elevated serum calcium level and back pain are the result of bone breakdown and osteoclast activating factor. Finally, the increased creatinine level indicates renal involvement.

- **What renal complications are associated with this condition?**

The large amount of **Bence Jones proteins** (free immunoglobulin light chains) found in the urine of patients with multiple myeloma causes azotemia. Other renal complications include inflammation with potential giant cell formation and metastatic calcification. The differential diagnosis of renal failure in myeloma includes amyloid kidney, myeloma kidney, light-chain deposition disease, uric acid stones, hypercalcemia, sepsis with acute tubular necrosis, and obstruction.

- **What other tests are useful in confirming the diagnosis?**

A complete blood count should be ordered. Patients with multiple myeloma may be anemic as a result of tumor cells overcrowding myeloid precursor cells. Electrophoresis with immunofixation will demonstrate **M protein,** the term given to the massively produced immunoglobulin. **Monoclonal gammopathy of undetermined significance** (MGUS) is the precursor lesion here if the M protein level is <3 g/dL, there are <10% plasma cells in the bone marrow, and if no clinical manifestations are present. Urinalysis of a 24-hour collection may reveal the presence of Bence Jones proteins. Bone marrow biopsy shows a 2- to 4-fold increase in plasma cells. Additionally, the total immunoglobulin levels may be low. Finally, as a result of the marked hyperglobulinemia, RBCs on peripheral blood smear will clump in a formation that resembles poker chips. This pattern is called **rouleaux formation.**

► Case 20

A mother brings her 4-month-old infant to the pediatrician because the child has had watery diarrhea almost daily for the past month. Previously a good eater, the baby is now refusing to feed and is irritable most of the time. While holding the baby, the mother also calls attention to a mass in his belly that has not resolved in several days.

What is the most common tumor occurring in infants?	Neuroblastoma.
What is the origin of this tumor?	Neuroblastoma is a malignancy of the sympathetic nervous system that arises during embryonic development. In the embryo, **neuroblasts** (pluripotent sympathetic stem cells) invaginate and migrate along the neuraxis to the adrenal medulla, the sympathetic ganglia, and various other sites. Figure 8-9 on the following page shows a large neuroblastoma occupying the left flank in an older child. The site of disease presentation depends on the area to which the neuroblasts migrate.
What prognostic factors are important in this tumor?	Tumor stage and the patient's age at diagnosis are the two most important diagnostic factors. Patients with localized disease, regardless of age, have a favorable prognosis (80%–90% 5-year survival). Overall, younger age at diagnosis carries a more favorable prognosis. The 5-year survival rate is 83% for infants, 55%–60% for children 1–5 years old, and 40% for children older than 5 years.
What are the likely findings on biopsy of this tumor?	Histologically, neuroblastoma presents as dense nests of small, round, blue tumor cells with hyperchromatic nuclei. **Homer-Wright pseudorosettes** are seen in 10%–15% of cases. These pseudorosettes are composed of neuroblasts surrounding neuritic processes and are pathognomonic of neuroblastoma.
What are the most appropriate treatments for this tumor?	For patients with localized disease, surgical excision is curative. For more advanced disease, treatment consists of surgical excision followed by chemotherapy. Chemotherapy for neuroblastoma consists of combination regimens, typically vincristine, cyclophosphamide, and doxorubicin. Other regimens include etoposide in combination with either cisplatin or carboplatin.

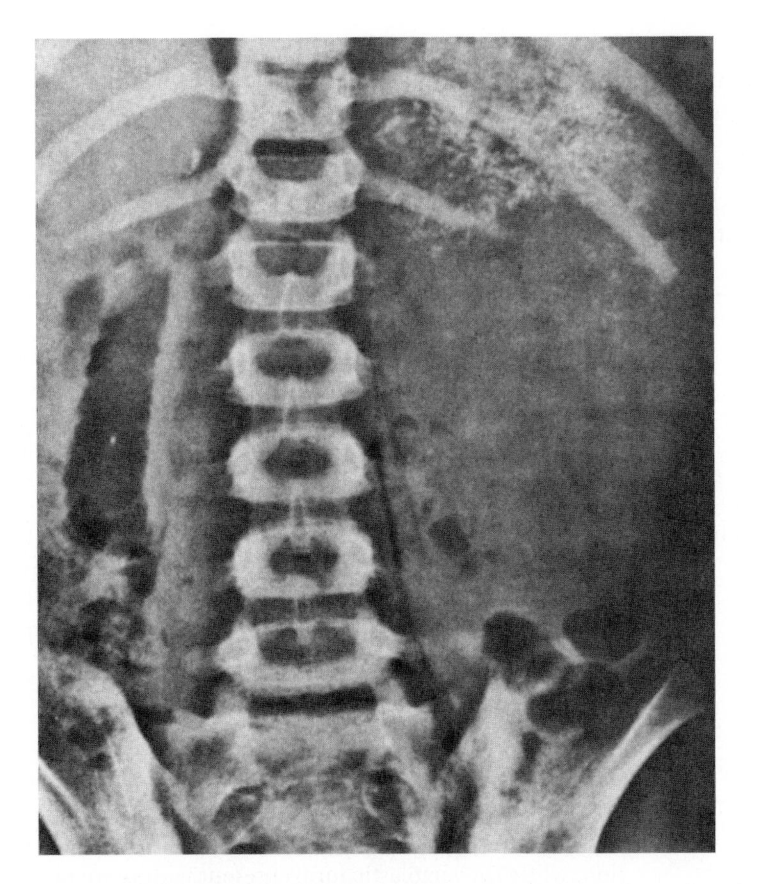

FIGURE 8-9. Chest x-ray of neuroblastoma of the adrenal gland. (Reproduced, with permission, from Tanagho EA, McAninch JW. *Smith's General Urology*, 16th ed. New York: McGraw-Hill, 2004: 506.)

▶ Case 21

A 30-year-old woman comes to her physician complaining of a headache that has affected her intermittently for the past 6 months. The headache is primarily in the front of her head, is present on most days, and is typically dull but sometimes piercing. Over the same time period, the woman has also had profound weakness in her right arm to the point at which she is sometimes unable to hold her 1-year-old daughter or to comb her hair. She also reports an intermittent sensation of "pins and needles" in her right hand.

What is the most likely diagnosis?	Oligodendroglioma. These relatively rare, slow-growing tumors occur at a rate of 0.3 per 100,000 individuals and are responsible for 2%–4% of primary brain tumors and 4%–15% of all intracranial gliomas. They occur with equal incidence in women and men, and the peak age incidence is 42 years. Primary brain tumors represent approximately 2% of all cancers.
Where do these tumors typically occur?	Oligodendrogliomas almost always (92% of cases) occur supratentorially and are most often found in the frontal lobes. Lesions are typically peripheral. Most oligodendrogliomas arise in the cortex and extend into the white matter of the cerebral hemispheres.
What symptoms are typically associated with these tumors?	As with most primary brain tumors, the clinical presentation of oligodendrogliomas is typically attributable to mass effects resulting from the compression of adjacent structures by the tumor. Oligodendrogliomas often cause headache, mental status changes, and paresis. Seizures may also occur. Because they are slow growing, these tumors may have a more insidious presentation, while the anaplastic forms present with more rapid neurologic decline.
What are the likely findings on histology?	**"Fried egg" cells** are typically seen on histologic section. These cells have characteristic round nuclei with clear cytoplasm (see Figure 8-10 below). The tumors often calcify (30% of cases), and calcifications may be apparent on histologic section.
What is the prognosis for patients with this tumor?	About 50% of patients with oligodendrogliomas survive longer than 5 years, and there is a 25%–34% 10-year survival rate. Mortality increases with features of increasing nuclear atypia, necrosis, and mitosis. Some oligodendrogliomas contain astrocytic components and are termed **mixed gliomas.** Patients with highly anaplastic oligodendrogliomas have a median survival of <2 years.

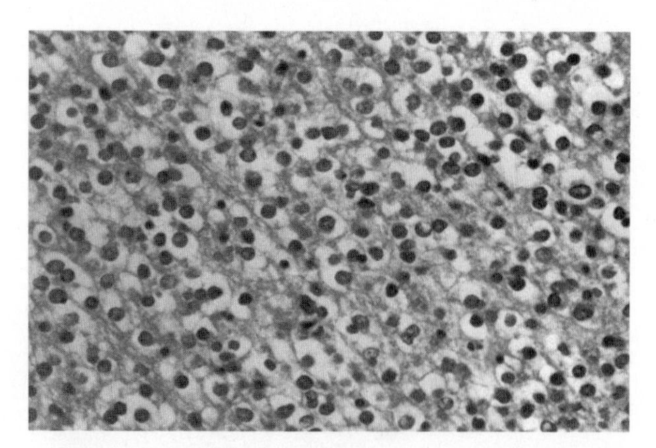

FIGURE 8-10. "Fried egg" cells on histologic exam in oligodendroglioma. (Reproduced with permission of the Pathology Education Instructional Resource Digital Library (http://peir.net) at the University of Alabama, Birmingham.)

▶ Case 22

A 49-year-old woman presents to her gynecologist because her menstrual periods have become irregular. The patient also reports she has hair growing on her face and has developed mild acne, which she hasn't had since she was a teenager. On physical examination, the patient's abdomen is somewhat distended and there is a palpable mass on the left adnexa.

- **What is the most likely diagnosis?**

A palpable adnexal mass in conjunction with abdominal swelling is suggestive of ovarian cancer, which is often accompanied by ascites. The patient's irregular periods may simply be normal menopause, but the triad of irregular periods, facial hair, and acne constitutes hirsutism. The **Sertoli-Leydig ovarian tumor,** also known as an androgenoma, is an androgen-producing neoplasm that presents with hirsutism in 50% of patients.

- **From what cell line does this tumor originate?**

The Sertoli-Leydig cell tumor is of sex cord–stromal origin. Tumors of this origin are relatively rare, and account for only 5% of ovarian neoplasm. They consist of mixtures of stromal fibroblasts, granulosa cells, theca cells, and cells that resemble testicular Sertoli cells and Leydig cells.

- **What other tumors have the same origin?**

Other stromal ovarian tumors include:

- **Fibromas,** solid tumors consisting of cells that resemble fibroblasts.
- **Thecoma** tumors, which contain fibroblasts plus lipid-containing cells.
- **Granulosa cell** tumors, which consist of estrogen-secreting granulosa cells and may present with abnormal vaginal bleeding or endometrial hyperplasia.

- **What are the likely findings on histology?**

The Sertoli-Leydig tumor typically is composed of large cells with large amounts of eosinophilic cytoplasm arranged into tubules and surrounded by a fibrous stroma. Sertoli cells are found lining the tubules, and Leydig cells may be found in the stroma.

- **What is the lymphatic drainage of the ovaries?**

Like that of the testicles, the ovaries' lymphatic drainage is to the lumbar and preaortic lymph nodes. The lymph vessels from the ovaries travel with the venous drainage in the broad ligament.

▶ Case 23

A 36-year-old diabetic African-American man presents to his primary care physician after his wife noted scleral icterus and a recent, unintentional, 11.4-kg (25-lb) weight loss. The patient denies abdominal pain. Physical examination reveals a mass in the right upper quadrant of the abdomen. Relevant laboratory findings are as follows:

Alkaline phosphatase: 127 U/L
Bilirubin: 2 mg/dL
Calcium: 10.6 mg/dL

What is the pathophysiology of this condition?	Pancreatic tumors form mostly in the head and neck of the pancreas from the endocrine and exocrine portions of the pancreas. The majority are exocrine and originate in the ductal epithelium, acinar cells, connective tissue, and lymphatic tissue.
What factors increase a person's risk for this condition?	▪ African-American race ▪ Cigarette smoking ▪ History of chronic pancreatitis ▪ History of diabetes mellitus ▪ Male gender
What are the common sites of invasion for this condition?	Pancreatic cancer can invade the duodenum, the ampulla of Vater, and the common bile duct. As a result, pancreatic cancer can often cause biliary obstruction. Figure 8-11 below shows pancreatic adenocarcinoma, which appears as a large, heterogeneously enhancing mass at the neck of the pancreas. In this case the mass is compressing the common bile duct, portal vein, splenic vein, superior mesenteric vein, and the inferior vena cava.
What is the most common form/ location for this condition?	Ninety percent of pancreatic tumors are adenocarcinoma, with 60% found in the head of the pancreas.
What are the common sites of metastasis?	Metastasis often begins in the regional lymph nodes and spreads to the liver or, less often, to the lungs. Pancreatic cancer can also directly invade the duodenum, stomach, and colon.

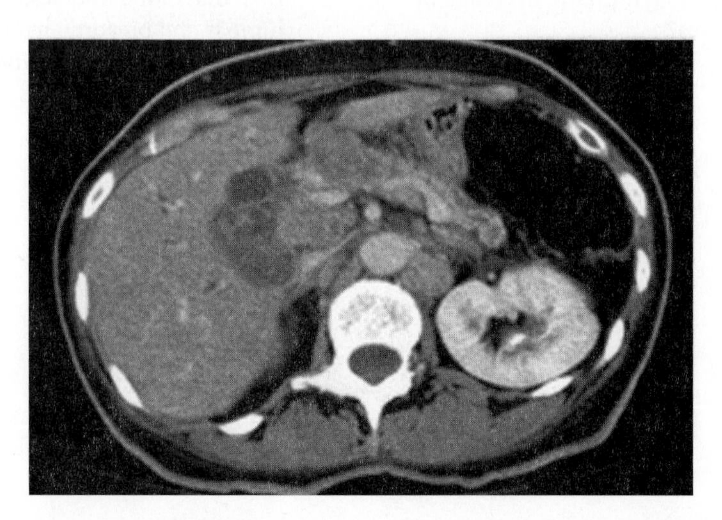

FIGURE 8-11. CT of pancreatic cancer. (Reproduced with permission of the Pathology Education Instructional Resource Digital Library (http://peir.net) at the University of Alabama, Birmingham.)

▶ Case 24

During the course of an annual physical examination, a previously healthy 70-year-old man mentions he has recently noted weakness and rib pain. His appetite has been good, and he has not experienced fevers, nausea, vomiting, or changes in bowel habit. Physical examination reveals splenomegaly. Results of a complete blood count are as follows:

WBC count: 10,000/mm^3
Hemoglobin: 22 g/dL
Hematocrit: 62%
Platelet count: 425,000/mm^3

■ **What is the most likely diagnosis?**	Polycythemia, also known as **erythrocytosis.** This patient's elevated hemoglobin concentration is a sign of increased RBC count. An increased RBC mass (>32 mL/kg in women and >36 mL/kg in men) is diagnostic of polycythemia in the absence of secondary causes of the disease.
■ **Levels of which hormone should be measured to establish the diagnosis?**	**Erythropoietin** can help the physician distinguish between primary and secondary causes of polycythemia. Erythropoietin levels will be decreased or normal in primary polycythemia **(polycythemia vera).** In secondary polycythemia, however, RBC precursors are responding to increased levels of erythropoietin secondary to an underlying pathology (eg, erythropoietin-secreting tumor, hypoxemia, altitude).
■ **Which two types of carcinoma are associated with this condition?**	**Renal cell carcinoma** and **hepatocellular carcinoma.** In a healthy adult, the kidneys produce a majority of the body's erythropoietin, and the liver is a secondary source.
■ **What mature cells descend from a myeloid stem cell precursor?**	Erythrocytes, platelets, basophils, eosinophils, neutrophils, and macrophages. Disorders of myeloid stem cell multiplication, as in polycythemia vera, can present with elevated cell counts of multiple myeloid descendants.
■ **How can an uncorrected ventricular septal defect (VSD) lead to this condition?**	In patients with uncorrected VSD, atrial septal defect, or patent ductus arteriosus, blood is shunted from the left side of the heart to the right side, which exposes the pulmonary vasculature to systemic blood pressures. Over time, the pulmonary vasculature adapts by increasing pulmonary resistance, and blood flow through the shunt is reversed to flow from right-to-left. This reversal of flow is known as **Eisenmenger's syndrome.** Right-to-left shunts cause hypoxemia and cyanosis, a potent stimulus for erythropoietin secretion and a cause of secondary polycythemia.
■ **What are the most appropriate treatments for this condition?**	Phlebotomy can reduce the risk of blood clots in patients with polycythemia to that of the normal population. In high-risk patients (the elderly, those with a history of clots), hydroxyurea may be useful for controlling the hematocrit; caution is advised, however, as this may be leukemogenic. Low-dose aspirin should be taken as primary prevention of arterial thrombosis.

▶ Case 25

A 20-year-old African-American woman visits her physician complaining of episodes of extreme pain and discomfort in her legs and lower back. She has been experiencing these recurrent episodes, accompanied by extreme fatigue, since she was a child. On physical examination, she appears jaundiced and has a hematocrit of 23% and a hemoglobin level of 7 g/dL. She reports she has family members who experienced the same symptoms.

What is the most likely diagnosis?	Sickle cell anemia.
What is the pathophysiology of this condition?	Sickle cell anemia develops at around 6 months of age when hemoglobin S (HbS) replaces hemoglobin F (HbF). The course of disease is punctuated by episodes of painful crises, which are believed to be a result of hypoxic tissue injury from microvascular occlusions. HbS is the result of a single missense mutation in the beta globin gene of hemoglobin. This causes RBCs to be susceptible to **sickling** in conditions of low oxygen or dehydration (see Figure 8-12 on the following page). Any organ can be affected by the vascular congestion, thrombosis, and infarction caused by sickling cells, so these patients tend to have multiple health problems. Microcytosis, sickled cells, and high reticulocyte counts are seen. The combination of sickle cell anemia and β-thalassemia is common and can also result in sickle crises.
What complications are common in patients with this condition?	Complications include painful (vaso-occlusive) crisis, aplastic crisis (cessation of erythropoiesis due to parvovirus B19 infection), and splenic sequestration crisis. Splenic sequestration eventually leads to autosplenectomy, which results in increased susceptibility to encapsulated organisms, including *Pneumococcus*. Other complications include increased susceptibility to *Salmonella* osteomyelitis for reasons not understood. Priapism, stroke, leg ulcers, acute chest syndrome (fat emboli, infection, vaso-occlusion), and dactylitis are important complications.
How prevalent is this condition among African-Americans?	Sickle cell anemia is an autosomal recessive disease with an 8% carrier rate in African-Americans. An estimated 0.2% of African-Americans have this disease.
What is the likely finding on radiology?	Erythropoiesis must increase in order to compensate for the decreased life span of RBCs (from 120 days to approximately 20 days). The resultant marrow expansion can lead to resorption of bone and subsequent new bone formation on the external aspect of the skull. This leads to a "crew cut" appearance on skull radiographs.
What is the most appropriate treatment for this condition?	Therapy includes hydroxyurea, which acts to increase HbF production, thereby reducing the number of cells with the potential to sickle. Exchange transfusion with normal RBCs may reduce the sickle RBC percentage and is used to treat the life-threatening complications of acute chest syndrome or stroke.

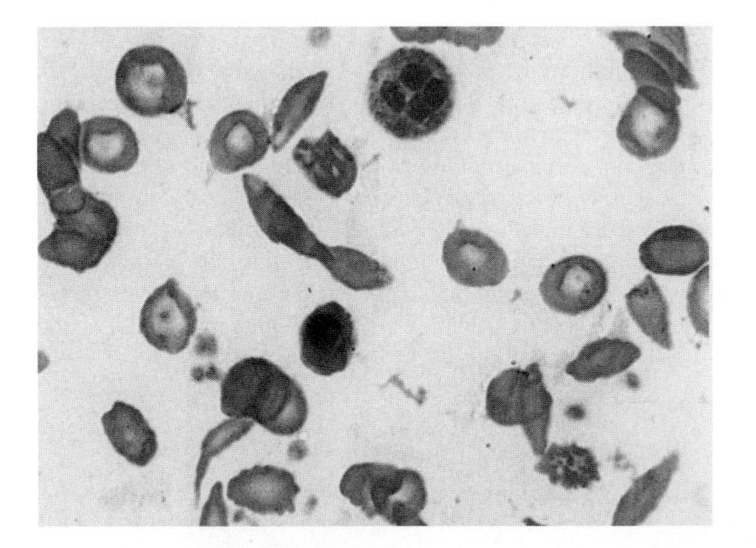

FIGURE 8-12. Peripheral blood smear of sickle cell anemia. (Reproduced with permission of the Pathology Education Instructional Resource Digital Library (http://peir.net) at the University of Alabama, Birmingham.)

▶ Case 26

A 3-year-old boy is brought to the pediatrician by his parents, who noticed that his right eye has turned "white" (see Figure 8-13 below). When they referred back to earlier photographs, the child's eyes were normally colored. The boy denies any pain or irritation in his eyes, and he does not complain of loss of vision. The parents deny any trauma to the area and there is no family history of ocular disease. On physician examination, the boy's extraocular movements are intact and symmetrical, his pupillary light reflexes are normal, and he has intact central and peripheral vision in both eyes. However, when he is asked to fixate at a point in the distance, the boy's right eye deviates toward his nose (esotropia). Fundoscopic examination reveals a chalky, white-gray retinal mass in the right eye.

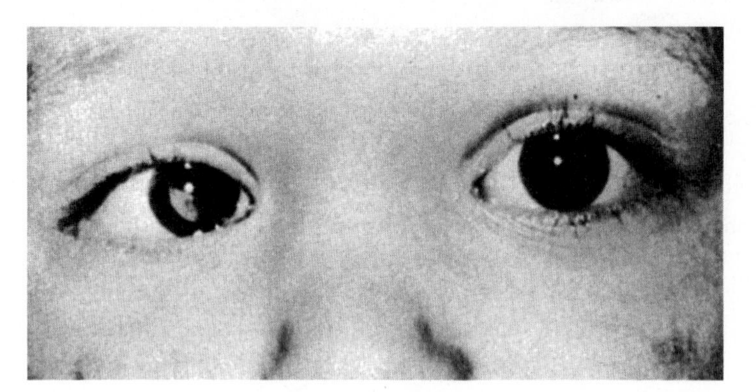

FIGURE 8-13. (Reproduced, with permission, from Riordan-Eva P, Whitcher JP. *Vaughan & Asbury's General Ophthalmology,* 16th ed. New York: McGraw-Hill, 2004.)

■ **What is the most likely diagnosis?**	Retinoblastoma. Other causes of leukocoria ("white pupil") include congenital cataracts, developmental anomalies of the vitreous and retina, and inflammatory conditions.
■ **What is the pathogenesis of this condition?**	Retinoblastoma results from mutations of both alleles of the ***Rb* gene,** on chromosome 13q14, which codes for a tumor suppressor protein. The Rb protein binds and sequesters transcription factors of the E2F family, to prevent the G1-to-S phase transition. Loss of this tumor suppressor protein promotes unregulated growth.
■ **What is the "two-hit hypothesis"?**	The **two-hit hypothesis** (Knudsen's hypothesis) suggests that two separate mutations are required for tumorigenesis involving a suppressor gene. In heritable disease, patients inherit a mutated germline allele from a parent, and acquire a second somatic mutation later in development. This often gives rise to binocular and multifocal disease. In noninherited disease, two spontaneous mutations arise in a single retinal cell during development, giving rise to uniocular, unifocal disease.
■ **What secondary malignancies is this boy at risk of developing?**	Osteogenic sarcoma, soft tissue sarcoma, and malignant melanoma commonly develop in patients with retinoblastoma. Metastatic spread occurs rapidly through direct infiltration or via the subarachnoid space, blood, and lymphatics.
■ **What is the most appropriate treatment for this condition?**	The treatment of choice for retinoblastoma is enucleation of the affected eye, with an effort to remove a large portion of the optic nerve, as this is the most common path for metastasis to the brain. Other treatment options include external beam radiation therapy, cryotherapy, and chemotherapy.

▶ Case 27

A 55-year-old woman presents to her physician complaining of a 2- to 3-month history of cough. The cough was initially nonproductive but has become progressively more productive of sputum and occasionally blood. She has a 50-pack-year history of cigarette smoking. Physical examination reveals marked wheezing, and an x-ray of the chest demonstrates hilar enlargement and a perihilar mass on the right side. The mass is biopsied, and the histologic specimen is shown in Figure 8-14 below.

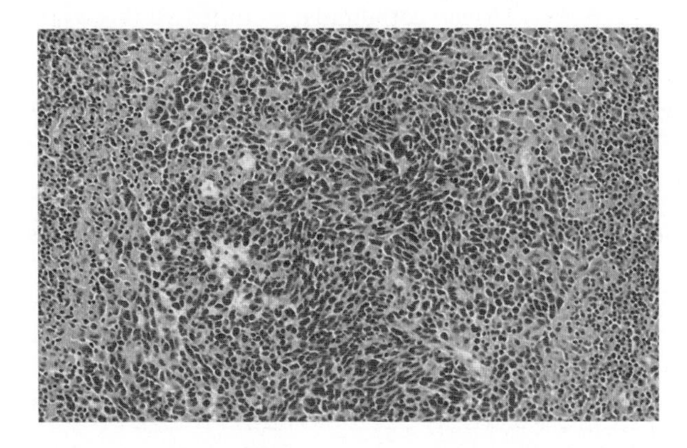

FIGURE 8-14. (Reproduced with permission of the Pathology Education Instructional Resource Digital Library (http://peir.net) at the University of Alabama, Birmingham.)

▪ **What is the most likely diagnosis?**	Small cell carcinoma of the lung (SCLC). SCLC often presents as a hilar or mediastinal mass.
▪ **What risk factors are associated with the development of this tumor?**	Smoking is the major risk factor for the development of most lung cancers, including small cell, squamous cell, and adenocarcinoma of the lung. Large cell lung cancer and bronchoalveolar carcinoma, however, are not thought to be related to smoking. Exposure to other substances, including asbestos, polycyclic aromatic hydrocarbons, and ionizing radiation, also increases the risk of certain lung cancers.
▪ **What other syndrome is this patient at greatly increased risk for developing?**	**Lambert-Eaton myasthenic syndrome.** This condition, which is very similar to myasthenia gravis, is caused by autoantibodies against the P/Q-type calcium channels in the presynaptic neuromuscular junction. It causes weakness of the proximal musculature, especially of the lower limbs. Cranial nerves are commonly affected, which often manifests as ptosis of the eyelids and diplopia.
▪ **What are the most common sites of metastasis for this tumor?**	Lung cancers metastasize to virtually every organ in the body. Brain metastases are common, with resulting neurologic deficits. Bone metastases result in bone pain or fractures and can cause spinal cord compression. Liver, supraclavicular lymph nodes, and adrenal metastases are also common.
▪ **What are the most appropriate treatments for this tumor?**	Most patients with SCLC have unresectable disease at the time of presentation. In patients with small peripheral lesions and no metastases, surgical resection may be an option. Treatment for SCLC involves chemotherapy, typically etoposide plus cisplatin, with or without radiotherapy. In patients who do not receive chemotherapy or radiation, mean survival ranges from 6 to 17 weeks.

▶ Case 28

Upon presentation to his family physician, an 8-month-old boy is noted to have jaundice and dyspnea. Physical examination reveals tachycardia and splenomegaly. The mother recalls a long family history of "blood disease." A Coombs' test is negative. Relevant laboratory findings are as follows:

Hemoglobin: 8.5 g/dL
Hematocrit: 29%
Mean corpuscular volume (MCV): 85 fl
Mean corpuscular hemoglobin concentration (MCHC): 400 g/L

■ **What is the most likely diagnosis?**	Hereditary spherocytosis, an autosomal dominant form of hemolytic anemia.
■ **What protein defect causes this condition?**	RBC membrane defects are the result of mutations in **spectrin** or **ankyrin** (erythrocyte skeletal proteins). This results in a decreased membrane:volume ratio, which makes the cells more fragile. Thus, a positive result on osmotic fragility testing is virtually pathognomonic for the disease. Cells are trapped in the spleen, where they are destroyed.
■ **What are the likely findings on peripheral blood smear?**	Small RBCs without central pallor **(spherocytes)** (see arrows in Figure 8-15 below).
■ **What blood test would be useful in establishing the diagnosis?**	An osmotic fragility test may confirm the presence of fragile sphere-shaped RBCs. The MCHC is increased due to a reduction in membrane surface area in the setting of a constant hemoglobin concentration. MCV remains normal because the overall volume remains stable. High reticulocyte counts (5%–10%) with elevated indirect bilirubin levels are also seen.
■ **What test could be used to differentiate this condition from autoimmune etiologies?**	A direct Coombs' test is used to distinguish hereditary spherocytosis from warm antibody hemolysis: Hereditary spherocytosis is Coombs' negative, while warm antibody hemolysis is Coombs' positive. A positive result on a direct Coombs' test indicates the presence of antibodies on RBCs. A positive result on an indirect Coombs' test indicates the presence of antibodies in the serum.
■ **What are the most appropriate treatments for this condition?**	Splenectomy is curative and should be considered in patients with more severe disease. Surgery also helps prevent gallstone (bilirubin) formation. Folate supplementation may also be useful.

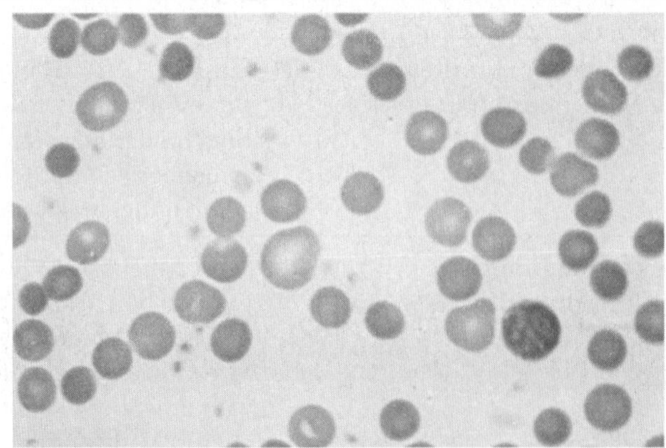

FIGURE 8-15. Histology of spherocytosis. (Reproduced, with permission, from Kasper DL, et al. *Harrison's Principles of Internal Medicine,* 16th ed. New York: McGraw-Hill, 2005: 609.)

▶ Case 29

A 27-year-old man is brought to the emergency department via ambulance after a motor vehicle accident. He was a restrained passenger in a two-car collision. He is complaining of left upper quadrant pain. On physical examination he appears restless and agitated, and he is noted to be tachycardic and tachypneic.

Damage to what organ is most likely involved in this case?	The spleen is an important organ in immune function and hematopoiesis. The primary functions of the spleen are synthesis of IgG, properdin, and tuftsin; clearance of abnormal RBCs; clearance of microorganisms and particulate matter from the bloodstream; and hematopoiesis (extramedullary hematopoiesis) in some diseases.
What is the normal size for this organ?	A normal spleen weighs 150 g. The spleen is approximately 11 cm in craniocaudal length, and is nonpalpable. Spleens that are prominent below the costal margin typically weigh 750–1000 g. An enlarged spleen below the costal margin may reach the right lower quadrant. Figure 8-16A below is a CT scan of a man with splenic injury due to blunt trauma. This scan, obtained soon after contrast administration, shows multiple large lacerations of the spleen, hematoma, and perihepatic free fluid. Figure 8-16B below, obtained after the contrast had cleared, more clearly shows a large laceration on the posterior surface of the spleen extending anteriorly to the hilum.
Where is the injured organ located?	The spleen is located under the rib cage in the left upper quadrant of the abdomen, below the diaphragm. Therefore, during palpation, descent of an enlarged spleen is felt on inspiration.
Where is the most common site of referred pain in this injury?	Left shoulder and trapezius ridge tenderness (C3–5 dermatomes, same as the roots of the phrenic nerve) may also be present as a result of subdiaphragmatic phrenic nerve irritation; referred pain is due to subdiaphragmatic pooling of blood.
Why is a blunt injury to this organ so concerning?	The spleen is a very vascular organ that filters up to 15% of the total blood volume per minute. The spleen can hold an average of 40–50 mL of RBCs in reserve and can pool significantly more blood.

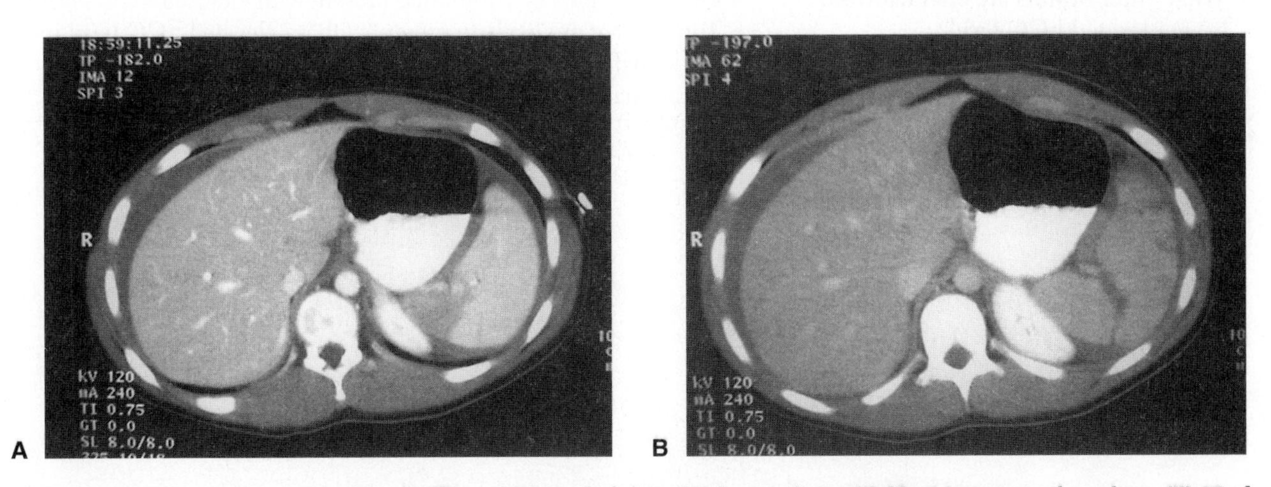

FIGURE 8-16. (A) CT of spleen early after contrast administration in a patient with blunt trauma to the spleen. (B) CT of spleen after contrast clears more clearly shows splenic laceration. (Reproduced, with permission, from Stone CK, Humphries RL. *Current Emergency Diagnosis & Treatment*, 5th ed. New York: McGraw-Hill, 2004: 471.)

ORGAN SYSTEMS

HEMATOLOGY AND ONCOLOGY

▶ Case 30

A 36-year-old sexually active man goes to his doctor after noticing that his left testicle has been swollen for the past few weeks. The patient has noticed a dull, achy sensation in this testicle, but no acute pain. On physical examination, the left testicle is larger than the right, and a nontender, round, firm, rubbery mass is palpated. Transillumination with a penlight reveals an opaque mass. Laboratory tests reveals a normal chemistry panel, normal complete blood count, an elevated lactate dehydrogenase (LDH) level, a normal serum human chorionic gonadotropin (hCG) level, and a normal α-fetoprotein (AFP) level.

What is the most likely diagnosis?	This is a testicular tumor, as suggested by the presence of a painless, nontransilluminating testicular mass. In a young man, the most likely diagnosis is a **seminoma,** which has a peak incidence of age 35 years and accounts for 40% of testicular tumors. This diagnosis is further supported by the elevated LDH level, normal hCG level (is elevated in 20% of seminomas), and normal AFP level. Seminoma can be differentiated from epididymitis or orchitis, which present with a painful testicle and an elevated WBC count. Elevated AFP levels would suggest a nonseminomatous germ cell cancer. A hydrocele would transilluminate.
What is the pathology of this tumor?	Seminoma cells resemble primary spermatocytes, and have large, vesicular nuclei and pale cytoplasm. The tumor cells occur in clusters, with a surrounding lymphoid infiltrate.
What is the analogous tumor in women?	The analogous ovarian tumor is the **dysgerminoma,** the most common germ cell tumor in women. It is usually malignant, and more common in younger patients. Like seminomas, they can produce LDH. They can also produce alkaline phosphatase.
What is the lymphatic drainage of this tumor?	Understanding the lymphatic drainage of the testicles is important in considering metastases. Because the testicles descend from the abdomen during development, the lymph vessels ascend to the lumbar and preaortic lymph nodes. Contrast this to the lymph drainage of the scrotum, which is an outpouching of skin. The lymph vessels of the scrotum drain to the superficial inguinal nodes.
What other tumors are characterized by an elevated hCG level?	Only 10%–20% of seminomas present with elevated hCG levels. Tumors that are likely to present with an elevated hCG level include hydatidiform moles, choriocarcinomas, and (in women) gestational trophoblastic tumors.

▶ Case 31

A 2-year-old boy is brought to his family physician by his parents, who are concerned about the multiple bruises on the boy's shins and hands. They report the child seems to get large bruises with minimal injury, and bleeds profusely when his teeth are brushed. They also relate that a month ago, he fell and hit his head on a coffee table and they could not stop the bleeding for hours. On questioning, they reveal the child has a grandmother with a bleeding disorder. The physician is concerned about child abuse, but orders laboratory tests; relevant findings are as follows:

Bleeding time: 14 min
Prothrombin time (PT): 12 sec
Partial thromboplastin time (PTT): 41 sec

▪ **What is the most likely diagnosis?**	von Willebrand's disease (vWD) is the most common inherited bleeding disorder. It is the result of a quantitative (type 1 or 3) or qualitative (type 2) defect in **von Willebrand's factor** (vWF). vWF is a large protein made by endothelial cells and megakaryocytes. It is a carrier for factor VIII and is a cofactor for platelet adhesion.
▪ **What clinical findings are commonly associated with this condition?**	vWD disturbs both primary and secondary hemostasis. Its role in adhesion of platelets to exposed subendothelium leads to increased bleeding time and an overall clinical picture of platelet dysfunction (mucous membrane bleeding, petechiae, and purpura) with vWF defects. The role of vWF as a carrier protein for factor VIII means that its deficiency leads to a clinical picture similar to a coagulation factor deficit: "deep bleeds" such as hemarthroses (bleeding into joints), easy bruising, and macrohemorrhages. Patients often have a positive family history.
▪ **What do the PT and PTT values reflect?**	PT: Reflects changes in factor II, V, VII, or X. PTT: Reflects changes in any of the coagulation factors except factors VII and XIII. Can be elevated in vWD.
▪ **How would the PT and PTT values differ with the administration of warfarin vs. heparin?**	**Heparin** affects the intrinsic pathway, causing increased PTT. **Warfarin** affects the extrinsic pathway, increasing PTT and PT. Therefore, PT should be monitored when patients with vWD receive warfarin. A useful mnemonic is "**WEPT**": Warfarin, Extrinsic, **PT.**
▪ **Which coagulation factors require vitamin K for synthesis?**	Factors II, VII, IX, and X and proteins C and S require vitamin K for synthesis. Warfarin interferes with vitamin K, leading to a similar clinical picture as vitamin K deficiency. The liver is important in the synthesis and metabolism of vitamin K and the coagulation factors (except VIII). Therefore, liver disease can also result in a similar clinical picture.
▪ **What are the most appropriate treatments for this condition?**	Treatment for mild bleeding in type 1 disease involves the use of desmopressin, which causes release of vWF from endothelial stores. Severe disease may be treated with cryoprecipitate.

NOTES

Musculoskeletal System and Connective Tissue

▶ Case 1

A 17-year-old male is brought to the emergency department by ambulance after a gunshot wound to the left flank. On survey, one entry site is noted with no exit wound; chest and abdominal x-ray films determine the bullet has lodged in the left flank. During assessment, the patient begins to go into hypovolemic shock with a steadily decreasing blood pressure. Because of his condition, the patient is rushed to the operating room for exploratory laparotomy. Relevant laboratory findings are as follows:

Hematocrit: 22%
WBC count: 17,000/mm^3
Blood pressure: 60/35 mm Hg

- **What retroperitoneal structures of the abdomen could the bullet have hit?**

- Ascending/descending colon
- Great vessels
- Kidneys
- Sympathetic trunk
- Suprarenal glands
- Ureters

- **What layers of the skin did the bullet pass through?**

- The **epidermis** is the thin outer layer; it contains
  - stratum corneum
  - keratinocytes (squamous cells)
  - basal layer
- The **dermis** is the middle layer; it is held together by collagen and contains
  - blood vessels
  - lymph vessels
  - hair follicles
  - sweat glands
- The **subcutaneous** is the deepest layer; it contains
  - mesh of collagen and fat cells

See Figure 9-1 on the following page for a schematic drawing of the layers of the skin.

- **Describe the blood supply to the kidney.**

Renal artery → segmental artery → lobar artery → arcuate artery → afferent arteriole → glomerulus → efferent arteriole → segmental vein → renal vein.

- **Describe the splenic blood supply.**

The main arterial blood supply is provided by the splenic artery, which is a branch of the celiac trunk. Branches of the splenic artery are the left gastro-omental and the short gastric arteries.

- **What organs supply the splenic vein?**

The splenic vein starts at the hilus of the spleen and receives blood from the stomach, pancreas, and inferior mesenteric vein.

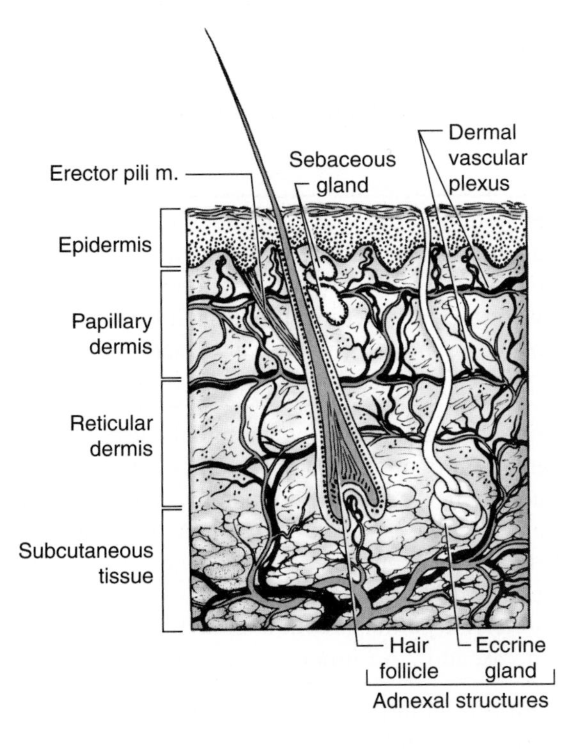

FIGURE 9-1. Schematic drawing of the layers of skin. (Reproduced, with permission, from Brunicardi FC, et al. *Schwartz's Principles of Surgery*, 8th ed. New York: McGraw-Hill, 2005: 430.)

► Case 2

A 62-year-old woman presents to her physician with a 2-day history of right-sided chest pain. She describes a sharp, nagging pressure lateral to her right breast. Physical examination reveals the chest wall is tender, and the pain is exacerbated by movement of her trunk and deep inspiration.

■ **What is the pathophysiology of this condition?**	Costochondritis, the inflammation of the costochondral or costosternal joints, causes localized pain and tenderness. Often more than one of the seven costochondral joints is affected, especially between the second and fifth joints. Repetitive minor trauma is the most likely cause, but bacterial and fungal infections can lead to costochondritis, as can thoracic surgery.
■ **What is the innervation of the intercostal space?**	The intercostal nerves (thoracic spinal and ventral rami) supply general sensory innervation to the skin of the thoracic and anterior abdominal walls. The dermatomes follow a girdle-like distribution. The sensory nerves also supply the parietal pleura and parietal peritoneum. The intercostal nerves also have motor innervation. The intercostal nerves are ventral rami of T1–12. Intercostal nerve 1 participates in the brachial plexus, 2–6 innervate the thorax, and 7–12 innervate the anterior abdominal wall.
■ **What are the three types of intercostal muscles?**	The intercostal muscles are divided into three groups of muscular and tendinous fibers running between the 11 intercostal spaces: ■ External intercostal muscles ■ Internal intercostal muscles ■ Innermost intercostal complex (transversus thoracis, innermost intercostals, subcostalis)
■ **How many ribs are there?**	The thoracic cage consists of 12 pairs of ribs. The first seven are true ribs because their cartilage articulates with the sternum, and the last five pairs are false ribs. The eleventh and twelfth ribs are floating ribs.
■ **What is the blood supply of the intercostal space?**	At each space there is a posterior and anterior set of arteries. The posterior artery originates from the descending thoracic aorta. Anterior intercostal arteries are smaller and include the supreme thoracic artery. The posterior intercostal vein, artery, and nerve run together as a neurovascular bundle along the lower border of each rib. Thus, it is important during thoracentesis that the needle is inserted above the lower rib in the intercostal space to avoid injury to the vessels and nerve.

▶ Case 3

A 2-week-old term boy is brought to his pediatrician because his parents have noticed he has a large, full right scrotum. The left scrotum and testicle are normal. On physical examination, the right scrotum appears to be filled with a volume of fluid that can be reduced by applying pressure. A small reducible bulging mass is also seen in the inguinal area on the right.

▪ **What is the most likely diagnosis?**	Right communicating hydrocele and right inguinal hernia. The fluid in the scrotum is a **hydrocele** that results from communication with the intraperitoneal fluid.
▪ **What structures define Hesselbach's triangle?**	**Hesselbach's triangle** is formed by the lateral border of the rectus abdominis muscle, the inguinal ligament, and the inferior epigastric vessels.
▪ **How is this condition classified?**	**Direct hernias** protrude through a weakness in the floor of the inguinal canal within Hesselbach's triangle (directly through the triangle) medial to the inferior epigastric vessels to enter the external ring into the scrotal sac. **Indirect hernias** enter the inguinal canal lateral to Hesselbach's triangle (lateral to the inferior epigastric vessels) indirectly through the internal inguinal ring (located in the fascia transversalis), then via the inguinal canal to the external inguinal ring located above and lateral to the pubic tubercle, and finally into the scrotal sac (see Figure 9-2 below).
▪ **Which type of this condition is more common in infants and children?**	Indirect inguinal hernias are more common in children, as they result from a congenital failure of the processus vaginalis to close.
▪ **What are the contents of the normal spermatic cord?**	The spermatic cord in the inguinal canal contains the testicular artery and veins, lymphatic vessels, and the vas deferens. The sheath of the cord is formed by the internal spermatic fascia, the cremasteric muscle, and the external spermatic fascia. The ilioinguinal nerve is in the sheath and exits at the external ring; it is vulnerable to injury in surgical repairs of hernias. The genital branch of the genitofemoral nerve supplies the cremaster muscle. The processus vaginalis is an extension of peritoneum that normally obliterates spontaneously between the upper pole of the testes and the internal inguinal ring. In some cases, however, this structure remains patent, increasing the risk of hydrocele and indirect hernia.

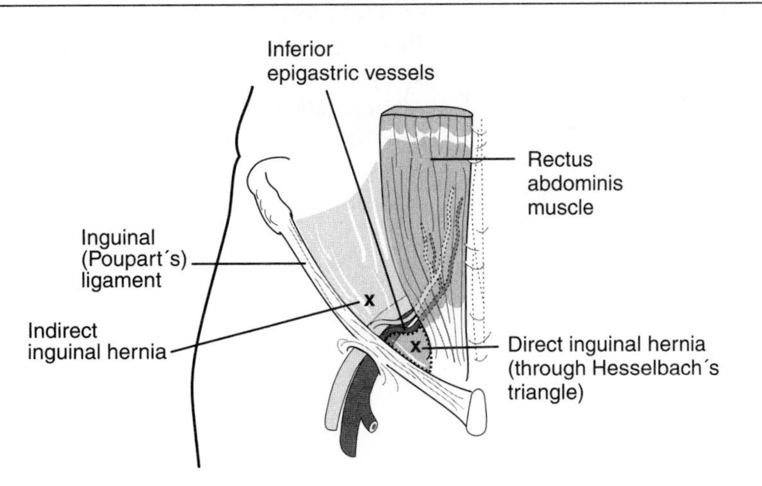

FIGURE 9-2. Direct and indirect inguinal hernia. (Reproduced, with permission, from Bhushan V, Le T, et al. *First Aid for the USMLE Step 1: 2006*. New York: McGraw-Hill, 2006: 273.)

► Case 4

A 72-year-old woman with a history of osteoporosis presents to her primary care physician after falling 2 days earlier on a slippery sidewalk and landing on her left side. Since the fall, she has been unable to walk due to severe pain in her left hip that is worse when she tries to move it. When asked to walk for assessment of her gait, she refuses, saying that it is too painful. Physical examination reveals extreme pain with both external and internal rotation of the hip, as well as tenderness over the anterolateral portion of the left hip.

What is the most likely diagnosis?	This is most likely a fracture of the neck of the femur, which is the portion of the femur that lies between the intertrochanteric line anteriorly and the intertrochanteric crest posteriorly (these run between the greater and lesser trochanter). Femoral neck fractures can be either incomplete or complete with either no, partial, or total displacement (types I–IV are shown in Figure 9-3 on the following page).
What is a potential complication of this type of injury?	Fracture of the neck of the femur may disrupt blood supply to the head of the femur. The major arterial supply to the head of the femur is the medial and lateral circumflex femoral arteries (branches of the deep femoral artery or femoral artery), and the artery of the ligament of the head of the femur (branch of the obturator artery). The circumflex arteries may be disrupted by a fracture of the femoral neck, leaving only the artery of the ligament (a branch of the obturator) as a supply. Disruption of the blood supply may result in **avascular necrosis** of the femoral head.
What bones form the hip joint?	The hip joint consists of the head of the femur articulating with the acetabulum. The acetabulum is formed by the ilium, the ischium, and the pubis. The fibrocartilaginous rim, the acetabular labrum, attaches to the acetabular margin and deepens the acetabular cup.
Six weeks later, an x-ray film in this patient shows a callus; where did the cells that form the callus originate?	The osteoprogenitor cells that form the callus are from the inner surface of the periosteum, not from the marrow or the epiphyseal plate.
What pharmacologic agents may be given to this patient to prevent similar injury in the future?	Bisphosphonates, such as alendronate and risedronate, are often first-line agents for both the treatment and prevention of osteoporosis. Raloxifene, a selective estrogen receptor modulator, is another frequently used pharmacologic therapy for treatment and prevention of osteoporosis. Intermittent administration of recombinant parathyroid hormone is also effective. Calcitonin and calcitriol are less effective treatments.

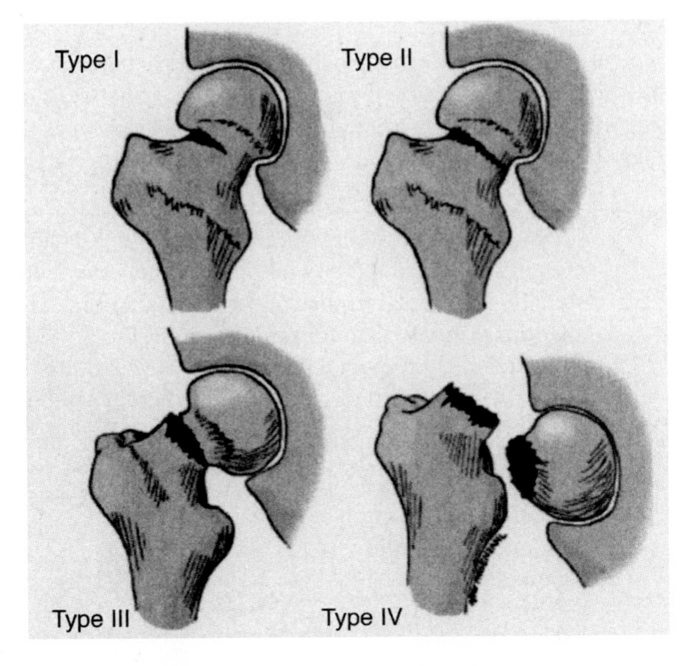

FIGURE 9-3. Types of fractures of the femoral neck. (Reproduced, with permission, from Brunicardi FC, et al. *Schwartz's Principles of Surgery*, 8th ed. New York: McGraw-Hill, 2005: 1685.)

▶ Case 5

A 19-year-old woman comes to the emergency department accompanied by her coach after the student injured her left knee during sports practice. She says she had made a quick turn when she developed a sharp pain on the lateral side of her knee, heard a "pop," and her leg "collapsed."

■ **What are the intracapsular ligaments in the knee?**	The **anterior cruciate ligament** extends from the anterior intercondylar area of the tibial plateau and traverses superior and lateral to the medial surface of the lateral femoral condyle. The **posterior cruciate ligament** extends from the posterior intercondylar area of the tibial plateau and traverses superior and medial to the lateral surface of the medial condyle of the femur (see Figure 9-4 below).
■ **What is the blood supply to the knee?**	Genicular branches of the following blood vessels: ■ Anterior recurrent tibial artery ■ Anterior tibial artery ■ Descending branch of the lateral circumflex artery ■ Femoral artery ■ Patellar plexus ■ Popliteal artery ■ Posterior tibial artery
■ **What is the role of the meniscus?**	The **meniscus** is cartilage in a half-moon shape that is found between the femur and tibia. The meniscus is responsible for absorbing the impact load of the joint and is involved in stability. The meniscus is mostly avascular and is divided into the anterior horn, body, and posterior horn.
■ **How do the collateral and cruciate ligaments differ in function?**	The cruciate ligaments remain tight in flexion and extension and relax at 30° of flexion. The collateral ligaments are tight in extension and relaxed in flexion. Also, the cruciate ligaments prevent anterior and posterior displacement of the tibia. The collateral ligaments prevent abduction/adduction of the knee.
■ **Which ligament of the knee is most often injured?**	The median collateral ligament is weaker than the anterior or the posterior cruciate ligaments, so medial collateral ligament injuries are more common.

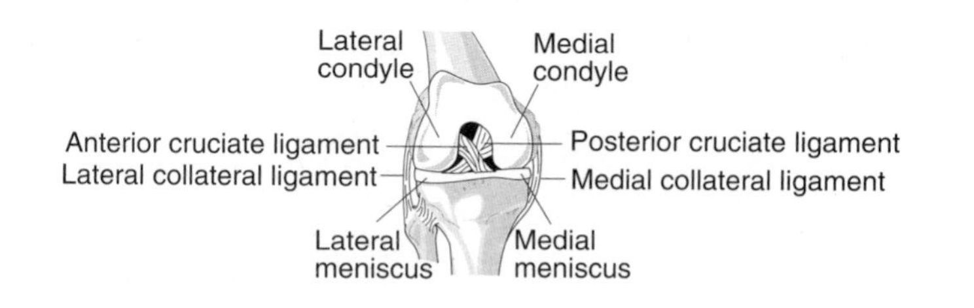

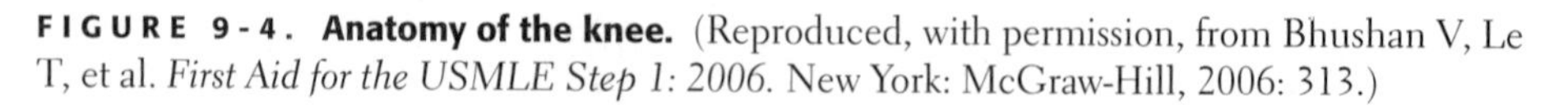
FIGURE 9-4. Anatomy of the knee. (Reproduced, with permission, from Bhushan V, Le T, et al. *First Aid for the USMLE Step 1: 2006*. New York: McGraw-Hill, 2006: 313.)

▶ Case 6

A 3-year-old boy is brought to the pediatrician by his parents because he has been having trouble getting up from a sitting or lying position, although he had previously done so with ease. His developmental history is notable for delayed motor skills; he began to walk at 18 months. The boy has a waddling gait, and when sitting he uses his arms to push himself into the upright position (Gower's sign; see Figure 9-5 below). Physical examination shows marked muscle weakness of the extremities, particularly of the proximal muscle groups, and hypertrophy of his calf muscles. Notably, the patient's maternal uncle, who died at age 16 years, suffered from similar symptoms when he was younger.

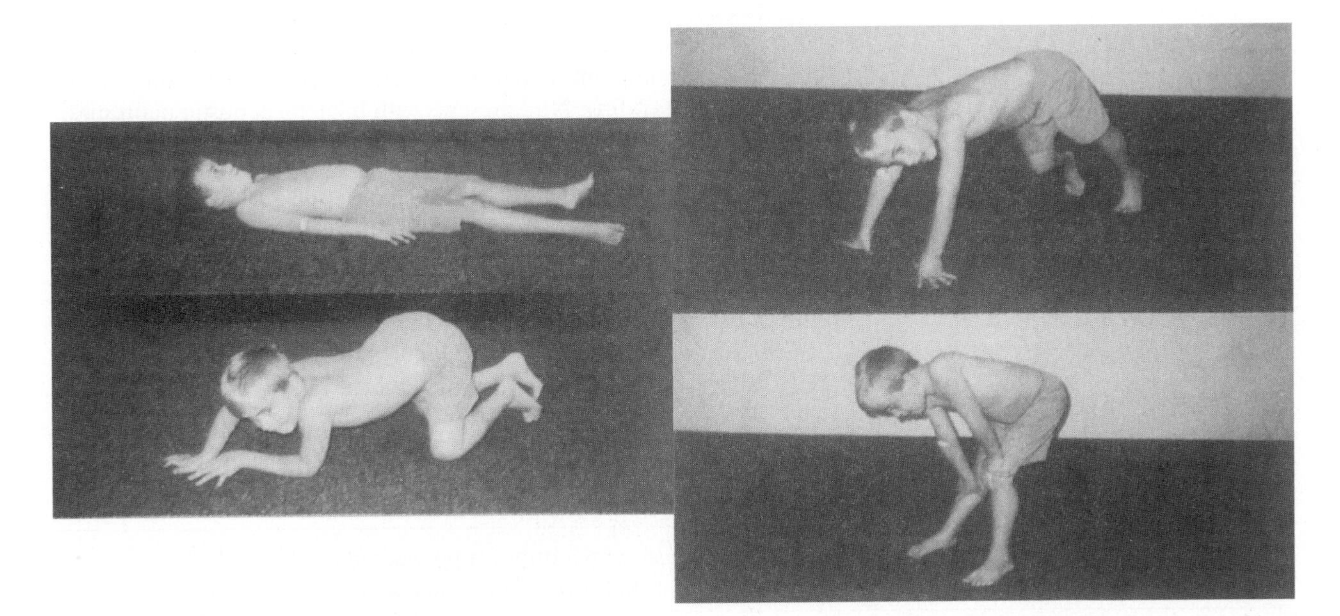

FIGURE 9-5. (Reproduced, with permission, from Kasper DL, et al. *Harrison's Principles of Internal Medicine*, 16th ed. New York: McGraw-Hill, 2005: 2526.)

▪ **What is the most likely diagnosis?**	Duchenne's muscular dystrophy (DMD). DMD is an X-linked recessive (Xp21) disorder in which there is a deficiency of functional **dystrophin,** a 23,000-kB protein involved in stabilization of muscle fibers. About one-third of cases are sporadic, due to spontaneous mutations (noninherited) that arise most commonly by a misalignment of chromosomes during a recombination event.
▪ **What is this patient's prognosis?**	Patients with DMD are usually unable to walk by the end of the first decade, and are confined to a wheelchair by age 12 years. Sadly, most afflicted patients die by the end of their second decade, usually due to extreme weakness of respiratory muscles or cardiomyopathy.
▪ **What findings would be likely on muscle biopsy?**	▪ Atrophic muscle fibers of various sizes in disarray ▪ Degeneration and necrosis of individual muscle fibers with fibrous replacement ▪ Inflammation
▪ **The couple has a second son who is now 6 months old. What is the chance that he will develop this disease as well?**	Fifty percent. Because the mother is a carrier of this disorder, this second son has a 50% chance of inheriting the X chromosome with the mutated allele from her.
▪ **Which band(s) in a sarcomere stays constant in length during muscle contraction?**	The A band, which corresponds to the length of the thick myosin filaments.

▶ Case 7

A young white couple seeks genetic counseling prior to conceiving their first child. The man is concerned because he has had bilateral tumors removed from his acoustic nerves. His mother suffered from similar tumors, but his father did not. The woman reports two previous surgeries for the removal of spinal cord tumors; her father and sister have had similar tumors. The woman's physical examination is significant for axillary freckles and approximately 15 light brown patches of skin averaging 3 cm in diameter.

What genetic syndromes do this man and woman have?	The woman has neurofibromatosis type 1 (NF1, or von Recklinghausen's neurofibromatosis), and the man has neurofibromatosis type 2 (NF2). NF1 is characterized by café au lait spots, meningiomas, **neurofibromas** (subcutaneous nodules), and axillary freckling. NF2 presents with bilateral acoustic neuromas.
What is their probability of having an asymptomatic child?	The probability is 25%. NF1 and NF2 are both autosomal dominant genes. On the basis of their family histories, the man and woman must be heterozygous for NF2 and NF1, respectively. Thus, each gene has a 50% chance of being passed on to the child. NF1 is on chromosome 17, and NF2 is on chromosome 22; thus, each gene's expression occurs independently of the other. The probability of two independent events occurring at once is the product of the probability of each event: 50% × 50% = 25%.
Which cell line is implicated in the formation of the woman's lesions?	**Neural crest cells.** Most clinical signs of NF1 are related to abnormal descendants of neural crest cells.
What is the mechanism of tumor formation for the woman?	The *NF1* gene is a tumor suppressor gene. Multiple loss-of-function mutations in this gene lead to tumor growth.
Describe the path of the eighth cranial nerve (CN VIII) from the periphery to its site of entry into the central nervous system.	From the cochlea and vestibular canals in the petrous bone, CN VIII enters the cranial vault through the internal acoustic meatus to enter the brain stem at the junction of the pons and the medulla.

▶ Case 8

An 8-year-old girl is brought to the pediatrician for evaluation of recurrent skeletal fractures. Although she avoids contact sports, she has already suffered three fractures of her femur, tibia, and elbow following seemingly minor trauma. The pediatrician notes the girl is short for her age and has mild scoliosis and blue sclerae. The girl's mother has blue sclerae as well.

■ **What is the differential diagnosis for recurrent fractures in children?**	■ Accidental injury ■ Birth trauma ■ Bone fragility (including osteogenesis imperfecta and rickets) ■ Child abuse (which accounts for the vast majority of cases)
■ **What is the most likely diagnosis?**	Osteogenesis imperfecta, which is an inherited disorder involving defects in type I collagen. It is also known as **brittle bone disease,** and its most common form has autosomal dominant inheritance. This disease is also associated with cardiac insufficiency and mitral valve prolapse. The most severe form is lethal in utero or soon after birth because of multiple fractures and pulmonary failure. The most severe forms are inherited in a recessive fashion.
■ **What are the four major types of collagen, and where are they predominantly found?**	■ **Type I:** bone, skin, tendon ■ **Type II:** cartilage ■ **Type III:** reticular, arterial walls, uterus ■ **Type IV:** basement membrane
■ **What steps are involved in collagen synthesis?**	Procollagen strands containing a repeating Gly-Pro-X sequence are synthesized in the ribosome, hydrolyzed by prolyl hydrolase, and glycosylated in the rough endoplasmic reticulum and Golgi complex. Three procollagen strands associate in a triple helix and are secreted into the extracellular space, where the propeptides are cleaved, allowing for polymerization with other collagen molecules to form collagen fibrils.
■ **What enzymes in collagen synthesis are dependent on ascorbic acid?**	Proline hydroxylase (which hydroxylates prolyl and lysyl residues) cross-links collagen and is dependent on ascorbic acid. Vitamin C deficiency can lead to **scurvy,** which causes ulceration of the gums, bruising, anemia, poor wound healing, and hemorrhage due to deficient collagen synthesis.

▶ Case 9

A 63-year-old woman goes to her primary care physician complaining that, since falling on her outstretched hands 3 weeks ago, she can no longer use her right arm to remove books from the overhead shelves in her office. Further questioning reveals that she also has pain in her right shoulder at night that occasionally wakes her up, and that she now avoids sleeping on her right side. Physical examination reveals tenderness to palpation below the right acromion; also, the patient has pain at 60° as she abducts her right arm, and is unable to abduct with resistance. When she is asked to hold her right arm abducted at 45°, then laterally rotate her forearm against resistance, she is unable to do so.

▪ **What is the most likely diagnosis?**

Rotator cuff tear, which presents with both pain and weakness. The subacromial bursa may also be involved, in which case pain is also felt at the insertion of the deltoid muscle in the middle of the upper arm. This is because the subacromial bursa is continuous with the subdeltoid bursa. Rotator cuff tendonitis would present with pain, but not weakness. A nerve injury would present with weakness, but not pain.

▪ **The tendons of which two muscles are most likely involved?**

Supraspinatus and infraspinatus.

▪ **What events commonly precipitate such an injury?**

Rotator cuff tears are rare in patients <40 years old, but quite common in patients >50 years with shoulder pain. However, sports injuries with rotator cuff tears are seen in young athletes. Other common causes of rotator cuff tears include:

- Direct blow to the affected shoulder
- Falling onto an outstretched hand (as this patient did)
- History of recurrent rotator cuff tendonitis
- Lifting a heavy object
- Shoulder dislocation

▪ **What other tendons are likely involved in this injury?**

The rotator cuff is made of the tendons of the "**SITS**" muscles: the **S**upraspinatus, **I**nfraspinatus, and **T**eres minor insert on the greater tuberosity, and the **S**ubscapularis inserts on the lesser tuberosity (see Figure 9-6).

▪ **What are the innervations and actions of these muscles?**

- Supraspinatus: the suprascapular nerve (C4–6), abduction of the arm beyond the initial 20° (the deltoid abducts the arm for the initial 20°)
- Infraspinatus: the suprascapular nerve (C4–6), external rotation of the arm
- Teres minor: the axillary nerve (C5–6), help in external rotation of the arm
- Subscapularis: the upper and lower subscapular nerves (C5–7), help with median rotation and adduction of the arm

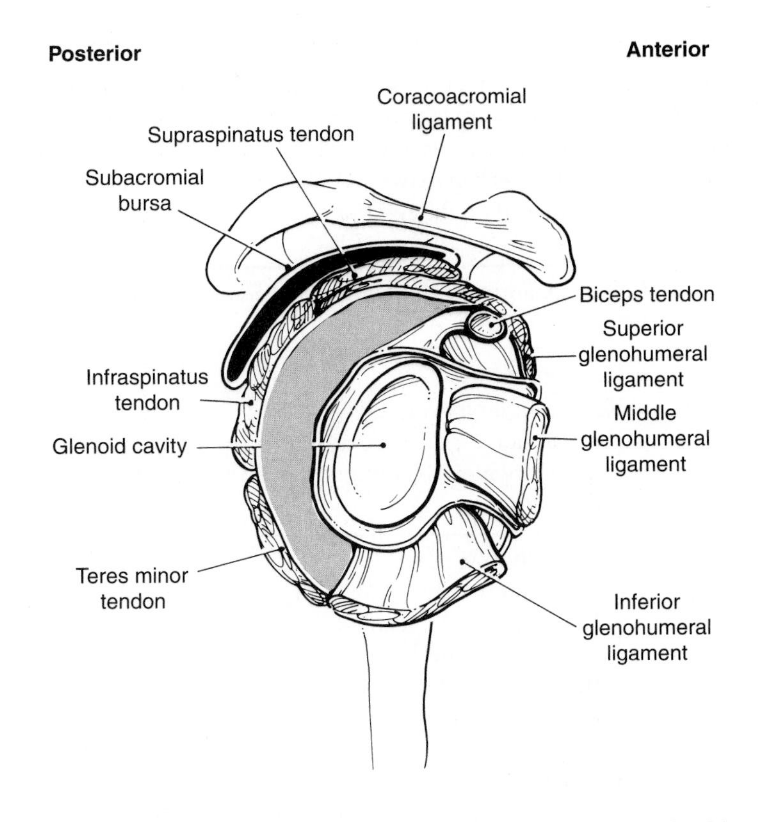

FIGURE 9-6. Lateral view of shoulder illustrating coracoacromial arch with rotator cuff and subacromial bursa. (Reproduced, with permission, from Tintinalli JE, et al. *Tintinalli's Emergency Medicine: A Comprehensive Study Guide*, 6th ed. New York: McGraw-Hill, 2004: 1780.)

▶ Case 10

A 15-year-old is brought to the emergency department via ambulance after a knife fight with his cousin. He has two stab wounds, one on the left immediately below his clavicle and the second on his right between the fifth and sixth ribs. Physical examination reveals the patient is tachypneic and hypotensive. A chest x-ray film indicates a hemothorax, and thus a chest tube is placed on the right.

▪ **What major vessels are at risk in a wound of this nature?**	Left lung, aorta, or right atrium, depending on how low the stab wound is found.
▪ **What nerves are at risk in a wound of this nature?**	▪ Cardiac plexus ▪ Recurrent laryngeal nerve ▪ Phrenic nerve ▪ Pulmonary plexus (contiguous with cardiac plexus) ▪ Vagus nerve

▪ **Describe the blood supply to this region.**	▪ Arterial supply:
	  ▪ Aortic arch
	  ▪ Brachiocephalic trunk
	  ▪ Common carotid
	  ▪ Internal thoracic
	  ▪ Left bronchial
	  ▪ Subclavian
	▪ Venous supply:
	  ▪ Azygos
	  ▪ Brachiocephalic
	  ▪ Internal thoracic
	  ▪ Jugular

▪ **Describe the lymphatic system of the thoracic cavity.**	The lymphatics in the lung arise from the superficial lymphatic plexus (located below the visceral pleura) and the deep lymphatic plexus (located along the bronchial tree except the alveoli). Both of the plexuses drain into hilar nodes (bronchopulmonary nodes). Lymph from the hilar nodes drains first into the carinal (tracheobronchial) nodes, then into the tracheal nodes. The tracheal nodes also receive lymph from the trachea, upper esophagus, and inferior larynx. Lymph from the tracheal nodes finally enters the bronchomediastinal lymph trunks.
▪ **What is the difference between the left and right mainstem bronchi?**	The mainstem bronchus passes inferolaterally from the bifurcation of the trachea at the sternal angle to the hilum. The **right main bronchus** is shorter and wider and runs more vertically, allowing for passage of aspirates more easily than the left bronchus. The **left main bronchus** is longer and travels anterior to the esophagus between the thoracic aorta and the left pulmonary artery.

Neurology and Psychiatry

▶ Case 1

A 73-year-old well-educated woman is brought to the physician by her daughter, who has become concerned about her mother's behavior. The mother volunteers at the local library shelving books, but for the past few months she has had trouble remembering where the books go. In addition, she often forgets to turn the stove off after cooking her family's long-time favorite dishes.

What is the most likely diagnosis?	This history is consistent with Alzheimer's disease, which is characterized by loss of short-term memory and general preservation of long-term memory.
What risk factors are associated with the development of this condition?	Advancing age and a family history of Alzheimer's disease are two well-known risk factors. Additionally, because the amyloid precursor protein (APP) is located on chromosome 21, patients with Down syndrome (trisomy 21) have increased APP levels; these patients often develop Alzheimer's disease at 30–40 years old.
What are the likely findings on gross pathology?	Neurofibrillary **tangles** and amyloid **plaques** (Figure 10-1A below; arrow points to tangles) are commonly seen on autopsy. A high degree of cerebral atrophy in the frontal, temporal, and parietal regions is also present, as can be seen in Figure 10-1B below.
What biochemical mechanism is believed to be involved in the pathogenesis of this condition?	A preferential loss of acetylcholine and choline acetyltransferase in the cerebral cortex may play a role in the development of clinical disease. The acetylcholinesterase inhibitor class of medications, including tacrine, donepezil, rivastigmine, and galantamine, have been shown to slow the progress of memory loss. Memantine, an N-methyl-D-aspartate (NMDA) receptor antagonist, may protect from Alzheimer's disease by blocking the excitotoxic effects of glutamate, independently of the effects of acetylcholinesterase inhibitors.
What is the most appropriate treatment for this condition?	Tacrine, which is an acetylcholinesterase inhibitor, is the only drug that is known to slow the progress of Alzheimer's-related memory loss.
What is the prognosis for the patient's daughter?	The familial form of Alzheimer's disease, which affects approximately 10% of patients with the disease, usually has an onset between the ages of 30 and 60 years. Given the mother's age and symptoms of early Alzheimer's disease, the mother likely does not have the familial form, and the daughter should not have an increased risk on the basis of family history alone.

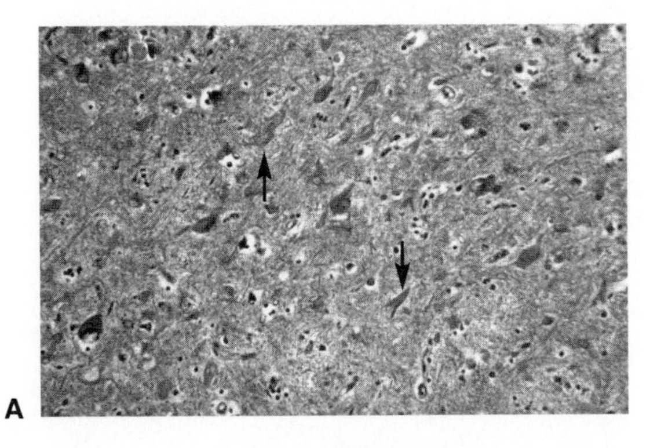

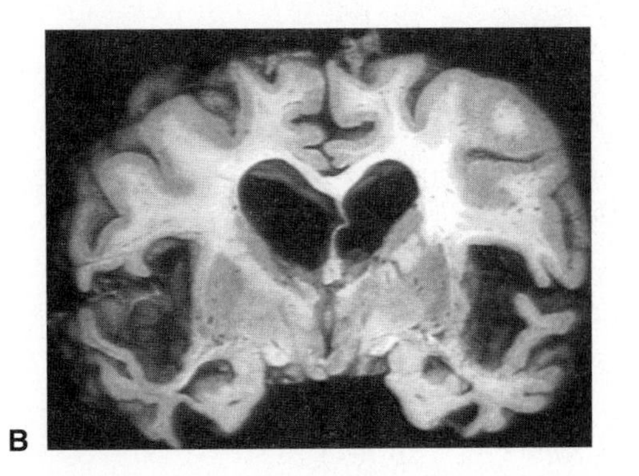

FIGURE 10-1. (A) Neurofibrillary tangles in Alzheimer's disease. (B) Coronal section showing atrophy in Alzheimer's disease. (Reproduced with permission of the Pathology Education Instructional Resource Digital Library (http://peir.net) at the University of Alabama, Birmingham.)

► Case 2

A mother brings her 3-year-old son to the physician because she believes he is not developing normally. She says he does not reach out for her with his arms, show joy, or follow her around like his siblings did. His language development is delayed and he often mechanically repeats other people. He needs to have "everything his way" and has many rituals. "He seems to be in a world of his own," she notes. Tests show a lower-than-average IQ.

What is the most likely diagnosis?

Autistic disorder. Autism is the most severe of the pervasive developmental disorders.

What is the classical triad of findings in this condition?

- Severe language disorder: delayed and abnormal speech, poor comprehension, no imaginative play, tendency to echo questions
- Profound difficulty relating to other people
- Marked routines and rituals associated with a poverty of imaginative play

Odd motor patterns such as hand flapping and walking on tiptoe are also common.

What is the epidemiology of this condition?

Autism is rare, with a prevalence of approximately 3 per 10,000 children. More common in boys, it presents in early childhood but is a lifelong handicap.

What is the etiology of this condition?

Autism is a behavioral syndrome, most cases of which are likely genetic and have no identifiable underlying cause.

What is the differential diagnosis of this condition?

Asperger's syndrome is a milder form of autism involving problems with social relationships and repetitive behavior. These children are of normal intelligence and lack social or cognitive deficits. The often have stiff, monotonous speech, are clumsy, and are obsessed by peculiar things.

▶ Case 3

A 22-year-old woman presents to the clinic with an 8-day history of insomnia and increased energy. Her roommate is concerned because the patient has been talking rapidly and has not been making much sense. The patient has made several expensive purchases recently and has been exhibiting bizarre behavior, dressing inappropriately for class, and drawing a lot of attention to herself.

What category of psychiatric disorder does this patient exhibit?	This patient is experiencing a manic episode (associated with bipolar disorder, which is a type of mood disorder). Other disorders in this class include major depressive disorder, dysthymic disorder, bereavement, and bipolar disorder.
How does the epidemiology differ between patients presenting with manic depression and those presenting with depressive disorder?	Manic depression is found in 1% of the population, affects women and men equally, and is usually found in younger patients. Depressive disorder is much more common (15%–25% lifetime prevalence), and is more commonly found in women and elderly patients.
What signs and symptoms are commonly associated with this disorder?	▪ Abrupt onset of increased energy ▪ Decreased attention span ▪ Decreased need for sleep ▪ Elevated or expansive mood ▪ Hyperreligiosity ▪ Hypersexuality ▪ Pressured speech ▪ Spending sprees
How is this disorder classified?	**Mania** presents a significant disability to the patient and usually is associated with psychotic symptoms and impairment in functioning. Episodes typically last >1 week. In contrast, **hypomania** is associated with a milder variety of similar symptoms as mania, but without gross functional impairment; this diagnosis requires only 4 days of symptoms. ▪ Bipolar I: requires distinct manic and depressive syndromes ▪ Bipolar II: requires distinct hypomanic and depressive syndromes ▪ Mixed: presence of both manic and depressive symptoms concurrently over a period of time (often described as dysphoric mania or agitated depression) ▪ Rapid cycling: presence of at least four distinct manic, depressive, or mixed mood episodes over a period of 1 year
What are the most appropriate treatments for this disorder?	Hospitalization can be necessary. First-line drugs include mood stabilizers (lithium, valproate, carbamazepine) and antipsychotic agents (olanzapine, haloperidol, risperidone).

▶ Case 4

A 35-year-old construction worker is taken to the emergency department following an accident in which a piece of metal became lodged in his back. In addition to experiencing excruciating pain at the site of his injury, the patient is unable to move his right leg. In the emergency department, a neurologic examination reveals the man's right leg is paralyzed, with an ipsilateral hyperactive patellar reflex and a positive Babinski's sign. The patient can move his left leg without difficulty and has a normal patellar reflex and no Babinski's sign. However, sensory testing reveals loss of temperature and pinprick sensation on the left leg up to the navel, along with loss of vibration sensation on the right leg up to the navel.

What is the most likely diagnosis?

Brown-Séquard syndrome due to a hemicord lesion. Brown-Séquard syndrome is characterized by ipsilateral spastic (upper motor neuron–type) paralysis ("1" in Figure 10-2 on the following page), ipsilateral loss of vibration and position sensation ("2" in Figure 10-2), and contralateral loss of pain and temperature sensation ("3" in Figure 10-2).

At what level is the lesion?

The loss of sensation up to the navel suggests that the lesion is near T10, because the dermatome that includes the navel is supplied by T10.

Damage to which tracts is causing the ipsilateral deficits in this case?

The motor deficits are due to damage to the **lateral corticospinal tract** (see Figure 10-3 on the following page), which carries motor neurons from the cortex that have decussated in the pyramids. The loss of vibration and position sense is due to damage to the **dorsal columns,** which carry information from sensory nerves that enter through the dorsal root, ascend to the caudal medulla (where the primary neuron synapses), and then cross to ascend to the contralateral sensory cortex. These deficits are ipsilateral because the tracts cross the midline high in the spinal cord.

Damage to which tracts is causing the contralateral deficits in this case?

The loss of pain and temperature sensation is due to damage to the **spinothalamic tract** (see Figure 10-3). The sensory neurons that travel in the anterolateral tract enter the spinal cord through the dorsal root, synapse almost immediately, and cross the midline (within one or two levels) via the anterior commissure to ascend to the cortex.

If the lesion were above T1, how would the presentation differ?

A hemicord lesion above T1, in addition to the findings above, will present as **Horner's syndrome,** which consists of ptosis, miosis, and anhidrosis (droopy eyelid, constricted pupil, and decreased sweating).

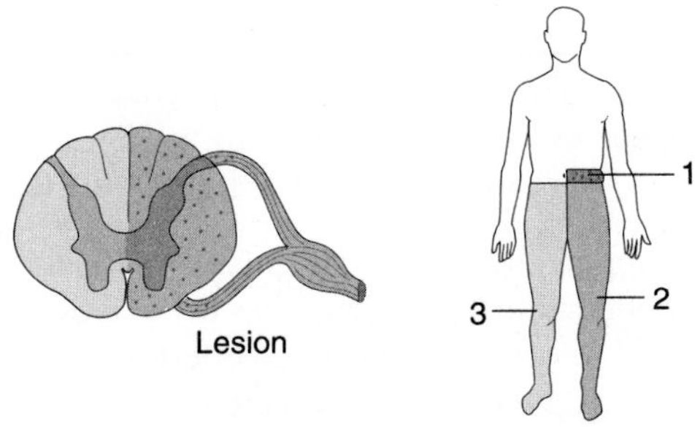

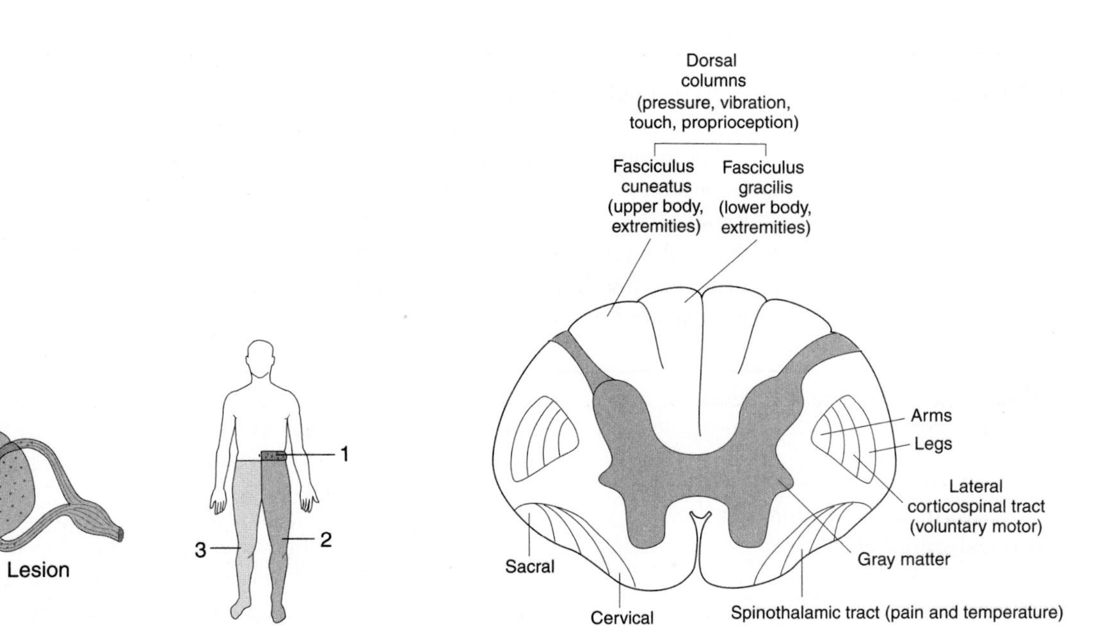

FIGURE 10-2. Brown-Séquard syndrome. (Reproduced, with permission, from Bhushan V, Le T, et al. *First Aid for the USMLE Step 1: 2006.* New York: McGraw-Hill, 2006: 354.)

FIGURE 10-3. Spinal cord and associated tracts. (Reproduced, with permission, from Bhushan V, Le T, et al. *First Aid for the USMLE Step 1: 2006.* New York: McGraw-Hill, 2006: 339.)

▶ Case 5

A 70-year-old man with a history of rheumatoid arthritis comes to his physician complaining of weakness 1 day after a motor vehicle accident. Physical examination reveals intact sensation and strength in the lower extremities along with bilateral upper extremity weakness. The patient is able to move his arms parallel to gravity but is unable to lift his arms, forearms, or hands upward against gravity; strength is rated 2/5. A cervical CT scan rules out the presence of a cervical spine fracture, and MRI demonstrates traumatic C6 disc herniation, buckling of the ligamentum flavum, and edema within the cervical cord in that area.

- **What is the most likely diagnosis?**

Central cord syndrome. This syndrome is characterized by upper extremity weakness that exceeds lower extremity weakness, along with varying degrees of sensory loss below the level of the lesion.

- **What is the arterial supply to the cervical spinal cord?**

The spinal cord is supplied by an anterior spinal artery (which is supplied by the vertebral arteries) that supplies the anterior two-thirds of the cord, and by two posterior spinal arteries (which are supplied by the vertebral posterior inferior cerebellar arteries) that supply the dorsal columns and part of the posterior horns.

- **What is a vascular watershed zone?**

A **watershed zone** is an area between two major arteries in which small branches of the arteries form anastomoses. Important watershed zones lie between the cerebral arteries (eg, between the middle and anterior cerebral arteries) and in the central spinal cord. These areas are particularly susceptible to infarction during times of hypotension or hypoperfusion. In this case, edema and trauma impair blood flow to the cervical cord, and the predominant symptoms result from damage within the central cord watershed zone.

- **What is supplied by the long tracts in the areas labeled "region A" in Figure 10-4 on the following page?**

Region A in Figure 10-4 indicates the most medial portions of the corticospinal tracts. These fibers supply the muscles of the upper extremity. Because they are medial structures, motor impairment of the upper extremities can occur following a smaller central cord lesion. The crosshatched pattern in Figure 10-5 on the following page indicates the area of impairment that would be associated with a central cord lesion.

- **What changes in the biceps, triceps, and brachioradialis reflexes would one expect to see following damage to the anterior horn cells supplying the C6 nerve root?**

The biceps reflex, which is regulated by fibers from C5 and C6, will be moderately diminished secondary to diminished lower motor neuron input. The triceps reflex is regulated primarily by C7 and should thus be unaffected by a C6 lesion. The brachioradialis reflex is primarily regulated by C6 and will thus be markedly diminished following a C6 lesion.

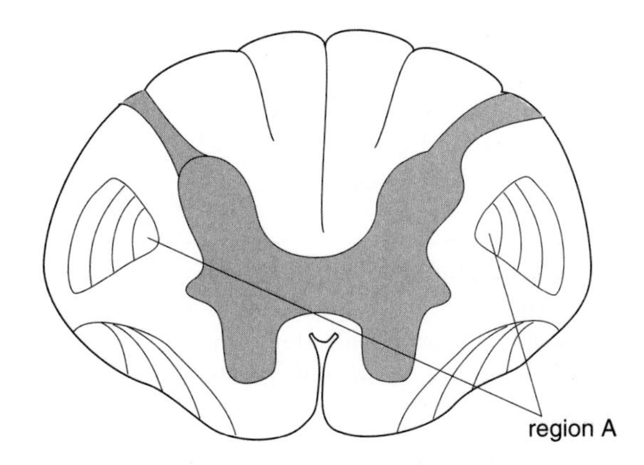

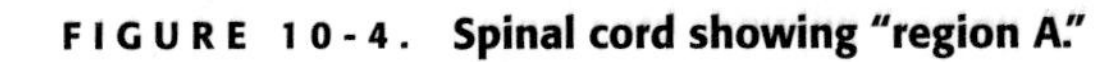

FIGURE 10-4. Spinal cord showing "region A."

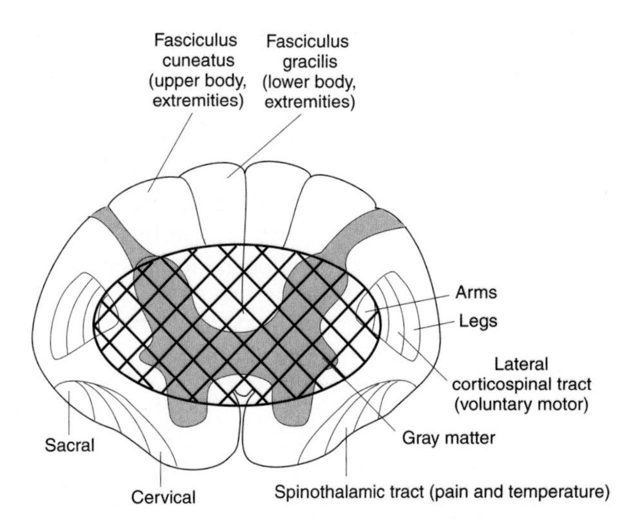

FIGURE 10-5. Spinal cord showing area of impairment associated with central cord lesion.

ORGAN SYSTEMS

NEUROLOGY AND PSYCHIATRY

► **Case 6**

A 16-year-old high school student goes to see the school nurse because of severe eye pain and a feeling that there is something "stuck" in his right eye. He does not wear contact lenses. He reports he was recently working with machines in shop class without wearing protective goggles. Ophthalmologic examination reveals no visible foreign body in the eye; visual acuity is slightly decreased at 20/30; pupils are equal, round, and reactive to light bilaterally; corneal reflex is intact; and extraocular muscles are intact, although the student says his right eye hurts when he moves it.

What is the most likely diagnosis?	The student has a corneal abrasion, which typically presents with significant eye pain and a foreign body sensation. The patient will also have photophobia. This patient also has a history suggestive of a source for his eye injury: working with machinery without wearing protective eyewear.
What is the pathway of the corneal blink reflex?	The excruciating pain being experienced by this patient is due to the rich innervation of the cornea by cranial nerve (CN) V, ophthalmic branch (V1). It is this same nerve that constitutes the afferent portion of the corneal blink reflex. After synapsing in the sensory nucleus of CN V, there is bilateral projection to the nucleus of CN VII. From there, motor neurons project to the orbicularis oculi muscles, causing a consensual blink response.
What space lies between the cornea and the lens?	The space between the cornea and the lens is the anterior compartment, which is subdivided by the iris into the anterior chamber and the posterior chamber (see Figure 10-6 below). The entire anterior compartment is filled with aqueous humor, which is secreted by the ciliary body.
What space lies behind the retina?	Behind the lens is the posterior compartment (see Figure 10-6), which is filled with vitreous humor, a gelatinous substance. At the anterior aspect of the posterior compartment, the lens is held in place by the suspensory ligament, which extends from the ciliary body of the choroid to the lens.
From what embryologic structures do the cornea, iris, ciliary body, lens, and retina develop?	The optic cup is an embryologic structure derived from neuroectoderm that gives rise to the retina, iris, and ciliary body. The lens is derived from surface ectoderm. The inner layers of the cornea are derived from mesenchyme, and the outer layer is from the surface ectoderm.

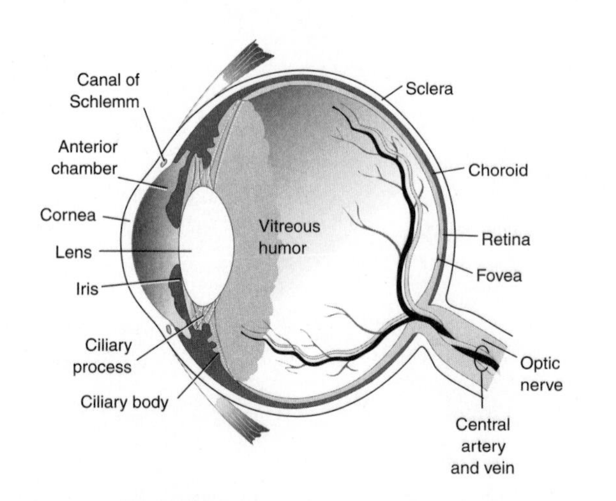

FIGURE 10-6. The eye and retina. (Reproduced, with permission, from Bhushan V, Le T, et al. *First Aid for the USMLE Step 1: 2006*. New York: McGraw-Hill, 2006: 345.)

► Case 7

A 45-year-old woman presents to her physician with a 3-month history of anxiety, tremor, hyperreflexia, hair thinning, and an unintentional weight loss of 4.5 kg (10 lb). She is treated surgically. After surgery, her symptoms have resolved, but the patient now complains of hoarseness.

What is the cause of the patient's hoarseness?	Damage to the recurrent laryngeal nerve may occur as the surgeon is ligating the inferior thyroid artery, which is adjacent to the nerve.
What cranial nerve is involved in this patient?	The recurrent laryngeal nerve is a branch of the vagus nerve (cranial nerve [CN] X).
This nerve provides motor innervation to which structures?	The recurrent laryngeal nerve innervates all intrinsic muscles of the larynx except for the cricothyroid, which is innervated by the external laryngeal nerve (also a branch of CN X).
Describe the course of this nerve.	The left recurrent laryngeal nerve branches off the vagus nerve at the level of the aortic arch, wraps posteriorly around the aorta, and ascends superiorly to the larynx (see Figure 10-7 below). The right recurrent laryngeal nerve branches off the vagus at the level of the right subclavian artery and vein, and wraps around the artery to ascend posteriorly to the larynx. Because the left recurrent laryngeal nerve has a long course arising from the vagus in the superior mediastinum, it is prone to injury from abnormal structures, such as enlarged lymph nodes, aneurysm of the arch of the aorta, a retrosternal goiter, or a thymoma.
What are other scenarios by which this nerve may be injured?	Left atrial enlargement (eg, from mitral regurgitation) and tumor in the apex of the right upper lobe of the lung can impinge on and injure the recurrent laryngeal nerve. Injury of the left recurrent laryngeal nerve may also result in compression by abnormal structures in the superior mediastinum (see above).

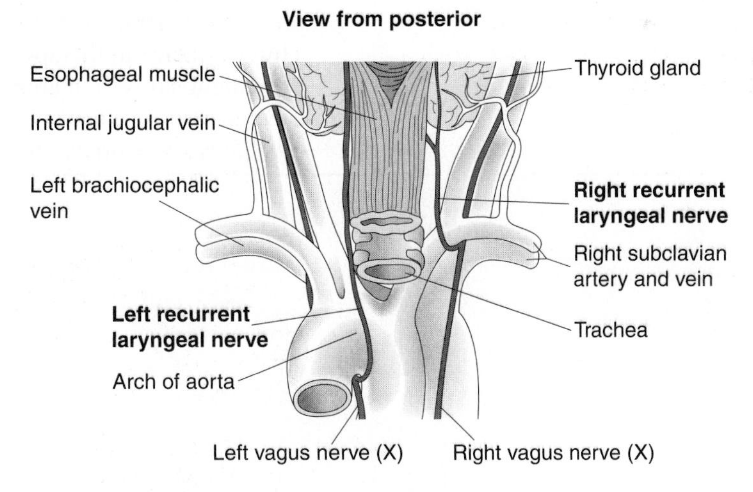

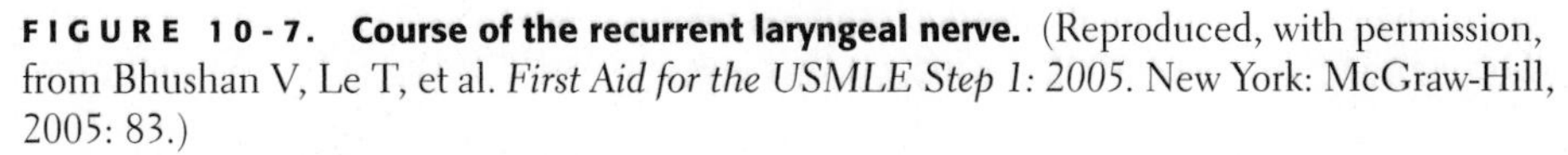

FIGURE 10-7. Course of the recurrent laryngeal nerve. (Reproduced, with permission, from Bhushan V, Le T, et al. *First Aid for the USMLE Step 1: 2005*. New York: McGraw-Hill, 2005: 83.)

▶ Case 8

A 37-year-old pianist visits her physician because of difficulty sleeping over the past 3 weeks. She has been waking up early in the morning, well before her usual waking time. In addition, she does not enjoy playing the piano as much as she used to. She has gained 4.5 kg (10 lb) in the past month. On questioning, she reveals she had a similar episode about 1 year ago.

What is the most likely diagnosis?	Major depressive disorder.
Which symptoms are most commonly associated with this condition?	The diagnosis of a major depressive disorder requires two or more episodes consisting of five of the following symptoms, present for at least 2 weeks (**"SIG E CAPS"**): **S**leep disturbances, decreased **I**nterest, **G**uilt, decreased **E**nergy, decreased **C**oncentration, change in **A**ppetite (usually decreased), **P**sychomotor retardation, **S**uicidal ideations, in addition to depressed mood. A diagnosis cannot be made in this patient without further questioning to elicit additional symptoms.
What other conditions can present with similar symptoms?	**Bereavement** can present similarly within 1 year of the loss of a loved one. In bereavement, the patient's symptoms are related to the loss of another person. Grief is characterized by shock, denial, guilt, and somatic symptoms. Depressive symptoms also raise the possibility of **dysthymia,** a milder form of depression with less intense symptoms, which lasts >2 years. Classically, patients with major depressive disorder exhibit melancholic features consisting of a profoundly sad or dysphoric mood along with the above neurovegetative symptoms.
What major neurotransmitter disturbances are characteristic of this condition?	Patients with major depressive disorder commonly have decreased levels of serotonin and norepinephrine. Dopamine may also be decreased in major depression. The reverse is thought to be true in mania.
What are the most appropriate treatments for this condition?	Antidepressant therapies, including selective serotonin reuptake inhibitors, monoamine oxidase inhibitors, and tricyclic antidepressants, generally take from 2 to 6 weeks for onset of action. Thus, a change in therapy should not be considered until after the patient has been taking these medications for at least 2 weeks. Electroconvulsive therapy can be used for major depressive disorder that is refractory to other treatments.

► Case 9

A 72-year-old woman falls while at home and lands face down. She is unable to get up and remains prone on the floor overnight, until a neighbor notices her missing and calls 911. She is taken to the emergency department (ED), where she is noted to have several hematomas on her face and a large hematoma on her right upper thigh. On physical examination, the ED resident discovers that the patient is unable to flex her right hip or extend her right lower leg. The resident cannot elicit a patellar reflex on the right. Leg adduction and abduction are intact bilaterally.

- **What is the most likely diagnosis?**

The patient has femoral neuropathy (L2–4), as suggested by weakness of the quadriceps muscles and hip flexors (which are innervated by the femoral nerve) and lack of patellar reflex. The cause of the neuropathy in this case is a hematoma (secondary to trauma) compressing the nerve. Because both the hip flexors (L2–3) and the quadriceps muscles (L3–4) are involved, the nerve is being affected above the inguinal ligament.

- **What sensory defects would be expected in this patient?**

The femoral nerve innervates the skin of the anterior and medial thigh; thus, light touch sensation would be decreased in these areas. The lateral aspect of the thigh is innervated by the lateral femoral cutaneous nerve (L2–3), and would be spared in an isolated femoral neuropathy. The **saphenous nerve** is a cutaneous branch of the femoral nerve that arises from the femoral nerve in the femoral triangle. It innervates the skin of the anteromedial knee, leg, and foot to the medial side of the big toe. Because this lesion is above the femoral ligament, the saphenous nerve distribution will also be involved.

- **What other structures are found with this nerve in the femoral triangle?**

The femoral nerve is the largest branch of the lumbar plexus and, after forming in the abdomen, runs posterolaterally to the inguinal ligament. It crosses under the inguinal ligament lateral to the psoas muscle and enters the femoral triangle. In the **femoral triangle** (which is bounded by the sartorius muscle, inguinal ligament, and adductor longus), it runs lateral to the femoral artery, which in turn is lateral to the femoral vein. The vessels are enclosed within the femoral sheath and the nerve is outside it.

- **Why is leg adduction spared in this patient?**

The major muscles responsible for thigh adduction are the adductor longus, adductor brevis, adductor magnus, and the gracilis, which are innervated by the obturator nerve (L2–4). Because this is a peripheral neuropathy, not pathology of the nerve root, the obturator nerve is spared, and so is thigh adduction.

- **What other clinical scenarios can be associated with this condition?**

- Diabetic vasculitic damage
- Direct penetrating trauma
- Hip fracture
- Iliac aneurysms
- Incorrect placement of femoral line
- Prolonged hip flexion during gynecologic or urologic procedures
- Tumor

▶ Case 10

A 51-year-old woman is brought to the emergency department by her husband because she has not left her house in 2 weeks without him. She says that she has worries almost every day, and her worrying has gotten worse over the past 8 months. She has uncontrollable anxiety, but cannot pinpoint what precipitates it. Six months ago, she sought treatment because she became convinced that her husband was going to leave her, and would follow him to work every day even though she realized this was not normal behavior. She is frequently irritable, tired, and unable to concentrate on her work.

▪ **What type of psychiatric disorder does this patient exhibit?**	Generalized anxiety disorder. This category, anxiety disorders, also includes panic disorder, agoraphobia (fear of open places), obsessive-compulsive disorder, and posttraumatic stress disorder (persistently reexperiencing a past traumatic event).
▪ **What signs and symptoms are commonly associated with this disorder?**	▪ Difficulty concentrating ▪ Fatigue ▪ Insomnia ▪ Irritability ▪ Restlessness ▪ Uncontrollable anxiety
▪ **What are the common sources of anxiety for these patients?**	▪ Cleanliness/contamination (washing hands, cleaning house) ▪ Doubt/mistrust ▪ Sex ▪ Symmetry (rituals around doorways, arranging objects)
▪ **What other disorders should be considered in this condition?**	"Normal" anxiety and adjustment disorder. In contrast to **normal anxiety,** individuals with generalized anxiety disorder have evidence of social dysfunction secondary to the disorder. **Adjustment disorder** is characterized by emotional symptoms following an identifiable stressor (ie, divorce, loss of job) and lasts <6 months. In contrast, symptoms in generalized anxiety disorder must have been present for >6 months.
▪ **What are the most appropriate treatments for this disorder?**	▪ Clomipramine ▪ Psychotherapy (cognitive behavioral therapy) ▪ Selective serotonin reuptake inhibitors (first-line treatment)

► Case 11

A 70-year-old man with a history of hypertension goes to his ophthalmologist for a routine eye examination. He has needed to wear eyeglasses while driving since he was 18 years old. Ocular examination reveals increased intraocular pressure in both of the patient's eyes. On a field test, there is significant loss of peripheral vision, and a funduscopic examination reveals cupping.

What is the most likely diagnosis?	Open-angle glaucoma.
What is the pathophysiology of this condition?	Open-angle glaucoma is caused by elevated intraocular pressure resulting from obstruction of flow of aqueous humor through the normal outflow channels.
What are the most appropriate treatments for this condition?	Pilocarpine and carbachol are the most appropriate drugs for the treatment of open-angle glaucoma. These direct cholinergic agonists act by stimulating ciliary muscle contraction, thereby relieving tension in the suspensory ligament. Cholinomimetics will also stimulate the sphincter pupillae of the iris, resulting in widening of the canal of Schlemm and pupillary constriction (miosis). Adverse effects include nausea, vomiting, diarrhea, salivation, sweating, vasodilation, and bronchoconstriction.
What effect does pilocarpine have on cardiac muscle?	Pilocarpine is an M3/M2 muscarinic receptor agonist. Cardiac cells have M2 receptors that, when activated, stimulate a G protein that inhibits adenyl cyclase and increases potassium conductance. Pilocarpine stimulation thus results in a decrease in heart rate and decreased force of contraction (**negative inotrope**).
What additional classes of drugs are useful in treating this condition?	▪ Adrenergic agonists such as epinephrine ▪ β-Blockers and acetazolamide (a carbonic anhydrase inhibitor), which decrease aqueous humor secretion ▪ Prostaglandins, which increase the outflow of aqueous humor

▶ Case 12

A 27-year-old man comes to his physician complaining of a tingling sensation in his toes and progressive weakness in both of his legs. On questioning, he recalls he had a minor cold 3 weeks ago that lasted for a few days. He has not traveled recently and has not eaten anything out of the ordinary. Physical examination reveals markedly decreased patellar and Achilles tendon reflexes bilaterally.

▪ **What is the most likely diagnosis?**	Guillain-Barré syndrome (GBS). GBS, or acute inflammatory demyelinating polyradiculoneuropathy, is characterized by symmetric ascending muscle weakness or paralysis that begins in the lower extremities. Hyporeflexia or areflexia is invariable but may not be present early in the course of disease.
▪ **What physical findings are commonly associated with this condition?**	Associated findings in GBS include ascending paresthesias, cranial nerve deficits leading to dysphagia, dysarthria, facial weakness, papilledema, autonomic dysfunction, and, in extreme cases, respiratory muscle paralysis. Figure 10-8 on the following page shows papilledema of the optic nerve head in GBS, along with the vascular congestion, elevation of the nerve head, and blurred disc margins often seen in papilledema, papillitis, and compressive lesions of the optic nerve.
▪ **In what settings does this condition usually occur?**	GBS often occurs 1–3 weeks after a gastrointestinal or upper respiratory tract infection, vaccination, or allergic reaction. Common associated infections include *Campylobacter jejuni* and herpesvirus. Although a preceding event is present in most patients, about one-third of patients with GBS report no such events during the preceding 1–4 weeks.
▪ **What is the etiology of this condition?**	GBS is thought to be an autoimmune reaction that develops in response to a previous infection or other medical condition. This process results in aberrant demyelination of peripheral nerves and ventral motor nerve roots. Cranial nerve roots can also be affected.
▪ **What laboratory finding is likely in this condition?**	The cerebrospinal fluid (CSF) reveals a markedly elevated protein concentration with a normal cell count, commonly referred to as **albuminocytologic dissociation.** This is in contrast to the increased cell counts typical of central nervous system infection. An increased CSF protein level can lead to papilledema.
▪ **If this man's symptoms worsened over the next few months with no signs of improvement, what alternative diagnosis might be considered?**	**Chronic inflammatory demyelinating polyradiculopathy** is a chronic progressive counterpart of GBS that often presents with similar symptoms.

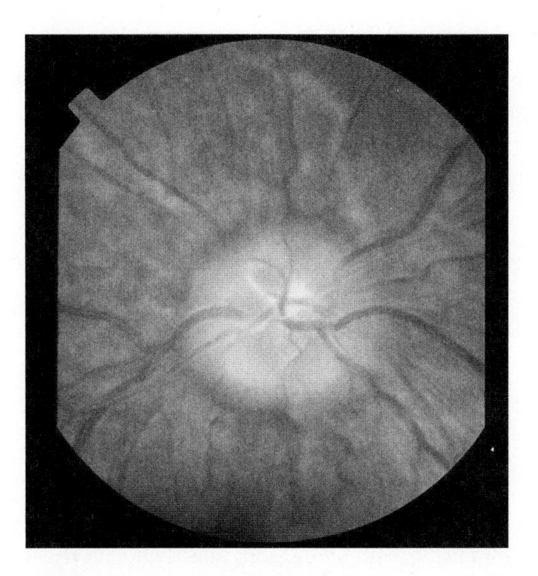

FIGURE 10-8. Papilledema of the optic nerve. (Reproduced, with permission, from Tintinalli JE, et al. *Tintinalli's Emergency Medicine: A Comprehensive Study Guide*, 6th ed. New York: McGraw-Hill, 2004: 1464.)

▶ Case 13

A 45-year-old man comes to the physician for a routine visit. On physical examination, his left eye appears abnormal (see Figure 10-9 below). In addition, his left pupil is constricted, although it reacts normally to light and accommodation. On questioning, he states the left side of his face has become abnormally dry.

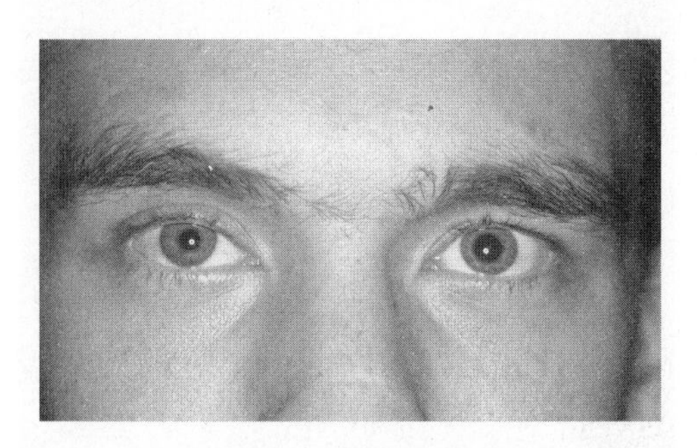

FIGURE 10-9. (Reproduced, with permission, from Tintinalli JE, et al. *Tintinalli's Emergency Medicine: A Comprehensive Study Guide*, 6th ed. New York: McGraw-Hill, 2004: 1463.)

What is the most likely diagnosis?	Horner's syndrome.
What is the pathophysiology of this condition?	Horner's syndrome results from a disruption in the sympathetic innervation of the face and subsequent uninhibited parasympathetic activity, producing the classic symptoms of ipsilateral **P**tosis (slight drooping of the eyelid), **A**nhidrosis (absence of sweating), and **M**iosis (pupillary constriction) (remember the mnemonic **PAM**).
What nerve pathway is disrupted in this condition?	The first neuron of the sympathetic pathway begins in the hypothalamus and synapses in the intermediolateral column of the spinal cord near T1 (see Figure 10-10 on the following page). The second, preganglionic neuron travels to the superior cervical ganglion. The third and final neuron of the pathway then innervates the pupil, the sweat glands of the face, and the smooth muscle of the eyelid.
If this patient presented with nystagmus to the left side and frequent falling, what acute condition should be considered?	**Wallenberg's syndrome,** which results from a stroke in the lateral medullary region supplied by the posterior inferior cerebellar artery, can present with ipsilateral Horner's syndrome, nystagmus to the side of the lesion, ipsilateral limb ataxia, and vertigo. Another distinguishing feature is impaired pain and temperature sensation in the ipsilateral face and contralateral hemibody.
What are other common causes of this condition?	Any pathology that causes interruption of the described pathway can cause Horner's syndrome. These include Pancoast's tumor, neck trauma, carotid dissection, cervical cord lesions, and multiple sclerosis. Additionally, many cases of Horner's syndrome are idiopathic.
What is Pancoast's tumor?	**Pancoast's tumor** is a carcinoma that usually affects the lung, occurring in the apex of the lung. It can cause Horner's syndrome and ulnar nerve pain.

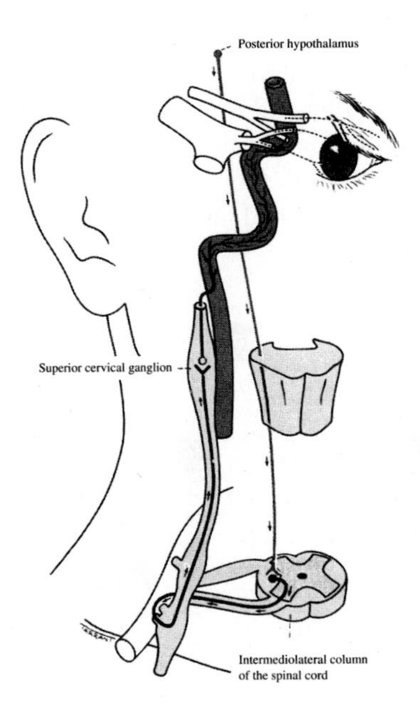

FIGURE 10-10. Nerve pathways disrupted in Horner's syndrome. (Reproduced, with permission, from Tintinalli JE, et al. *Tintinalli's Emergency Medicine: A Comprehensive Study Guide,* 6th ed. New York: McGraw-Hill, 2004: 1463.)

▶ **Case 14**

A 39-year-old man is concerned about his health because his father died at the age of 45 years after several years of dementia and uncontrollable twitching and dancelike movements in his extremities. On further questioning, the patient reports many members of his family have had similar symptoms. The patient's knowledge of his family history allows the physician to construct a detailed family tree (see Figure 10-11 below; the asterisk represents the patient).

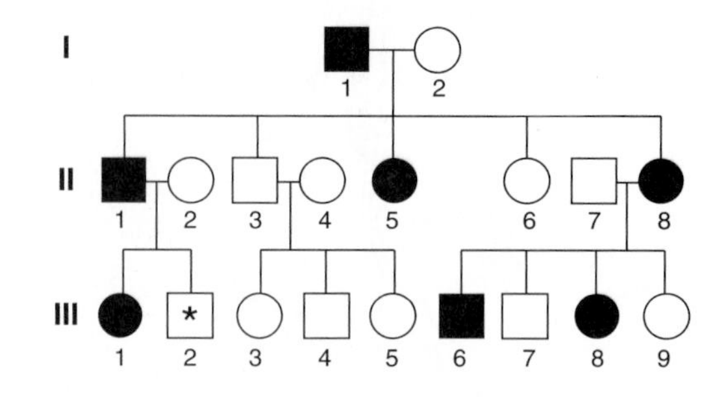

FIGURE 10-11.

▪ **What condition is the patient at risk for developing?**	Huntington's disease, which is characterized by dementia, choreoathetoid movements of the face and extremities, and early death. Huntington's disease has an autosomal dominant inheritance.
▪ **What is the genetic basis of this condition?**	A mutation in chromosome 4 results in expansion of trinucleotide CAG repeats, which may result in decreased transcription of a striatal neurotrophic factor, brain-derived neurotrophic factor.
▪ **What neuronal pathology in patients with this condition makes CT imaging useful?**	Patients with Huntington's disease have marked atrophy of the striatum, including the caudate and putamen, representing degeneration and loss of γ-aminobutyric acid (GABA)-ergic and cholinergic neurons.
▪ **What other conditions often present with similar movement abnormalities?**	Sydenham's chorea in rheumatic fever, tardive dyskinesia, and Wilson's disease are among other diseases associated with choreoathetoid movements.
▪ **What is the prognosis for this patient?**	Expansion of trinucleotide repeats over successive generations leads to earlier manifestations of disease in offspring; this is called **anticipation.** The patient's father died at age 45 years and likely developed Huntington's disease many years earlier. If this patient had the genetic mutation, then he might already be expected to show symptoms.
▪ **What other conditions are associated with trinucleotide repeats?**	Fragile X syndrome, myotonic dystrophy, and spinocerebellar ataxia types I and II are also associated with trinucleotide repeats.

▶ Case 15

The parents of a term, 1-year-old girl are concerned because the child's head seems abnormally large. Their pediatrician notes the child's head circumference has accelerated beyond her established growth curve over the past month. An axial CT of her head (see Figure 10-12 below) demonstrates dilated atria of the lateral ventricles and a rounded third ventricle.

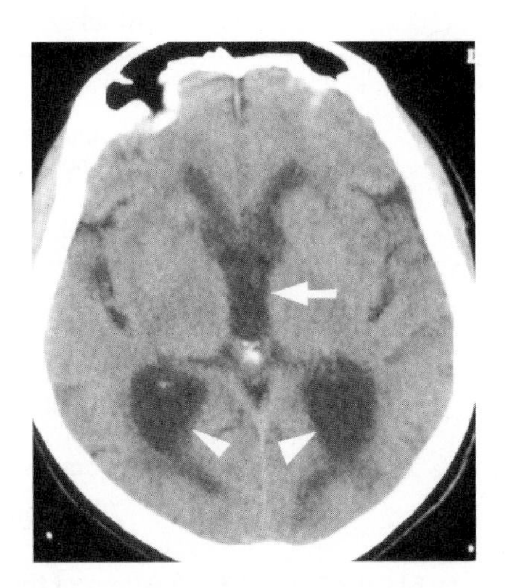

FIGURE 10-12. (Reproduced, with permission, from Brunicardi FC, et al. *Schwartz's Principles of Surgery*, 8th ed. New York: McGraw-Hill, 2005: 1650.)

▪ **What is the most likely diagnosis?**	Hydrocephalus, which is defined as an excessive volume of cerebrospinal fluid (CSF) within the ventricles of the brain. Because CSF is trapped within the ventricular system in this case, this is an example of a **noncommunicating hydrocephalus.** A **communicating hydrocephalus** can occur in states of excess CSF production. In this CT showing a dilated ventricular system (Figure 10-12 above), note the dilated atria of the lateral ventricles (arrowheads) and rounded third ventricle (arrow).
▪ **Where is CSF produced?**	CSF is produced by the choroid plexus epithelium within the cerebral ventricles. The anatomy of the ventricular system is shown in Figure 10-13 on page 244. The lateral ventricle communicates with the third ventricle via the foramen of Monro. The third ventricle communicates with the fourth ventricle via the aqueduct of Sylvius. The fourth ventricle communicates with the subarachnoid space via the foramen of Luschka (laterally) and the foramen of Magendie (medially).
▪ **How is CSF reabsorbed?**	Arachnoid villus cells, which are located in the superior sagittal sinus, return CSF to the bloodstream within vacuoles (via a process called **pinocytosis**).
▪ **What forms the blood-brain barrier?**	Capillary and choroid endothelium form the **blood-brain barrier.** Tight junctions of capillary endothelium within the brain impede the passage of water and solutes. Within the choroid plexus, the choroid endothelium regulates the transport of water and solutes.

- **What is the pathophysiology of this condition?**

Hydrocephalus results from a mismatch of CSF production and reabsorption in which the rate of production exceeds reabsorption. Thus, causes of the condition include:

- Excess CSF production (eg, choroid plexus papilloma)
- Impaired CSF reabsorption (due to obstruction or disruption of arachnoid villi)
- Blockage of the flow of CSF

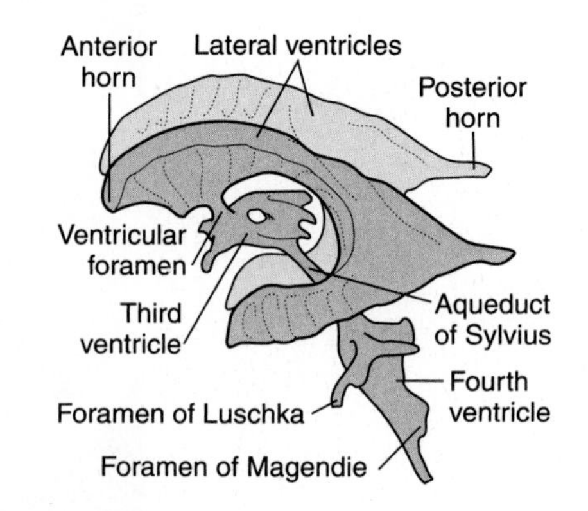

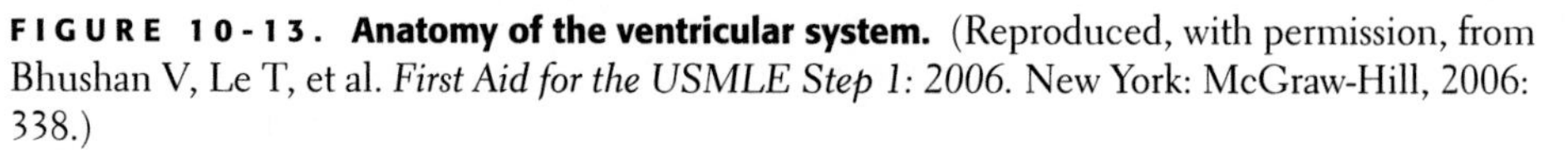

FIGURE 10-13. Anatomy of the ventricular system. (Reproduced, with permission, from Bhushan V, Le T, et al. *First Aid for the USMLE Step 1: 2006*. New York: McGraw-Hill, 2006: 338.)

▶ Case 16

A 75-year-old woman visits an ophthalmologist because she has noticed a gradual decline in both her distance and near vision over the past 2 years. In particular, she has difficulty reading and focusing on objects in front of her and has trouble adjusting her vision to the dark. She denies pain in her eye or any associated trauma. Funduscopic examination reveals deposits in the macula (see Figure 10-14 below) and abnormal vision as assessed by the Amsler grid (see Figure 10-15 below; normal grid [A], patient's view [B]). Her peripheral vision and extraocular movements are intact.

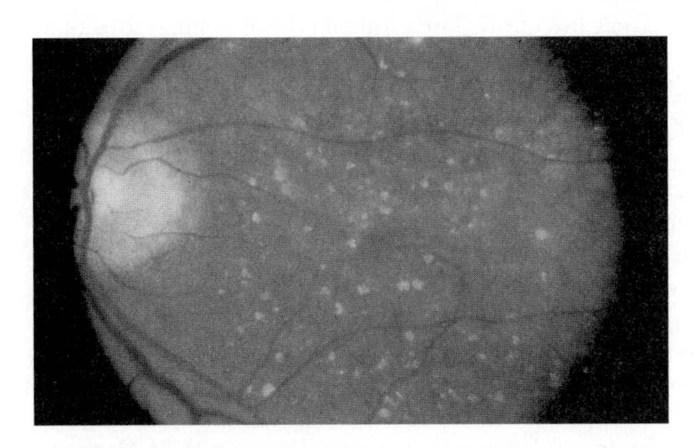

FIGURE 10-14. (Reproduced, with permission, from Knoop KJ, Stack LB, Storrow AB. *Atlas of Emergency Medicine,* 2nd ed. New York: McGraw-Hill, 2002: 77.)

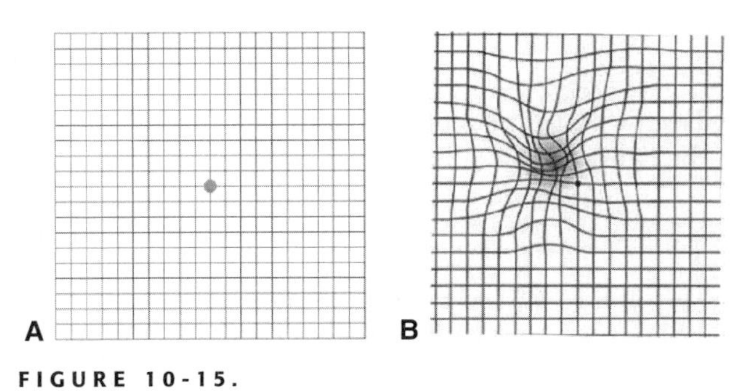

FIGURE 10-15.

- **What is the abnormality in this patient's vision as assessed by the Amsler grid?**

The **Amsler grid** assesses the degree of central vision loss (see Figure 10-15A). Patients are asked to cover one eye and, with the open eye, focus on the dot at the center of the grid. Patients with vision deficits in their macula will see a distortion of the grid (see Figure 10-15B).

- **What is the most likely diagnosis?**

The most likely diagnosis is age-related macular degeneration (ARMD), a significant cause of vision loss in the elderly, in which central vision is blurred. In contrast, glaucoma typically affects peripheral vision while sparing central vision.

- **What are the two variants of this condition?**

There are dry and wet forms of macular degeneration. The **dry form** (representing 85% of cases) typically progresses more slowly and occurs earlier in the disease process. The **wet form,** although rarer (representing 15% of cases), causes the vast majority of significant blindness in patients.

- **What are the histologic features of the retina in this condition?**

Drusen are extracellular protein and lipid deposits in the retina, which appear on funduscopic examination as yellow or white spots in the eye (see Figure 10-14 above). Irregularity and, in later stages, atrophy of the retinal pigmented epithelium also occur. In wet ARMD, new vessels from the choroid may grow into the subretinal space, causing **metamorphopsia** (a wavy distortion of vision), hemorrhage, and scarring.

- **What is the macula?**

The **macula,** which is located temporal to the optic disc, is the area of the retina that is specialized for fine-detail vision. The center of the macula is the **fovea,** which has the highest density of cone photoreceptor cells in the retina and the smallest amount of convergence to bipolar cells. This provides for exquisite detail in visual perception.

▶ Case 17

A 10-year-old boy is brought to his pediatrician because of a painful ear. The pain began 1 week previously concurrent with a runny nose and sinus pressure that progressed to ear pain and dizziness. On otoscopic examination, the child's tympanic membrane is red and bulging. He has a low-grade fever of 37.8° C (100.1° F), but no other physical findings.

What is the most likely diagnosis?	Acute otitis media. The bulging, red tympanic membrane is a sign of middle ear infection. The clinical course is suggestive of a viral upper respiratory infection that led to secondary involvement of the middle ear due to inflammation and congestion of the eustachian tube, which connects the middle ear to the nasopharynx.
From what embryologic structure is the tympanic membrane derived?	The tympanic membrane is derived from the first pharyngeal membrane. The **pharyngeal membranes** are the tissue between the pharyngeal groove, or cleft, and pharyngeal pouch. Only the first pharyngeal membrane is retained in the adult; the rest are obliterated during development.
What three bones are located in the middle ear, and from what embryologic structures do they derive?	The three bones located in the middle ear (auditory ossicles) are the malleus, incus, and stapes (see Figure 10-16 on the following page). They function to transmit sound from the tympanic membrane to the internal ear. The **malleus,** which articulates with the tympanic membrane, is derived from the first branchial arch. The **incus,** which lies between the malleus and the stapes, is derived from the first branchial arch. The **stapes,** which articulates with the oval window of the inner ear, is derived from the second branchial arch.
What two muscles control the movement of the bones of the middle ear, and what is their innervation?	The tensor tympani inserts on the malleus, and dampens the amplitude of the tympanic membrane oscillations, which prevents damage when the inner ear is exposed to loud sounds. Innervation is by the mandibular nerve (cranial nerve [CN] V3). The stapedius inserts onto the neck of the stapes, and dampens movement of this ossicle. It is innervated by the facial nerve (CN VII).
What organisms commonly cause pediatric ear infections?	In order of prevalence, common bacteria that cause middle ear infection are: *Streptococcus pneumoniae, Haemophilus influenzae* (although rarely type B since the introduction of the conjugated vaccine), and *Moraxella catarrhalis.* Less common organisms are group A streptococci, *Staphylococcus aureus, Pseudomonas,* and, in newborns, gram-negative bacilli. Approximately 15%–20% of middle ear infections are due to viruses, including respiratory syncytial virus, rhinovirus, influenza viruses, and adenovirus.

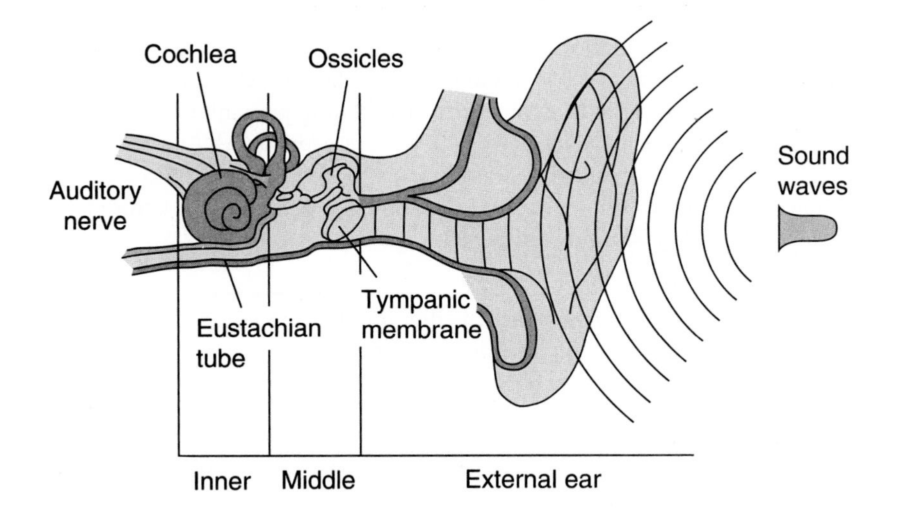

FIGURE 10-16. Anatomy of the ear. (Reproduced, with permission, from Lalwani AK. *Current Diagnosis & Treatment in Otolaryngology—Head & Neck Surgery*. New York: McGraw-Hill, 2004.)

ORGAN SYSTEMS

NEUROLOGY AND PSYCHIATRY

▶ Case 18

An 18-year-old woman goes to her family physician for an evaluation of severe headaches. She describes her headaches as unilateral, beginning with a dull and steady ache and increasing in severity to a throbbing, debilitating pain after several hours. No aura is associated with the headaches, but they are exacerbated by motion and light. Consequently, the patient prefers to remain in a dark room when her headaches occur. She also states this is the second episode she has had; the first episode occurred approximately 4 weeks ago and dissipated within a few days.

- **What is the most likely diagnosis?**

Migraine headache. Further questioning may reveal that the 4-week interval coincides with menstruation, which is a typical trigger of migraine in young women.

- **What signs and symptoms are commonly associated with this condition?**

Migraines are unilateral in 60%–70% of cases, while the remaining cases are typically bifrontal or, less frequently, bioccipital. The pain often begins with the gradual onset of a deep, steady ache that crescendos within several hours to a pulsatile, severe pain. Migraines are typically worsened by movement, loud noises, and bright lights. Although **auras** (temporary neurologic symptoms such as light flashes, zigzag lines, or numbness and tingling in the arms and face) are commonly associated with migraine headaches, they are actually seen in only 20% of cases.

- **How is this condition differentiated from other, more serious pathologic conditions of the head?**

Warning signs that a headache may be serious include:

- Absence of similar episodes in the past
- Association with vigorous exercise or trauma (suggestive of carotid dissection)
- Change in mental status
- Concurrent infection
- Sudden onset within seconds to minutes (suggestive of subarachnoid hemorrhage)

Physical findings pointing to potentially serious pathology include nuchal rigidity (meningitis), poor general appearance, or papilledema (elevated intracranial pressure).

- **How can this woman's headache be differentiated from cluster or tension headaches?**

Tension headaches are typically bilateral and are often described as a bandlike tightness or pressure (as if the patient were wearing a tight hat). They are typically not debilitating, and the pressure waxes and wanes over an unpredictable time course. Tension headaches are closely associated with stress.

Cluster headaches typically occur in males and are always unilateral. The pain often begins around the eye or temple; is sudden in onset (and could thus be mistaken for subarachnoid hemorrhage); and is described as deep and persistent. The pain often lasts for several hours and can be associated with tearing of the eyes and sweating.

- **What are the most appropriate treatments for this condition?**

Possible treatments include nonsteroidal anti-inflammatory agents (especially indomethacin), acetaminophen, triptans (ie, sumatriptan, a serotonin agonist), and less typically ergotamine agents (ie, dihydroergotamine). For more frequent, chronic migraines, daily treatment with β-blockers such as propranolol or calcium-channel blockers such as verapamil can be effective in prevention.

▶ Case 19

A 25-year-old woman presents to her physician with difficulty chewing and swallowing her food. She also complains of occasional double vision. She states her symptoms are often absent in the morning and appear to worsen as the day progresses.

What is the most likely diagnosis?	Myasthenia gravis.
What risk factors are more commonly seen in older men and younger women?	Myasthenia gravis is more commonly seen in men than in women, and most patients are >50 years old when diagnosed.
What signs and symptoms are commonly associated with this condition?	Patients may present with a variety of findings, including ptosis, diplopia, dysarthria, difficulty chewing, and difficulty swallowing. Proximal muscle weakness is usually greater than distal muscle weakness. Weakness increases with use of the muscles.
What is the pathophysiology of this condition?	Patients develop antibodies directed toward **acetylcholine** receptors. Because of a higher threshold of activation by acetylcholine, signal transmission across the neuromuscular junction is decreased. This process leads to muscle weakness.
What tumor is commonly associated with this condition?	Myasthenia gravis has been associated with an increased frequency of **thymomas.** It is thought that the thymus is the site of production of autoantibodies against acetylcholine receptors. Even in patients with no thymus neoplasm, **thymectomy** has been shown to improve symptoms in 85% of cases.
How would the clinical presentation differ in a patient with autoantibodies against presynaptic voltage-gated calcium channels?	**Lambert-Eaton syndrome** presents in a similar manner and is associated with small cell lung cancer. However, symptoms usually **decrease** with muscle use as more calcium is released. This is in contrast to myasthenia gravis, in which weakness **increases** with muscle use.

▶ Case 20

A 28-year-old previously healthy woman comes to the physician complaining of weakness in her legs, urinary incontinence, and difficulty speaking. She has also noticed a slight tremor in her hand when she attempts to eat. She says her symptoms have worsened over the previous 4 weeks. She denies any history of fever or vomiting and has no other health problems. Upon questioning, she recalls her mother had similar symptoms when she was young. Physical examination reveals left-sided facial droop, left tongue deviation, and lateral gaze weakness. An MRI is shown in Figure 10-17 below. Relevant laboratory findings are as follows:

WBC count: 9100/mm^3
Hemoglobin: 13.3 g/dL
Hematocrit: 37.1%
Platelet count: 287,000/mm^3
Cerebrospinal fluid (CSF) IgG index: 0.89 (normal <0.66)

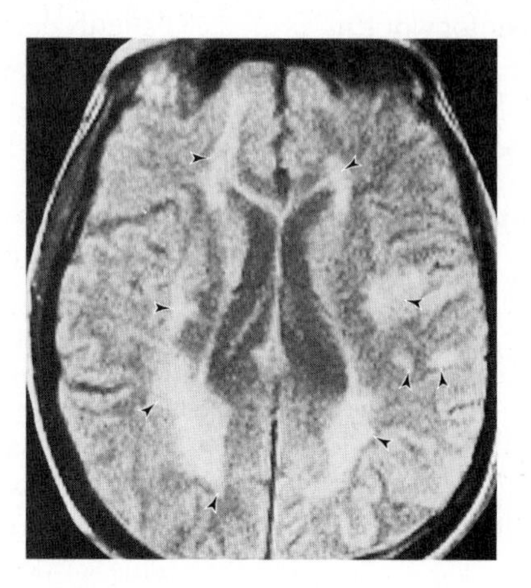

FIGURE 10-17. (Reproduced, with permission, from Waxman SG. *Clinical Neuroanatomy*, 25th ed. New York: McGraw-Hill, 2003.)

▪ **What is the most likely diagnosis?**	Multiple sclerosis (MS). The arrowheads in Figure 10-17 above show the lesions of MS.
▪ **What risk factors are associated with this condition?**	▪ Being 20–50 years old (mean age of onset 30 years) ▪ Being a woman (female:male ratio 1.77:1.00) ▪ Being raised in a temperate climate ▪ Having a family history of MS
▪ **What anatomical finding could explain the findings on physical examination?**	A **medial brain stem lesion** involving cranial nerves VI, VII, and XII (see Figure 10-18 on the following page) would lead to the constellation of facial droop, tongue deviation, and lateral gaze weakness. The intention tremor indicates cerebellar involvement.
▪ **What are the typical CSF findings in this condition?**	**Oligoclonal bands** are seen in 85%–95% of cases. The presence of these immunoglobulins reflects the autoimmune nature of the disease. Similarly, the **IgG index** is elevated in >90% of patients with definite MS. The total CSF WBC count is normal in most patients, so an elevated WBC count is nonspecific.
▪ **What is the likely finding on imaging of the brain?**	Multiple **demyelinating plaques** are usually present in the brain of patients with MS, especially in the periventricular region, corpus callosum, and centrum semiovale.

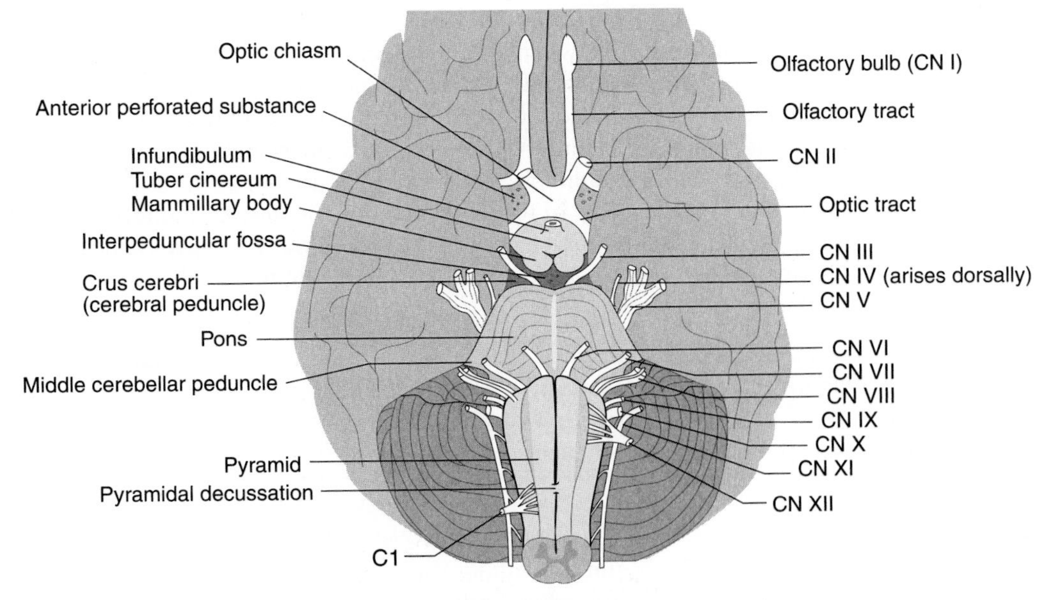

FIGURE 10-18. Brain stem anatomy. (Reproduced, with permission, from Bhushan V, Le T, et al. *First Aid for the USMLE Step 1: 2006*. New York: McGraw-Hill, 2006: 342.)

▶ Case 21

A 29-year-old well-groomed man, with no prior medical or psychiatric history, consults a psychiatrist for evaluation. The patient has noticed that over the past 6 months he has been preoccupied with counting items, such as bricks in his driveway, raisins in his cereal, and tiles in the ceiling. Moreover, he says he feels compelled to count particularly to the number 30; for example, he must do 30 push-ups in the morning, jog for 30 minutes, and chew his food 30 times. He has not told anyone about his recent habit, and does not believe it is interfering with his work. However, he is troubled by his own behavior and feels unable to stop. During the medical history, the patient reveals his 30th birthday is next week.

What is the most likely diagnosis?	Obsessive-compulsive disorder (OCD), as suggested by the patient's obsessions (recurrent thoughts) and compulsions (recurrent acts).
What is the epidemiology of this condition?	OCD occurs in about 3% of the general population. Males are much more frequently afflicted than females. The disorder often runs in families, and may be associated with tic disorders (eg, Tourette's syndrome).
What is cognitive behavioral therapy?	**Cognitive behavioral therapy** is a time-limited type of psychotherapy, in which the patient's obsessive thoughts are seen as the source of symptoms such as anxiety, phobias, depression, and somatization (the compulsions are a way to temporarily relieve the anxiety). The goal of therapy is to identify the irrational beliefs and illogical thinking patterns (such as fear of turning 30) and how these altered cognitions contribute to and perpetuate anxious or depressive feelings. After recognition of such irrational beliefs, behavioral strategies are used to minimize symptoms. Cognitive therapy often involves "homework" such as behavioral assignments or reading material.
What are the most appropriate pharmacologic treatments for this condition?	Clomipramine and selective serotonin reuptake inhibitors are first-line treatments for OCD.
What is the difference between OCD and obsessive personality disorder?	In OCD, the patient recognizes that his/her beliefs are irrational, and is disturbed by them. An individual with obsessive personality disorder believes that his/her beliefs are rational and logical.

▶ Case 22

A 48-year-old man visits his physician for a routine physical examination. During the interview, he mentions he is having some difficulty at work. His boss claims he is unable to finish tasks within a reasonable amount of time. Yet the patient maintains that his coworkers "don't do things the way I tell them to," and he doesn't feel he can delegate tasks because "they don't do things right." He also admits to frequent arguments with his wife, who does not put things away in the places they are supposed to go. He cannot tolerate anything that is not orderly. During the office visit, the patient takes copious notes.

- **What is the difference between a personality trait and a personality disorder?**

A personality **trait** is a typical pattern of relating to or thinking about the world that is exhibited in various social and personal contexts. A personality trait becomes a **disorder** when the traits are extreme and become maladaptive, leading to problems with social behavior and functioning and personal distress. A person is usually not aware of a personality disorder.

- **How are these disorders classified?**

The *Diagnostic and Statistical Manual of Mental Disorders, 4th edition*, classifies personality disorders into three clusters:

- Individuals in cluster A are described as odd or eccentric ("weird").
- Individuals in cluster B are described as dramatic or erratic ("wild").
- Individuals in cluster C are described as anxious or fearful ("worried").

This patient falls into cluster C, obsessive-compulsive personality disorder (OCPD).

- **How can this disorder be differentiated from obsessive-compulsive disorder?**

Obsessive-compulsive disorder (OCD) is a disease with the presence of obsessions and compulsions, both of which are unable to be resisted and are experienced as abnormal by patients **(ego-dystonic). Compulsions** are repetitive behaviors performed usually to lessen the anxiety associated with **obsessions,** which are repetitive thoughts or images that the patient cannot resist. Symptoms worsen in times of stress and are particularly debilitating due to time consumption and interference with daily, social, and occupational functioning. OCD is not to be confused with OCPD, in which patients lack true obsessions and compulsions, but instead have a rigid preoccupation with order. Patients with OCPD find little to be abnormal with their beliefs and order **(ego-syntonic)**; their behaviors may bother the people around them, but they do not bother the patient him- or herself.

- **What is the first-line treatment of OCPD?**

Symptoms of OCPD often do not respond to medication. Cognitive behavioral therapy can be useful in these patients. Also, because OCPD is often accompanied by depression, antidepressant agents may be helpful in some patients. Selective serotonin reuptake inhibitors (fluvoxamine, paroxetine, sertraline, and fluoxetine) and clomipramine (the most serotonergic tricyclic antidepressant) are often used.

▶ **Case 23**

A 20-year-old woman complains to her physician that she is unable to drive her car because she frequently panics while driving. She describes several episodes of palpitations, nausea, sweating, breathlessness, and an intense fear of dying in these situations. These episodes started about 8 months ago, but are increasing in frequency. The episodes begin suddenly at variable times during the car ride and intensify over the course of 5 minutes, so that she must stop the car to calm down. She finds the symptoms confusing and frustrating, stating that she has "never had any problems with cars before" and that she now avoids travel where a car might be involved. Recently, these episodes have become more common, and can occur even while she is at home.

What is the most likely diagnosis?	Panic disorder. However, organic causes of her symptoms, including hyperthyroidism, hyperparathyroidism, pheochromocytoma, hypoglycemia, seizures, and drug use, must be ruled out before panic disorder can be diagnosed.
How are "panic attacks" related to this condition?	Panic disorder requires repeated **panic attacks** (or episodes), with relevant behaviors or attitudes between attacks, such as worry about not being able to control the panic attacks. Patients with panic disorder usually also have unprovoked panic attacks periodically, but often these episodes are generalized to a particular situation.
What anatomic abnormality can trigger a panic attack?	Medial temporal lobe **seizures** can produce fear and autonomic phenomena. This is thought to occur because the amygdala, located in the temporal lobe, is often associated with responses to fear.
What are the most appropriate treatments for this condition?	Panic disorder is often treated with selective serotonin reuptake inhibitors (SSRIs), tricyclic antidepressants, and monoamine oxidase (MAO) inhibitors. These drugs influence the central nervous system levels of norepinephrine, serotonin, and γ-aminobutyric acid. Benzodiazepines are also useful in the short-term management of patients with panic disorder.
What syndrome can develop when SSRIs are used with MAO inhibitors?	**Serotonin syndrome** may result from the use of drugs that enhance serotonin signaling. Since MAO inhibitors and SSRIs both enhance serotonin signaling through different mechanisms, the risk of serotonin syndrome is higher when these drugs are taken together. Serotonin syndrome is more likely to occur with this combination of drugs because most MAO inhibitors irreversibly inhibit MAO. Thus, the risk of accumulated serotonin is increased with coadministration of SSRIs. Symptoms of serotonin syndrome fit into three main categories: ▪ Autonomic dysfunction (eg, hyperthermia, tachycardia, unstable blood pressure, diarrhea, sweating) ▪ Cognitive and behavioral changes (eg, agitation, confusion, coma) ▪ Neuromuscular abnormalities (eg, hyperreflexia, shivering, myoclonus, ataxia)

▶ Case 24

A 66-year-old man presents to his physician with a new-onset tremor in his right hand that worsens when he is watching television. He has also been experiencing some difficulty walking, and his friends complain that he has not been able to keep up with them on the golf course. His wife has noticed he does not seem to get excited about anything.

What is the most likely diagnosis?	Parkinson's disease. Parkinson's disease typically presents with symptoms described by the mnemonic **TRAP: T**remor that is worse at rest, **R**igidity, **A**kinesia or bradykinesia, and **P**ostural instability.
What neuropathologic findings are associated with this condition?	Parkinson's disease is marked by significant neuronal loss in the **substantia nigra,** which leads to decreased dopaminergic input into the basal ganglia. Characteristic findings include depigmentation of neurons in the substantia nigra and concentric eosinophilic cytoplasmic inclusions called **Lewy bodies** (see Figure 10-19 below).
How does a loss of dopamine release from the substantia nigra lead to a decrease in movement?	Dopamine activates the direct motor pathway in the basal ganglia and inhibits the indirect pathway. Normally, dopamine inhibits the inhibitory motor output from the globus pallidus interna (GPi) via these pathways. Decreased dopamine levels in Parkinson's disease due to substantia nigra compacta (SNc) degeneration result in increased inhibitory output from the GPi and substantia nigra reticulata (SNr) and subsequent bradykinesia.
What symptoms are likely to develop over time in this patient?	As the disease progresses, additional symptoms that may develop include shuffling gait, masked facies, and dementia.
What are the most appropriate treatments for this condition?	Carbidopa can be used with levodopa in the treatment of Parkinson's disease. Carbidopa, a peripheral dopa decarboxylase inhibitor, reduces peripheral conversion of levodopa. This augments its action in the central nervous system and reduces its action outside the central nervous system (where levodopa can cause arrhythmias and dyskinesias). Pramipexole and bromocriptine, which are direct dopaminergic agonists, can also be used to augment dopamine signaling.
What other etiologies might result in a similar presentation?	Typical antipsychotic agents have antidopaminergic activity. Thus, patients taking these medications for schizophrenia can exhibit Parkinson-like symptoms. 1-Methyl-4-phenyl-1,2,3,6-tetrahydropyridine (MPTP) and antiemetic agents can also induce parkinsonian symptoms.

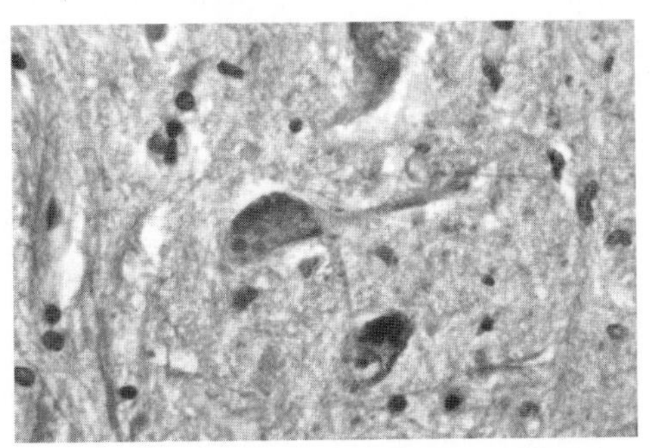

FIGURE 10-19. Lewy bodies in Parkinson's disease. (Reproduced with permission of the Pathology Education Instructional Resource Digital Library (http://peir.net) at the University of Alabama, Birmingham.)

▶ Case 25

The parents of a 22-year-old man bring him to the family physician because they have noticed a distinct change in their son's behavior over the past 4 months. He appears unkempt, does not have any friends at school, and his grades have started to drop. The young man believes that their neighbor has been sent to spy on him, and his parents have heard him carrying on conversations with imaginary partners. The son denies any history of substance use.

■ **What is the most likely diagnosis?**	The constellation of symptoms suggests the diagnosis of **schizophreniform disorder,** which is the presence of psychotic symptoms for >2 weeks, but <6 months. This is in contrast to a diagnosis of **schizophrenia,** which requires the presence of symptoms for at least 6 months. Many patients with schizophreniform disorder ultimately develop schizophrenia.
■ **What symptoms are associated with this condition?**	Positive symptoms include formal thought disorder (disorganized speech, loosening of associations), delusions, hallucinations, and **ideas of reference** (beliefs or perceptions that irrelevant, unrelated, or innocuous things are referring to a person directly, or have a special significance for that person). Negative symptoms include flat affect, social withdrawal, and **avolition** (inability to initiate and maintain goal-directed activities).
■ **What is the epidemiology of this condition?**	The lifetime prevalence of schizophrenia is approximately 1%. It occurs equally often in males and females (although it is often present earlier in males), and its incidence does not differ according to race. Most patients with schizophrenia (75%) present between 15 and 25 years old. Genetic factors are thought to be important in its etiology. Some evidence suggests patients with schizophrenia are more likely to have been born in the winter and early spring. Viral hypotheses are thought to explain these findings.
■ **What neurotransmitter abnormalities are associated with this condition?**	An excess of dopamine and serotonin are thought to contribute to the development of schizophrenia.
■ **What are the most appropriate pharmacologic treatments for this condition?**	Typical antipsychotic agents (such as thioridazine, haloperidol, fluphenazine, and chlorpromazine) block dopamine$_2$ receptors. Atypical antipsychotic agents (clozapine, olanzapine, and risperidone) block serotonin receptors and multiple subtypes of dopamine receptors.
■ **What personality disorders are commonly associated with this condition?**	There is a familial association between schizophrenia and **cluster A personality disorders,** ie, paranoid, schizoid, and schizotypal personality disorders.

▶ Case 26

An emergency medical team is called to help a 30-year-old woman who is unconscious at work. Her coworkers state that before she became unconscious, for the first 10 seconds or so she pointed to her right hand as it began twitching rhythmically, then stiffened every muscle and fell down. After about 15 seconds, she became incontinent and started jerking her arms and legs rhythmically for a few minutes. She then lay still, unresponsive and unconscious, for about 3 minutes. The medical team notes she is now breathing deeply but remains unresponsive.

- **What is the most likely diagnosis?**

Seizure. Involvement of the left motor cortex is implicated, because the seizure started with a right-handed motor activity.

- **How is this condition classified?**

This is a simple partial seizure with motor signs secondarily generalizing into a tonic-clonic seizure. During the first 10 seconds, the patient maintained consciousness, pointing to a **"simple" seizure** ("complex" seizures require a loss of consciousness) After the first 10 seconds, her simple partial seizure evolved into a generalized tonic-clonic seizure. The **tonic phase** is characterized by the immobile contraction of all muscles, and the **clonic phase** is characterized by the bilateral rhythmic jerking of the extremities.

- **Why is the woman breathing deeply after her incident?**

The patient is likely responding to acidosis. A **respiratory acidosis** can develop from the loss of coordinated respirations during the seizure, and a **metabolic acidosis** can develop as muscles contract under anaerobic conditions and produce lactic acid.

- **What is the most appropriate treatment for this condition?**

Popular antiseizure medications include valproic acid, phenytoin, phenobarbital, primidone, and carbamazepine. Many antiseizure medications work by enhancing γ-aminobutyric acid (GABA) binding on chloride channels. GABA binding allows chloride ions to flow into neurons, thereby inhibiting neuronal firing. Barbiturates act on the same chloride channel as does GABA and enhances GABA signaling by increasing the **duration** of chloride channel opening. Benzodiazepines act on the same channel and enhance GABA signaling, but they do so by increasing the **frequency** of chloride channel opening.

- **What are the most common adverse effects of these medications?**

- Valproate: hepatotoxicity, neutropenia, thrombocytopenia, teratogenicity (neural tube defects in fetus)
- Carbamazepine: hepatotoxicity (must check liver function), aplastic anemia, agranulocytosis
- Phenytoin: gingival hyperplasia, teratogenic
- Ethosuximide and lamotrigine: Stevens-Johnson syndrome (a bullous form of erythema multiforme that involves mucous membranes and large areas of the body)
- Carbamazepine and phenobarbital: induction of cytochrome P450, resulting in drug interactions

▶ Case 27

A 28-year-old woman presents to her physician with abdominal pain that has persisted for the past several weeks. The patient reports she is unable to sleep at night and has "tried everything for the pain but it won't go away." She reports nausea and diarrhea. Her last menstrual period was 3 months ago. Review of her chart shows she has been seen several times over the past few months for similar symptoms without any significant laboratory findings. She wonders whether she should have surgery to find out what is wrong.

What is the most likely diagnosis?

Somatoform disorder. These disorders include body dysmorphic disorder, conversion disorder, hypochondriasis, pain disorder, and somatization disorder.

What are common symptoms of this disorder?

Patients present with multiple somatic complaints often including various organ systems:

- Gastrointestinal complaints include nausea, diarrhea, or abdominal pain.
- Neurological complaints include weakness and sensory loss.
- Sexual complaints include irregular menses, pain associated with sexual activity, or problems with any phase of the sexual response.

How are these disorders categorized?

- **Body dysmorphic disorder:** patients are excessively concerned with an imagined or slight physical defect, to the point where social, occupation, or academic functioning is adversely affected.
- **Conversion disorder:** patients unconsciously mimic medical disorders (often neurologic and solitary in nature) for the purposes of acquiring the sick role.
- **Hypochondriasis:** patients persistently believe they have a particular disease, despite multiple pieces of evidence suggesting absence of that illness.
- **Pain disorder:** patients have complaints of pain, but psychological factors contribute to the onset, severity, maintenance, and exacerbation of these complaints.
- **Somatization disorder**: patients have several recurring, clinically significant physical complaints, which cannot be fully explained by physical findings.

These somatoform disorders must be distinguished from **factitious disorders** (patients consciously induce or mimic medical disorders, perhaps by contaminating urine specimens or surreptitiously injecting insulin, for the purposes of acquiring the sick role) and **malingering** (patients consciously feign medical disorders for the purposes of acquiring tangible goals such as money, shelter, or food).

What are the most appropriate treatments for this disorder?

Continuity of care is very important with these patients. Frequent appointments with the same primary care provider during which the patient can express his/her symptoms and concerns are important. The patient should receive a physical examination to rule out a medical cause, but diagnostic testing should be limited once it is determined that no medical cause underlies the condition. A psychiatric referral should be made when the patient is ready.

▶ Case 28

A 35-year-old woman presents to the emergency department complaining of back pain. Six years ago, she was diagnosed with a 2.5-cm primary breast tumor with metastases to one axillary lymph node. At that time, she underwent a mastectomy and adjuvant chemotherapy. She had been feeling well until 3 months ago, when she began to develop back pain. The pain has become progressively worse, particularly when she lies down. She also notes some weakness in both legs but no leg pain. She denies fever, night sweats, weight loss, or headache. Physical examination reveals no cervical lymphadenopathy; 4/5 muscle strength in the lower extremities bilaterally; normal pain, vibration, and position sensation; 3+ patellar reflexes bilaterally; a positive Babinski's reflex on the right; and normal anal sphincter tone.

▪ What are common causes of back pain?

- Disk herniation
- Metastases
- Musculoskeletal (eg, muscle strain, osteoarthritis, compression fracture, ankylosing spondylitis)
- Osteomyelitis
- Referred pain from visceral disease (eg, gallstones or kidney stones, pancreatitis, aortic aneurysm)

▪ What is the likely cause of this patient's back pain?

The patient's history of breast cancer raises concern for the development of metastases resulting in epidural **spinal cord compression.** Her leg weakness, hyperreflexia, and positive Babinski's signs indicate upper motor neuron lesions, which are likely the cause of her weakness as well. Her pain at rest and lack of sciatica argue against disk herniation.

▪ How would signs of upper motor neuron lesions contrast with those of lower motor neurons lesions?

As in this patient, upper motor lesions are characterized by spastic paralysis, hyperreflexia, and a positive Babinski's sign. In contrast, lower motor neuron lesions are associated with flaccid paralysis, muscle atrophy, muscle fasciculations and fibrillations, and hyporeflexia.

▪ What are the most common metastases to bone?

The most common sources of bone metastases are cancers of the breast, prostate, lung, and kidney (renal cell carcinoma).

▪ What are the most appropriate treatments for this condition?

Treatment options include steroids such as dexamethasone, radiation therapy, and surgical decompression. Spinal cord compression is an oncologic emergency because neurologic dysfunction, if present, may become permanent if it is not immediately addressed.

▶ Case 29

A 72-year-old woman is at home with her husband when he notices she sounds confused even though she had been speaking clearly just moments before. He brings her into the emergency department, where she is unable to follow commands. Her speech is fluent but does not make any sense. A CT scan of the head is shown in Figure 10-20 below.

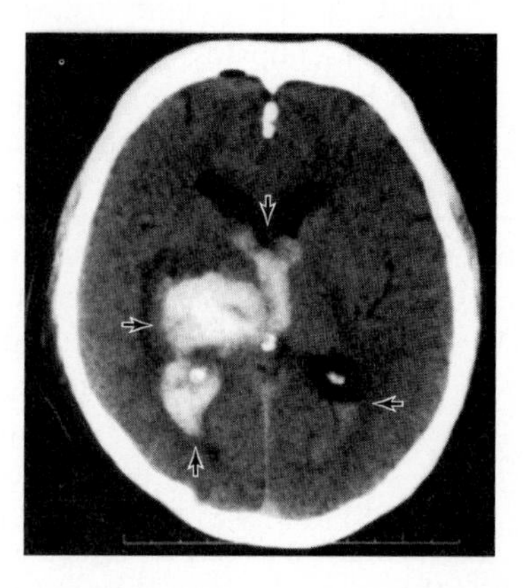

FIGURE 10-20. (Reproduced, with permission, from Aminoff MJ, Greenberg DA, Simon RP. *Clinical Neurology*, 6th ed. New York: McGraw-Hill, 2005: 315.)

What is the most likely diagnosis?	Stroke. Figure 10-20 above shows extensive hemorrhage in the thalamus (left arrow) and its extension into the third (top arrow), ipsilateral (bottom arrow), and lateral ventricles (right arrow).
What risk factors are associated with this condition?	▪ Advanced age ▪ Cardiovascular disease ▪ Carotid disease ▪ Diabetes mellitus ▪ Dyslipidemia ▪ Family or personal history of transient ischemic attack or stroke ▪ Hypertension ▪ Smoking
What type of aphasia does the patient exhibit?	The combination of fluent but nonsensical speech with poor comprehension is characteristic of **Wernicke's aphasia** (sensory aphasia). These patients also display poor repetition and naming ability. Other findings commonly associated with Wernicke's aphasia include contralateral visual field cut (due to ischemia of optic radiation) and **anosognosia** (unawareness of one's deficit).
A lesion in what anatomical area would cause these findings?	Wernicke's aphasia is usually the result of ischemia in the superior temporal gyrus, which is supplied by the inferior division of the left middle cerebral artery.
What speech pattern would result if this condition affected the inferior frontal gyrus?	The inferior frontal gyrus controls motor aspects of speech. A stroke in this area would cause **Broca's aphasia** (motor aphasia), which is characterized by nonfluent, agrammatic speech. Due to the proximity of the primary motor cortex for the face and arm, **dysarthria** (difficulty in articulating words) and right face and arm weakness are often associated with Broca's aphasia. Comprehension is intact in these patients.

- **If the patient had nail-bed hemorrhages, nodules on her fingers and toes, and retinal hemorrhages, what diagnosis should be considered?**

This constellation of symptoms suggests the diagnosis of **infective endocarditis,** which is characterized by splinter hemorrhages, Osler's nodes on the pads of the fingers and toes, and Roth's spots on the retina. Infective endocarditis can lead to the release of thrombi from the valvular vegetations, resulting in embolic events.

▶ Case 30

A 43-year-old woman with a history of hypertension presents to her physician with a severe headache. She says this is the most painful headache she has ever experienced. The headache began this morning while she was watching television. She also had two episodes of vomiting earlier in the day. She denies any traumatic events. Cardiac examination reveals a midsystolic click with a late systolic murmur at the apex. A CT scan of the head is shown in Figure 10-21 below.

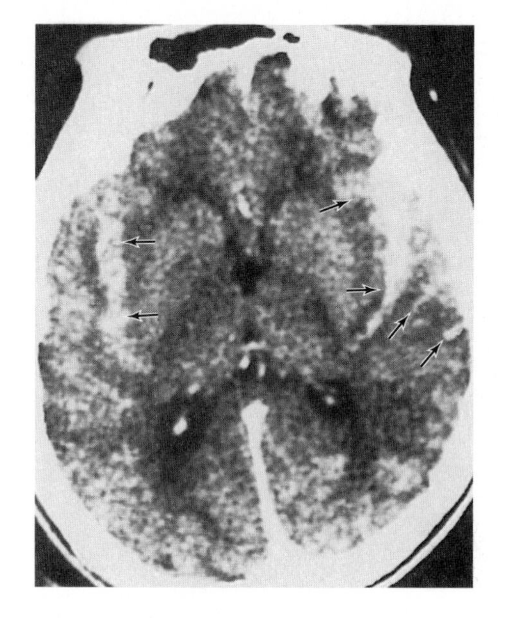

FIGURE 10-21. (Reproduced, with permission, from Waxman SG. *Clinical Neuroanatomy*, 25th ed. New York: McGraw-Hill, 2003.)

■ **What is the most likely diagnosis?**	Subarachnoid hemorrhage (see arrows in Figure 10-21 above).
■ **What are some common etiologies of this condition?**	Most spontaneous subarachnoid hemorrhages occur in the **circle of Willis** (commonly at the bifurcation of the middle cerebral artery) as a result of the rupture of a berry aneurysm (see Figure 10-22 on the following page, arrowhead points to berry aneurysm) or an arteriovenous malformation. The risk is increased by a history of hypertension. The most common location of **berry aneurysm** is the anterior communicating artery, then the posterior communicating artery, followed by the middle cerebral artery. Trauma causes more subarachnoid hemorrhages than spontaneous ruptures do.
■ **Given this patient's symptoms, what is the pathophysiology of this condition?**	The murmur on cardiac examination is characteristic of mitral valve prolapse, which is commonly seen in **Marfan's syndrome.** Berry aneurysms have been associated with Marfan's syndrome, Ehlers-Danlos syndrome, adult polycystic kidney disease, and coarctation of the aorta.
■ **What are the typical findings on cerebrospinal fluid (CSF) analysis?**	The CSF is usually bloody with a xanthochromic or yellow supernatant, reflecting bilirubin release from the breakdown of hemoglobin.
■ **Why was the patient vomiting?**	Vomiting is a common sign of increased intracerebral pressure, which in this patient would be secondary to the hemorrhage.

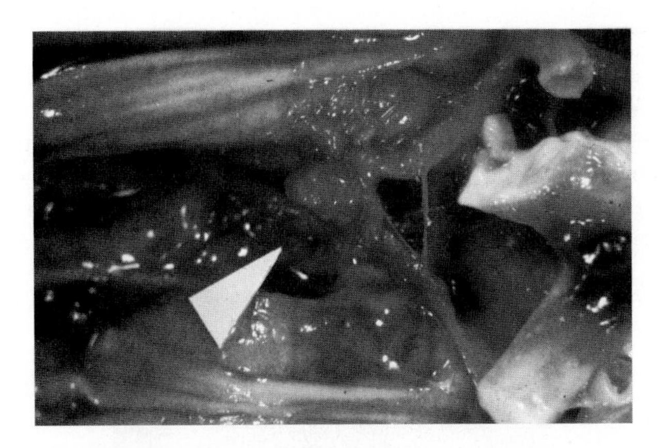

FIGURE 10-22. Berry aneurysm. (Reproduced with permission of the Pathology Education Instructional Resource Digital Library (http://peir.net) at the University of Alabama, Birmingham.)

► **Case 31**

A 77-year-old man falls while climbing the stairs to his apartment. He temporarily loses consciousness and awakens with a mild headache. His relatives do not notice any problems until 3 weeks later, when they begin to note a change in his mental status. Typically a personable man, he starts to yell at his family members for no reason and does not recognize people he knows well. He is brought to the emergency department, where a CT scan of the head is obtained (see Figure 10-23 below).

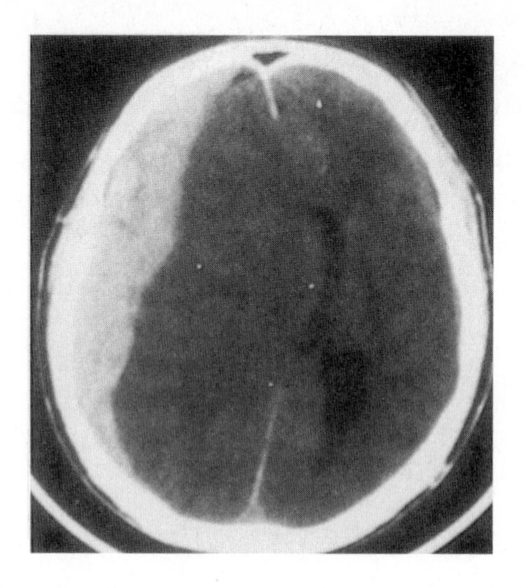

FIGURE 10-23. (Reproduced, with permission, from Aminoff MJ, Greenberg DA, Simon RP. *Clinical Neurology*, 6th ed. New York: McGraw-Hill, 2005: 329.)

▪ **What is the most likely diagnosis?**	This is a common history for a chronic subdural hematoma. The diagnosis is confirmed by CT scan (see Figure 10-23 above), which shows a crescent-shaped area of hemorrhage that crosses cranial suture lines.
▪ **What is the source of bleeding in this type of injury?**	Subdural hematomas result from head trauma that causes venous bleeding, most commonly from bridging veins within the dura, which then bleed into the space between the arachnoid and dura mater.
▪ **What would explain the delayed onset of symptoms?**	Symptoms in chronic subdural hematoma result from an expanding blood accumulation, which slowly and progressively compresses the cerebrum. Deficits in central nervous system functioning may be delayed depending on when specific intracranial areas are affected by the compression.
▪ **What would one expect to see on CT scan if the patient experienced no loss of consciousness, followed shortly thereafter by mental status changes?**	This scenario is more consistent with an **epidural hematoma.** The CT scan of an epidural hematoma (see Figure 10-24 on the following page) usually shows a biconcave disk formation that does not cross suture lines. The most common source of bleeding in epidural hematoma is lacerations of the middle meningeal artery.

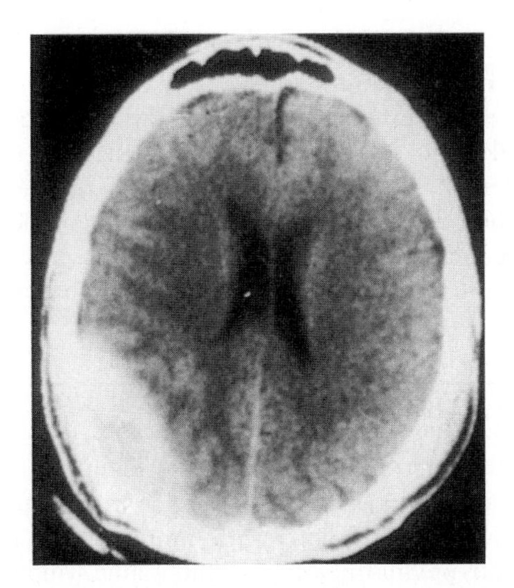

FIGURE 10-24. Epidural hematoma. (Reproduced, with permission, from Aminoff MJ, Greenberg DA, Simon RP. *Clinical Neurology*, 6th ed. New York: McGraw-Hill, 2005: 329.)

▶ Case 32

A 38-year-old man with human immunodeficiency virus (HIV) infection presents with pneumonia after decreased compliance with his HIV medications. He has a 2-month history of anorexia and weight loss and appears tachypneic. He is admitted to the hospital and given an albuterol inhaler, which helps to resolve his breathing difficulties. During physical examination 2 days later, he reports insomnia and appears agitated with grandiose plans for the future. He has rapid and pressured speech and appears to have a euphoric affect. He is also tachycardic. When asked about his mood, he reports he feels "sunny."

▪ **What is the most likely diagnosis?**	Steroid-induced mania.
▪ **What drugs are most commonly associated with these symptoms?**	Drug-induced mania can be secondary to ingestion of cocaine or amphetamines. Cortiocosteroids are the most common iatrogenic cause of manic symptoms. Although more likely to cause depression, prednisone can result in manic symptoms when acutely prescribed.
▪ **What signs and symptoms are commonly associated with this condition?**	▪ Dilated pupils ▪ ECG arrhythmia or ischemia ▪ Hypertension ▪ Manic syndrome ▪ Tachycardia
▪ **What tests are useful in confirming the diagnosis?**	Urine or serum toxicology screening can identify specific drugs the patient may have ingested. If the patient is in the hospital, the medication list should be reviewed for possible iatrogenic cause.
▪ **What are the most appropriate treatments for this condition?**	The dose of steroids should be reduced as much as clinically possible. If agitation or psychotic symptoms are present, haloperidol is useful, sometimes also with lorazepam. Calcium-channel blockers can be used for the acute autonomic symptoms.
▪ **These symptoms could also be seen in which other psychiatric disorders?**	These symptoms are also common in patients with delirium, bipolar disorder (manic type), or schizophrenia.

▶ Case 33

A 61-year-old man with a history of chronic diarrhea presents to the emergency department after fainting. He reports he suddenly collapsed after getting up to go to the bathroom. He did not note any prodromal symptoms or vertigo. The patient has spent the past few days recovering from the flu, during which time he has had a poor appetite. He denies a history of seizures and has no known cardiac or valvular abnormalities. On admission, his blood pressure is 115/80 mm Hg supine and 90/70 mm Hg standing. His pulse is 88/min, and his respiratory rate is 20/min.

What is the most likely diagnosis?	Syncope.
What signs of volume depletion are evident on physical examination?	Orthostatic hypotension, tachycardia, tachypnea, dry mucous membranes, and decreased skin turgor are evident on physical examination.
What are the major causes of this condition?	In order of decreasing frequency: ▪ Vasovagal reflex ▪ Cardiogenic causes (including arrhythmias, aortic stenosis, tamponade, pulmonary embolism, and aortic dissection) ▪ Neurogenic causes (including transient ischemic attack, migraine, and seizure) ▪ Orthostatic hypotension ▪ Medications No cause can be determined in many cases.
What is the most likely cause of this condition in this patient?	The most likely cause of syncope in this patient is orthostatic hypotension secondary to poor food and water intake and chronic diarrhea.
What is the Bezold-Jarisch reflex?	An increase in sympathetic tone induces a vigorous ventricular contraction, leading to a reflex increase in vagal tone. This reflex reaction (the so-called **Bezold-Jarisch reflex**) leads to a decrease in heart rate and/or blood pressure via the vagus nerve.
How does the vascular system compensate for the decrease in venous return following an orthostatic change?	Mechanoreceptors in the heart react to the decrease in blood pressure and compensate by increasing sympathetic tone, which decreases vagal tone and increases ADH release. This results in increased peripheral vascular resistance (increasing venous return) and an increase in cardiac output, thereby minimizing the drop in blood pressure.

► Case 34

A 57-year-old obese, right-handed man with a history of atrial fibrillation and mitral valve repair is brought to the emergency department by a coworker, who noticed a sudden onset of slurred speech and hand clumsiness. The coworker states the man's speech suddenly became slow, as if he had trouble finding words, as well as slurred. The coworker also notes the patient was generally confused but able to understand and follow commands, and he denied seeing any seizure-like activity or loss of consciousness. The patient denies any recent head trauma. Physical examination reveals an irregularly irregular heartbeat and a left carotid bruit. Neurologic examination reveals the patient's cranial nerves are grossly intact with the exception of mildly decreased facial sensation on the right. He has 4/5 muscle strength in his extremities and diminished sensation in the right arm. A CT scan of the head is negative for bleeding or mass lesion. The patient's symptoms resolve spontaneously within 2 hours of their onset.

- **What is the most likely diagnosis?**

Transient ischemic attack.

- **What is the most likely cause of this condition in this patient?**

This is most likely an **embolic stroke,** as the patient has several risk factors for emboli:
- Carotid stenosis, presumably from atherosclerosis, which can be a source of emboli
- History of atrial fibrillation, which can predispose to embolus formation
- Mitral valve repair, which can harbor vegetations that may embolize

- **What findings on CT scan of the head suggest the presence of cerebral edema?**

Signs of cerebral edema include loss of the gray matter-white matter junction; loss of prominence of sulci; and evidence of a mass effect, such as midline shift, decreased size of the lateral ventricles, and uncal herniation.

- **What artery supplies the affected area of the brain in this patient?**

The patient experienced right hand clumsiness, suggesting a left hemisphere event (motor fibers cross at the pyramidal decussation at the level of the midbrain; see Figure 10-25 on the following page for a review of the circle of Willis). His speech deficit also suggests a compromise of blood to his left hemisphere, as the verbal center in most right-handed individuals is in the left hemisphere. The left middle cerebral artery, supplying the motor cortex and verbal centers, is the most likely culprit in this patient.

- **What are the components of a neurologic language examination?**

- **Comprehension:** This is disrupted in patients with Wernicke's aphasia
- **Speech production, or fluency:** This is disrupted in patients with Broca's aphasia
- **Repetition**
- **Naming**

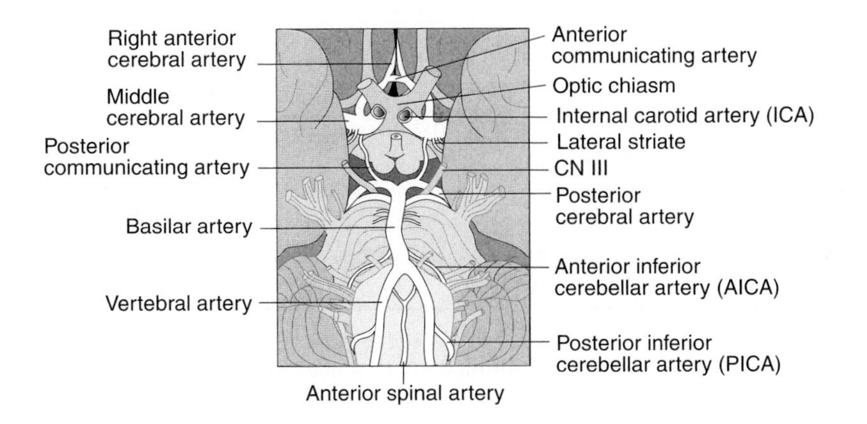

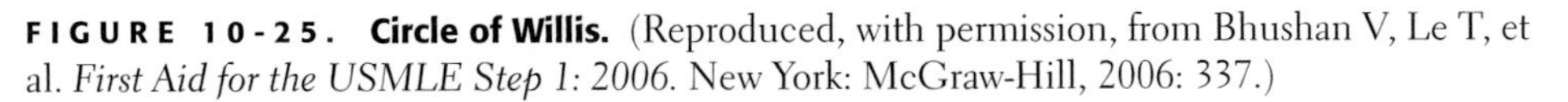

FIGURE 10-25. Circle of Willis. (Reproduced, with permission, from Bhushan V, Le T, et al. *First Aid for the USMLE Step 1: 2006*. New York: McGraw-Hill, 2006: 337.)

▶ Case 35

A 45-year-old man visits his primary care physician because he has noticed that his hearing has progressively worsened. Otologic examination reveals the patient's external ear canals are occluded with cerumen. The physician instructs the patient to use a ceruminolytic preparation overnight and to return the next day. On the following day, the physician performs a test that includes placing warm water into the patient's right ear canal. This causes the patient's eyes to move in an unusual way, rhythmically moving slowly toward the right and then jumping quickly back to the midline.

- **What reflex is being demonstrated here?**

This is the vestibulo-ocular reflex, which is responsible for keeping the eyes stabilized on an object while the head or body is in motion.

- **What are the patient's eye movements called?**

These rhythmic eye movements are called **nystagmus.** Nystagmus consists of two alternating phases: the slow phase, in which the eyes move slowly and smoothly as if they were following a moving object, and the fast phase, during which the eyes return to midline with rapid, saccadic movements. By convention, nystagmus is labeled according to the direction of the fast phase; this patient thus has a leftward nystagmus.

- **What is the pathway of this reflex?**

When warm water is introduced to the external ear canal, it induces convection currents that stimulate the semicircular canals. When a patient's head is tilted to about 60°, the horizontal canals are most stimulated. Input from the semicircular canals travels via the vestibular nerve to the vestibular nuclei in the brain stem. From there, projections travel along the medial longitudinal fasciculus to the nuclei of cranial nerves III, IV, and VI (see Figure 10-26 on the following page). From these nuclei, inhibitory and excitatory motor projections coordinate the eye movements of nystagmus.

- **How do the semicircular canals sense movement?**

Each semicircular canal has an ampulla at its base that contains hair cells embedded in the crista ampullaris. When the endolymph within the semicircular canals moves as a result of movement of the head, it displaces the hair cells, and this mechanical disruption is translated into **depolarization** if the flow of fluid is one direction, or **hyperpolarization** if the fluid moves in the opposite direction.

- **If the physician had used cold water to irrigate the ear canal, would the reflex have been elicited?**

Both warm water and cold water can stimulate the vestibulo-ocular reflex. However, because the direction of endolymph flow depends on convection currents set up by the temperature of the water in the external canal, warm water stimulates nystagmus toward the side of stimulation, while cold water stimulates nystagmus away from the side of stimulation. This can be remembered by the mnemonic **COWS** (**C**old = **O**pposite, **W**arm = **S**ame). Note, however, that this maneuver is rarely performed in an awake patient, as it can be associated with nausea. When performed in a comatose patient, the maneuver may elicit only the slow phase.

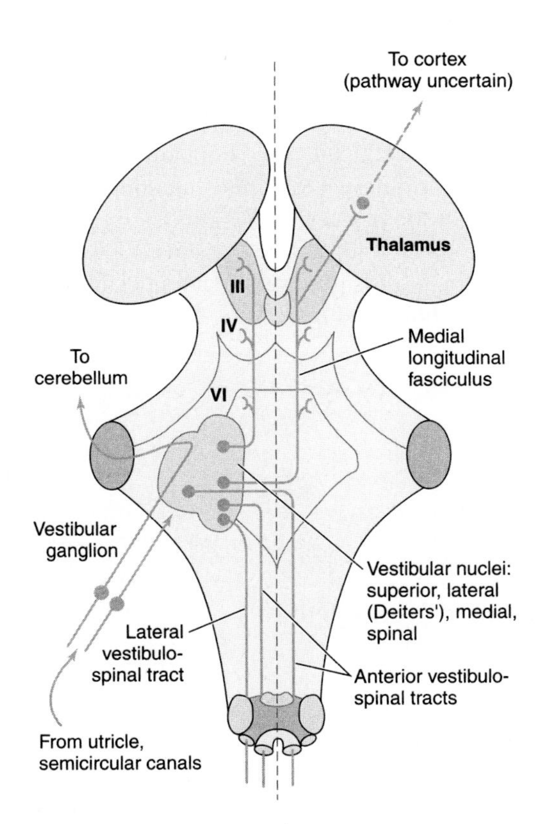

FIGURE 10-26. Principal vestibular pathways superimposed on a dorsal view of the brain stem. (Reproduced, with permission, from Ganong WF. *Review of Medical Physiology*, 19th ed. Stamford, CT: Appleton & Lange, 1999. Copyright © The McGraw-Hill Companies, Inc.)

▶ **Case 36**

A 14-year-old boy is sent to the emergency department (ED) by the nurse at his summer camp after he experienced a 1-minute seizure earlier that day. The boy has no previous history of seizure activity. In the ED, the boy complains of lethargy, vomiting, myalgias, severe headache, and neck stiffness. On further questioning, he reveals he has had many of these symptoms for the past few days. A lumbar puncture is performed, and a Gram stain of the cerebrospinal fluid (CSF) is negative. However, polymerase chain reaction (PCR) analysis of the CSF is positive for viral nucleic acid sequences. The cells found in the boy's CSF are shown in Figure 10-27 below.

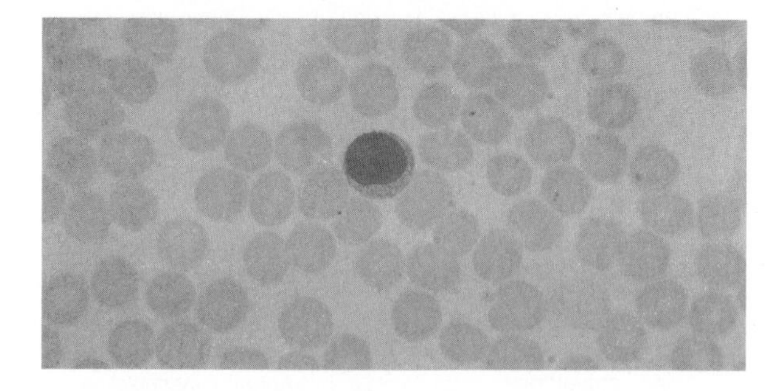

FIGURE 10-27. (Reproduced, with permission, from Berman I. *Color Atlas of Basic Histology*, 3rd ed. New York: McGraw-Hill, 2003: 107.)

■ **What is the most likely diagnosis?**	This likely represents a viral meningitis.
■ **What organisms are most likely to cause this condition?**	The most common causative organism of viral meningoencephalitis is **echovirus**, which is part of the enterovirus subgroup of the picornavirus family. Other causative organisms include coxsackievirus (another enterovirus), adenovirus, human immunodeficiency virus, cytomegalovirus, Epstein-Barr virus, and herpes simplex virus.
■ **Detection of the most likely viral agent with PCR requires modification of the standard PCR strategy. What type of enzyme is essential to this modification?**	Reverse transcriptase. Because enteroviruses are RNA viruses, detection proceeds with "reverse transcript PCR." Basically, viral RNA is transcribed into DNA, and that DNA is amplified using the standard PCR DNA amplification strategy.
■ **What changes in this patient's glucose and protein levels in CSF are most likely to be seen?**	As with most cases of viral meningitis, CSF glucose concentration should be normal and CSF protein concentration should be normal to slightly increased. This is in contrasted to CSF findings in bacterial meningitis, in which protein is increased, glucose is decreased, and polymorphonuclear leukocytes are prominent in the CSF. Table 10-1 on the following page compares CSF findings in bacterial, viral, and fungal meningitis.
■ **Some viruses capable of causing this patient's symptoms are sensitive to acyclovir. What is the mechanism of action of this drug?**	Acyclovir targets viral DNA polymerase. Herpesviruses are DNA viruses that are sensitive to acyclovir. Picornaviruses, however, are RNA viruses that do not contain DNA polymerase, and therefore they are not sensitive to acyclovir.
■ **What type of cells is shown in Figure 10-27 above?**	The cell in Figure 10-27 is a **lymphocyte**, which is characterized by its small size, with most of the cell volume occupied by the darkly stained and round nucleus. Lymphocytes play a key role in cellular immunity, particularly in the combating of viral infection. Lymphocytosis of the CSF is commonly seen in viral meningitis.

TABLE 10-1. CSF Findings in Meningitis

	Pressure	Cell Type	Protein	Sugar
Bacterial	↑	↑ PMNs	↑	↓
Fungal/TB	↑	↑ lymphocytes	↑	↓
Viral	Normal/↑	↑ lymphocytes	Normal	Normal

Reprinted, with permission, from Bhushan V, Le T, et al. *First Aid for the USMLE Step 1: 2006.* New York: McGraw-Hill, 2006: 161.

▶ Case 37

A 30-year-old woman presents to the emergency department (ED) with complaints of involuntary twitching of her lips and tongue. Upon questioning, she reveals she was diagnosed with schizophrenia in her early twenties and has achieved fairly good control of her psychotic symptoms with both oral and intramuscular depot antipsychotic agents. She recalls one prior visit to the ED shortly after she was diagnosed with schizophrenia for evaluation of a neck spasm that was painful and "locked my neck to the left."

What is the most likely diagnosis?	Tardive dyskinesia. Extrapyramidal symptoms, such as stereotypic oral, buccal, or lingual movements and choreiform or athetoid movements, can be seen after several months or years of therapy with antipsychotic agents. These symptoms are often irreversible.
What is the pathophysiology of this condition?	Dopamine$_2$ receptor supersensitivity after long-term use of antidopaminergic drugs is the likely cause.
What risk factors are associated with this condition?	▪ Diabetes mellitus ▪ History of movement disorders ▪ Tobacco use ▪ Typical antipsychotic agents (strong risk factor, especially higher doses for longer periods)
What other movement abnormalities are associated with the use of antipsychotic agents?	▪ Acute dystonia (sustained muscular spasms—facial, torticollis, oculogyric crisis) is the earliest to present (within hours) ▪ Akathisia, characterized by extreme restlessness, is the most common extrapyramidal disorder and is one of the most likely causes of medication nonadherence ▪ Akinesia (characterized by extreme restlessness)
What can be done to minimize the future risk of developing these symptoms?	Lowering the dose of typical antipsychotic agents can result in resolution of symptoms, but this may produce a transient worsening of dyskinesia, because of dopamine receptor supersensitivity. Switching patients to atypical antipsychotic agents is advised, as they are associated with fewer extrapyramidal symptoms. Clozapine is the least likely of all antipsychotic drugs to cause tardive dyskinesia, but may be difficult to administer because of the need for routine hematologic monitoring. High doses of vitamin E have been used with variable success; its effect is thought to be a result of its antioxidant properties.

▶ Case 38

A 26-year-old man is being evaluated by a neurologist for recurrent headaches and changes in vision. A careful ophthalmologic examination reveals multiple hemangiomas of the retina in both eyes, and an MRI of the brain demonstrates three hemangioblastomas of the cerebellum.

What is the most likely diagnosis?	von Hippel–Lindau (VHL) disease. This disease is characterized by diffuse hemangioma formation, including cavernous hemangiomas, as well as by an increased incidence of renal cell carcinoma (RCC).
What is the pattern of inheritance for this condition?	VHL disease is inherited in an autosomal dominant fashion in 75% of cases. It is associated with deletion of the *VHL* gene, a tumor suppressor gene on the short arm of chromosome 3. Twenty-five percent of cases occur sporadically. In the United States, the incidence of VHL disease is about 1 in 36,000 individuals.
What is Knudsen's two-hit theory of carcinogenesis?	Dr. Alfred Knudsen described the recessive nature of target genes involved in the development of retinoblastoma in infancy. The two-hit theory of carcinogenesis describes a gene product whose normal function is to inhibit cell growth (a **tumor suppressor gene**). An individual may inherit one inactive allele (the first "**hit**"), but the remaining allele can suppress cell growth. If a second hit is acquired in the somatic cell, there is no longer any tumor suppressor activity, and there is a tendency toward growth and malignant progression. The *VHL* gene on chromosome 3 acts as a classic tumor suppressor gene.
What is the leading cause of death in patients with this condition?	RCC, predominantly the clear cell type, is the leading cause of death in patients with VHL, with some case series reporting a prevalence as high as 40%–75% at autopsy. In patients with VHL, RCC develops from malignant degeneration of renal cysts and is usually bilateral. The average age for development of RCC in patients with VHL is 44 years. Because of the high incidence of renal cysts and RCC in patients with VHL, periodic imaging of the kidneys is key in patients and at-risk relatives.
What other tumors and lesions are patients with this condition at increased risk of developing?	Patients with VHL disease are at risk for developing multiple cysts in the liver, epididymis, pancreas, and kidneys. Pheochromocytomas, rare pancreatic carcinomas, and endolymphatic sac tumors are also part of the spectrum of VHL. Hemangioblastomas are typically in the cerebellum or medulla but may also occur in the spinal cord. Hemangiomas of the retina are common and are often bilateral.

► Case 39

A 55-year-old man is brought to the emergency department by a friend who has noticed the patient has had memory lapses and difficulty with walking and balance. The patient has a 26-year history of excessive alcohol use. On further questioning, the patient is unable to relate a consistent history. When asked about his location, the patient states he is at home. Physical examination reveals his left eye does not adduct on rightward gaze, and his gait is ataxic.

What is the most likely diagnosis?	These symptoms are suggestive of Wernicke's encephalopathy, which classically presents as the triad of **ophthalmoplegia** (paralysis of one or more eye muscles), ataxia, and encephalopathy. This may progress to Korsakoff's syndrome, which consists of memory lapses, confusion, and confabulation.
What type of memory deficit is likely to be seen in this condition?	Patients with Wernicke-Korsakoff syndrome usually suffer from **anterograde amnesia,** which is characterized by an inability to form new memories with general preservation of long-term memories. This is in contrast to **retrograde amnesia,** in which the only memories that are lost are long-term memories that precede the precipitating event.
What is the pathophysiology of this condition?	This disease is seen in alcoholics with thiamine deficiency due to poor nutrition and absorption. The thiamine deficiency results in periventricular hemorrhage and degeneration in a symmetric pattern in multiple cerebral areas, including the cerebellum, brain stem, and bilateral mammillary bodies (see Figure 10-28 below; arrows show abnormal enhancement of the mammillary bodies).
What specific cranial nerve pathway is responsible for the abnormality noted on lateral gaze?	Inability to adduct the left eye on rightward gaze suggests a left medial longitudinal fasciculus (MLF) lesion. Normally, the abducens nucleus projects neurons both to the ipsilateral lateral rectus muscle via cranial nerve (CN) VI and to the contralateral medial rectus muscle via the MLF and CN III. In this case, the contralateral MLF pathway must be damaged, resulting in inability to adduct the contralateral (left) eye during lateral gaze.
For which essential biochemical pathways is thiamine required?	Thiamine is needed for the oxidative carboxylation of α-keto acids and is a cofactor for the transketolase hexose monophosphate shunt.
What other disease can result from thiamine deficiency?	**Beriberi** is a deficiency of thiamine (vitamin B_1) secondary to malnutrition. It is characterized by peripheral neuropathy and axonal demyelination.

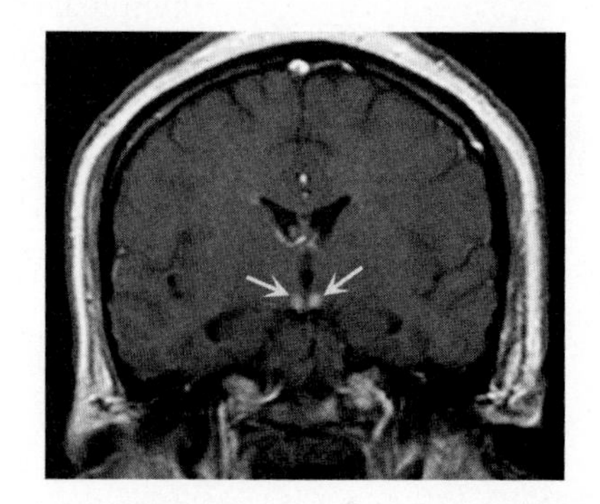

FIGURE 10-28. MRI of mammillary bodies in Wernicke's disease. (Reproduced, with permission, from Kasper DL, et al. *Harrison's Principles of Internal Medicine,* 16th ed. New York: McGraw-Hill, 2005: 1636.)

▶ Case 40

A 14-year-old boy is brought to his family physician complaining of weakness of his left hand and wrist. He is a varsity tennis player and has been having difficulty playing, and over the past week he has developed a burning sensation and numbness of the fourth and fifth fingers of his left hand. He says he woke up with the change in sensation/strength after falling asleep with his left arm over the side of his bed. Physical examination reveals no evidence of fracture, but there is significant edema of his elbow and a generalized weakness of the medial digits.

▪ **What is the most likely diagnosis?**	Injury of the ulnar nerve. Ulnar nerve injuries often present in a partial "clawlike" deformity. There is typically weakness of wrist and little and ring finger flexion at the metacarpophalangeal (MP) joint, and difficulty abducting and adducting the fingers at the MP joints. Flexion of the index and the middle finger at the MP joint will be normal. The typical sensory changes in the ulnar territory are felt in the medial hand and medial 1.5 fingers. The median nerve targets (both motor and sensory) will be preserved.
▪ **Describe the function of the radial and ulnar nerves.**	The **radial nerve** supplies arm extension at the elbow, wrist extension, metacarpal extension, interphalangeal joint extension, and thumb extension and supination. It provides sensory information for the back of the upper arm below the insertion of the deltoid, the forearm, and the hand. The **ulnar nerve** causes flexion of the medial wrist and flexion of the MP, proximal interphalangeal (PIP), and distal interphalangeal (DIP) joints of the ring and little fingers (it supplies the flexor carpal ulnaris muscle and the medial part of the flexor digitorum profundus muscles—the extrinsic muscles of the hand). It also innervates all intrinsic muscles of the hand except the thenar muscles and the first two lumbricals. Its functions in the hand, therefore, are adduction at the carpometacarpal joint of the thumb and adduction and abduction at the MP joints of all fingers. The ulnar nerve also is responsible for flexion at the MP joint and simultaneous extension of the PIP and DIP joints. It provides sensory information to the medial palm and dorsum of the hand and the medial half of the ring and little fingers (both palmar and dorsal surfaces).
▪ **What movements of the hand will be weakened by this injury?**	Wrist adduction or ulnar deviation (flexor carpi ulnaris) and adduction and abduction at the MP joints will be affected. Patients are unable to hold anything between their fingers, and thumb adduction will also be affected. The ulnar nerve regulates sensation in the medial 1.5 fingers and the medial border of the hand.
▪ **What are the most common causes of this injury?**	Injuries include direct trauma and prolonged pressure or compression of the nerve. Ulnar nerve damage is a distal neuropathy. The symptoms occur because the myelin sheath is destroyed, which slows or prevents nerve conduction. The most common site of ulnar nerve injury is at the elbow, because the nerve lies superficially in the groove between the medial epicondyle and the olecranon. A hit on the medial epicondyle often hits the nerve, causing tingling in the territory of the ulnar nerve and the so-called "funny bone."
▪ **What is the most appropriate treatment to reduce the swelling at this patient's elbow?**	Corticosteroids.

NOTES

Renal System

▶ Case 1

A 29-year-old woman who was involved in a motor vehicle accident is brought to the emergency department, where she is found to be hypotensive with severe internal bleeding. She is given several units of blood by transfusion and is sent to the intensive care unit for monitoring. Within 36 hours, a slight decrease in urine output and an increase in blood urea nitrogen (BUN) are noted, and by 72 hours there is a dramatic drop in urine output. Laboratory studies at 72 hours demonstrate the following:

Serum
- Potassium: 5.1 mEq/L
- BUN: 25 mg/dL
- Creatinine: 2.5 mg/dL

Urinalysis: mild hematuria, mild proteinuria, granular casts, renal tubular epithelial cells in sediment

Fractional excretion of sodium (Fe_{Na}): 2.2%

What is the most likely diagnosis?	The patient is most likely suffering from acute tubular necrosis (ATN) secondary to renal ischemia as a consequence of shock following the accident. ATN is the most common cause of acute renal failure and is a result of direct injury to the renal tubular epithelia.
What are common causes of this condition?	Common causes include renal ischemia (shock), crush injury (myoglobin is nephrotoxic), and various toxins, including some chemotherapeutic agents and aminoglycoside antibiotics.
What is the cause of the patient's azotemia?	ATN involves direct damage to renal tubular epithelial cells. The loss of intact tubule cells in addition to the blockage of the tubular lumen by necrotic cellular debris serve to block the collecting system. This leads in turn to fluid backflow across the tubule and, consequently, to a decreased glomerular filtration rate (GFR).
How do the laboratory findings assist in establishing the diagnosis?	Epithelial cells and granular casts in the urine are pathognomonic for ATN. Hematuria and proteinuria may also be found. The urine is typically isotonic. With ATN, the serum creatinine level rises rapidly, but the BUN:creatinine ratio remains nearly normal. Additionally, the Fe_{Na} is often >2% (in contrast with prerenal azotemia, where Fe_{Na} is <1% and the BUN:creatinine ratio rises to >20:1). This is due to sodium wasting as a result of tubular damage and is also a normal response to volume expansion due to decreased GFR.
What is the prognosis for patients with this condition?	ATN goes through an initiatory phase within 36 hours of injury with a slight decrease in urine output and an increase in BUN. Within 2–6 days, there is a dramatic fall in urine output that can last for weeks. During this maintenance phase, there is a significant risk of death without proper management. Recovery typically occurs within 2–3 weeks.

▶ Case 2

A 27-year-old man visits his physician because he is concerned about the large amounts of blood he has noticed in his urine over the past week. He denies increased frequency or dysuria but does admit to intermittent aching back pain over the past few months, which he attributes to sitting at his desk for long periods of time each day at work. Ultrasound shows massively enlarged kidneys bilaterally. The surface of the right kidney is studded with several dozen well-circumscribed cysts, and ultrasound of the left kidney demonstrates similar lesions.

What is the most likely diagnosis?	Autosomal dominant polycystic kidney disease (ADPKD).
What is the mode of inheritance of this condition?	Roughly 90% of cases of ADPKD are due to a mutation in the *APKD1* gene on chromosome 16. The disease is inherited in an autosomal dominant fashion. The juvenile form of the disease, which is exceedingly rare, is inherited in an autosomal recessive fashion.
How do patients with this condition typically present?	ADPKD may present at any age but is most frequently diagnosed in the third to fifth decades. Patients experience chronic flank pain as a result of massively enlarged kidneys, and microscopic or massive hematuria is common. Nocturia may be present if renal concentrating ability is impaired. Hypertension at presentation is not uncommon.
What are the extrarenal manifestations of this condition?	Colonic diverticular disease is the most common extrarenal effect of ADPKD. Hepatic cysts (see Figure 11-1 below) are present in 50%–70% of patients and are generally asymptomatic with little effect on liver function. There is an association between ADPKD and berry aneurysms, with a potential for significant injury or death from subarachnoid hemorrhage. Mitral valve prolapse is found in 25% of patients with this disease.
What is the prognosis for patients with this condition?	Progression to chronic renal failure is common, with 50% of patients developing **end-stage renal disease** by age 60 years. There is great variability in the progression of the disease even within families. Early age at diagnosis, male sex, recurrent infection, and hypertension are all associated with an early onset of renal failure.

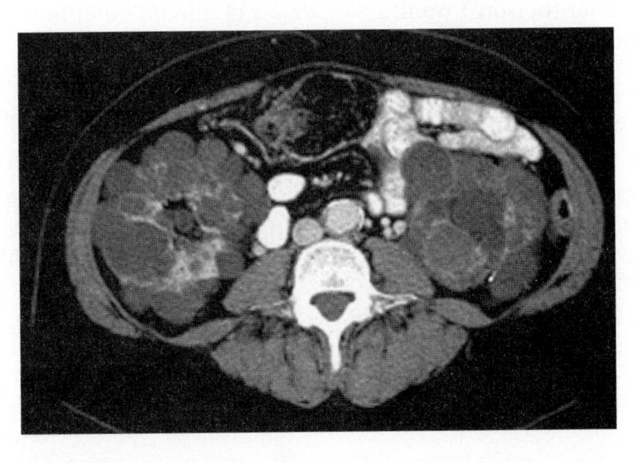

FIGURE 11-1. **Bilateral kidney cysts in polycystic kidney disease.** (Reproduced with permission of the Pathology Education Instructional Resource Digital Library (http://peir.net) at the University of Alabama, Birmingham.)

► Case 3

A 10-year-old boy is brought to his pediatrician for evaluation of bloody urine. A urine sample is positive for hemoglobin and RBC casts. The boy's maternal grandfather suffered from deafness and died of renal failure. The boy also has a 25-year-old male maternal cousin who currently uses a hearing aid and requires dialysis for end-stage renal disease. The family pedigree is shown in Figure 11-2 below; the boy is indicated by the arrow, his maternal grandfather by the number 1, and his maternal cousin by the number 2. Darkened symbols represent people with known renal disease.

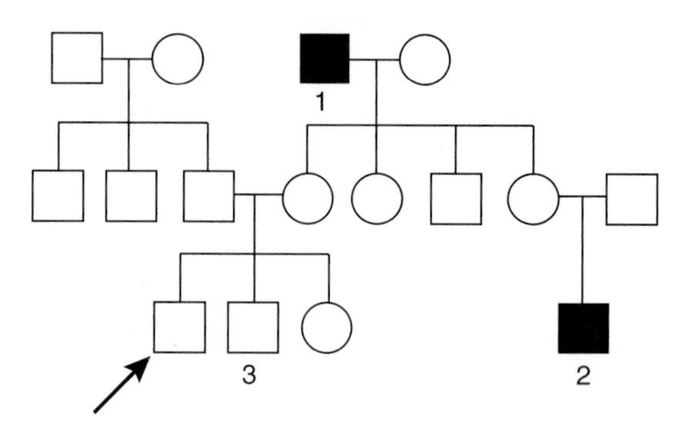

FIGURE 11-2.

What is the most likely diagnosis?	The likely diagnosis is hereditary nephritis, or Alport's syndrome, which consists of glomerular disease, nerve deafness, and ocular abnormalities such as lens dislocation and cataracts. These patients often progress to end-stage renal disease by age 30 years.
This condition is due to a mutation in a gene coding for which protein?	The defective gene codes for the α_5 subunit of type IV collagen. Tissue from patients with this mutation fails to stain for this protein.
Because of this mutation, the glomerulus loses the ability to selectively filter on the basis of what property?	Size. The glomerular basement membrane is primarily a size-selective filter, and thus damage to the basement membrane leads to loss of size selectivity.
What is the probability that this patient's brother (person 3 on the pedigree above) has the same disease?	The probability is 50%. The pedigree represents X-linked dominant inheritance. Since the boy's mother is a carrier, each son has a 50% chance (one of two X chromosomes in the mother) of inheriting the mutation. There are also autosomal recessive and autosomal dominant variants of Alport's syndrome.
What other screening tests, in addition to urinalysis, should be performed on this patient?	Because Alport's syndrome is associated with ocular abnormalities and deafness, sensitive vision and hearing tests should be performed, as deficits may be subtle. Skin biopsies can also be useful in diagnosing Alport's syndrome.

▶ Case 4

A 4-year-old boy presents with a rash of 2 days' duration that has spread from his legs to his buttocks. He is not febrile and has no sick contacts or other pertinent exposures. The rash consists of nonclustering, nonblanching, raised spots of more than 2 mm spread over the boy's lower body. The boy also complains of knee and ankle stiffness and diffuse abdominal pain. His vital signs are stable, and a urinalysis is unremarkable. His laboratory findings are as follows:

Hematocrit: 35%
WBC count: 7000/mm^3
Platelet count: 200,000/mm^3
International Normalized Ratio (INR): 1.0
Prothrombin time: 12 sec
Partial thromboplastin time: 25.2 sec

What is the most likely diagnosis?

Henoch-Schönlein purpura (HSP). In children, the combination of rash (as described above), arthralgias, abdominal pain, and renal disease is pathognomonic for HSP, although only 63% of patients with HSP actually present with abdominal pain and only 40% with renal disease. An additional 33% of patients also have evidence of gastrointestinal bleeding. Less common symptoms include intussusception, pancreatitis, cholecystitis, and protein-losing enteropathy. Some 1% of children with HSP progress to end-stage renal disease. HSP is more common in children than in adults.

What are the distinguishing characteristics of this condition?

Purpura is characterized by nonblanching, flat lesions measuring more than 2 mm in diameter. Related findings are **petechiae,** which are nonblanching, flat lesions measuring <2 mm in diameter. Both are signs of bleeding occurring in the skin. Both purpuric and petechial lesions may be seen in HSP.

What is the pathophysiology of this condition?

HSP is a small vessel vasculitis. Although the precipitating factor is unknown, anecdotal evidence points to upper respiratory infection for children. With HSP, IgA deposition in blood vessels causes leaking, which leads to purpura and petechiae. This is pathophysiologically similar to IgA nephropathy.

Which conditions should be considered in the differential diagnosis of this patient's rash?

The main concerns, in addition to HSP, are clotting disorders and sepsis; as a result, coagulation studies should be performed. A similar rash can be caused by rickettsial infections, although this patient is afebrile. It is very important to distinguish HSP from **hemolytic-uremic syndrome** (HUS), as both present similarly and both can cause extensive renal disease. However, HUS is not likely in this patient, as there are no signs of hemolytic anemia. In adults, HSP must be distinguished from systemic diseases such as hypersensitivity vasculitis and systemic lupus erythematosus.

What are the most appropriate treatments for this condition?

Treatment is based on the severity of symptoms, as the disease is typically self-limiting. An asymptomatic patient requires no treatment. However, severe symptoms, including signs of renal involvement, require intravenous steroids. Regardless of the severity of symptoms, patients with HSP require urinalysis every 3 months for 1 year, as HSP has a high rate of recurrence. Patients have been known to experience recurrence from 6 months to 80 years after the initial diagnosis.

▶ Case 5

A 45-year-old man is brought to the emergency department by his mother after 2 days of worsening confusion, diuresis, polydipsia, and constipation. His past medical history is significant only for chronic osteomyelitis of the right arm secondary to a burn injury sustained in a house fire 5 years ago. Physical examination is unremarkable with the exception of uniformly depressed deep tendon reflexes. The patient is also visibly uncomfortable and disoriented and is uncooperative during much of the examination. ECG reveals a QTc interval of 390 msec. Relevant laboratory findings are as follows:

Serum calcium: 8.26 mEq/L
Serum albumin: 1.45 mEq/L
Ionized calcium: 7.06 mg/dL
Blood urea nitrogen (BUN):creatinine ratio: 29:1.4

The patient is immediately started on 1 L of normal saline with a goal of 4–6 L over 24 hours, with furosemide added shortly thereafter.

- **What other symptoms are common in this condition?**

Symptoms of hypercalcemia include lethargy, hyporeflexia, confusion, depression, headaches, psychosis, bradycardia, a shortened QT interval, nausea, vomiting, constipation, muscle weakness, polyuria, polydipsia, and gastroduodenal ulcer disease.

- **How does hypoalbuminemia affect this condition?**

Hypoalbuminemia can decrease serum calcium levels independently of any net change in ionized calcium levels. One should anticipate a drop of approximately 0.8 mg/dL in total serum calcium for each decrease of 1.0 g/dL in serum albumin below normal.

- **What is the importance of ionized calcium and albumin in the diagnosis of this condition?**

The fraction of ionized calcium determines the activity of cellular and membrane functions. The proportion of ionized calcium can vary without any concordant change in overall calcium concentration secondary to variations in plasma protein concentration. Additionally, changes in serum pH alter the fraction of ionized calcium. For example, alkaline pH decreases the fraction of ionized calcium.

- **What are pseudohypercalcemia and pseudohypocalcemia?**

Pseudohypercalcemia and the converse, **pseudohypocalcemia,** refer to perturbations in net calcium concentration in the setting of a normal ionized fraction. Given a normal ionized fraction, the clinical picture is normal. They are usually caused by alterations in plasma protein concentration.

- **What is hypercalcemic crisis?**

This patient was in hypercalcemic crisis. Calcium acts as a direct toxin to the renal tubules and thereby blocks ADH activity, causing vasoconstriction and decreasing the glomerular filtration rate. This results in polyuria but increases calcium reabsorption and serum calcium, thereby exacerbating nephrotoxicity.

- **What are the most appropriate treatments for this condition?**

Symptomatic hypercalcemia, as seen in this patient, should first be treated with a saline infusion to expedite renal calcium excretion. Furosemide may be initiated in these patients to promote calciuresis only after the patient is volume repleted. Furosemide serves both to promote natriuresis and to increase calcium excretion. Care must be taken to ensure the patient does not become hypovolemic during calciuresis. Bisphosphonates inhibit osteoclast activity and are efficacious in the treatment of hypercalcemia secondary to this mechanism. Given this patient's past history of chronic osteomyelitis, there is a high clinical suspicion for underlying soft tissue malignancy.

▶ Case 6

A 57-year-old man with a history of coronary artery disease presents to the emergency department with a 1-week history of progressive weakness, fatigue, and shortness of breath on exertion. On physical examination, the man's heart rate is irregularly irregular, and his lung examination is notable for bilateral crackles that are most pronounced at the bases. An x-ray of the chest demonstrates pulmonary edema, and an ECG reveals he is in atrial fibrillation. The patient is started on digoxin and furosemide. Three days later, he complains of rapid onset of shortness of breath and light-headedness with progressive weakness. His laboratory values are significant for a serum sodium level of 142 mEq/L and a serum potassium level of 2.7 mEq/L. An ECG demonstrates torsades de pointes.

- **What is the most likely diagnosis?**

Hypokalemia.

- **What are the two main factors that predisposed the patient to torsades de pointes?**

The patient was started on digoxin to increase cardiac output and to treat the atrial fibrillation, and the furosemide was added to treat the pulmonary edema. However, furosemide in the setting of congestive heart failure can lead to severe hypokalemia (serum potassium level <2.5 mEq/L). Digitalis use in the setting of hypokalemia can predispose a patient to possibly fatal arrhythmias.

- **What are the most common causes of this condition?**

There are three broad etiologies of hypokalemia: decreased intake, increased losses, and increased translocation into cells.

- Decreased intake is a very rare cause of hypokalemia.
- Increased losses can either be gastrointestinal (eg, from vomiting, diarrhea, or laxative abuse) or, more commonly, urinary (eg, secondary to diuretic use, primary aldosteronism, loss of gastric secretions, metabolic acidosis, or polyuria).
- Increased translocation into cells occurs with alkalosis, increased insulin availability, β-adrenergic stimulation, and hypothermia.

- **How does alkalosis lead to this condition?**

The Na^+-K^+-ATPase pump keeps intracellular potassium levels much higher than the serum/extracellular level. However, in the setting of alkalosis, hydrogen ions leave cells to minimize pH change. In the process, hydrogen ions function in an apparent exchange for potassium that can lead to hypokalemia.

- **How is metabolic acidosis associated with this condition?**

Metabolic acidosis leads to an apparent exchange of hydrogen ions into the cells and potassium out of the cells, which would seem to cause hyperkalemia. However, in the setting of metabolic acidosis (notably diabetic ketoacidosis), urinary potassium excretion is also increased. This leads to a situation in which potassium is being moved from the cells only to be excreted in the urine; so while the serum potassium level is normal or even high in metabolic acidosis, the total body stores are actually low. The hypokalemia will often reveal itself once the acidosis is corrected.

- **What are the most appropriate treatments for this condition?**

Potassium can be repleted either directly (ie, with potassium chloride) or through the use of a potassium-sparing diuretic such as amiloride, spironolactone, or triamterene. Amiloride is often the diuretic of choice, as it lacks the hormonal adverse effects of spironolactone (gynecomastia, amenorrhea).

► Case 7

A 6-year-old boy is brought to his pediatrician after his mother notices that his limbs seem swollen and his stomach distended. She says the boy received an influenza shot 1 week ago. Physical examination reveals generalized pitting edema and shifting dullness of the abdomen suggestive of ascites. Urinalysis reveals 4+ proteinuria, and laboratory findings show a decreased serum albumin level, hypertriglyceridemia, and a decreased serum ionized calcium level. Blood urea nitrogen (BUN) and serum creatinine values are within normal limits.

■ **What is the most likely diagnosis?**	The boy likely has minimal change disease (lipoid nephrosis), the most common manifestation of nephrotic syndrome in children (approximately 90% of cases occur in children younger than 10 years of age).
■ **What are the four classic symptoms of this condition?**	Nephrotic syndrome classically presents with massive proteinuria, hypoalbuminemia, generalized edema, and hyperlipidemia.
■ **What pathologic change at the glomerular level are associated with this condition?**	The glomerular basement membrane contains heparin sulfate, which acts as a negative charge barrier that keeps small proteins such as albumin from crossing the membrane. Minimal change disease is sometimes associated with recent infection or vaccination; it is believed that T cells release cytokines that injure glomerular epithelial cells. Consequently, the negative charge barrier is damaged, while the size filter provided by nephrin deposits between foot processes remains intact. This leads to renal albumin wasting.
■ **What are the likely findings on histology?**	Glomeruli appear normal on light microscopy; hence the name "minimal change." However, when the glomeruli are viewed under electron microscopy, effacement or flattening of foot processes can be seen. The electron micrograph in Figure 11-3 below shows both a normal foot process (full arrow) and effacement of foot processes (arrowhead).
■ **What is the most appropriate treatment for this condition?**	Given the high incidence of minimal change disease in children with nephrotic syndrome, presentations such as these are assumed to be minimal change disease. Treatment consists of an empiric trial of corticosteroids.

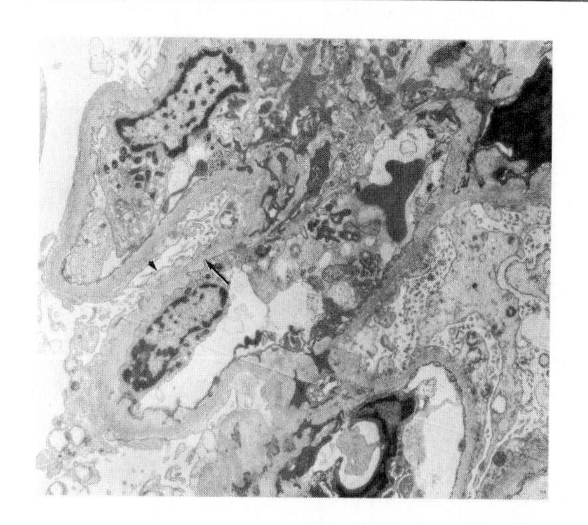

FIGURE 11-3. Electron micrograph showing glomeruli in minimal change disease. (Reproduced, with permission, from Bhushan V, Le T, et al. *First Aid for the USMLE Step 1: 2006*. New York: McGraw-Hill, 2006.)

▶ Case 8

A 6-year-old boy is sent to his school nurse after his gym teacher notes that he was unusually short of breath while playing soccer. After noticing that the boy's socks left deep indentations in his calves and shins bilaterally, the nurse obtains a urine sample that demonstrates proteinuria, but no glucose, no RBCs, and no WBCs. He is then brought to the emergency department for further workup. Relevant laboratory test results are as follows:

Sodium: 55.2 mEq/L
Potassium: 0.9 mEq/L
Serum albumin: 2.3 g/dL
Cholesterol levels: elevated

What is the most likely diagnosis?	The boy's presentation suggests nephrotic syndrome, which is characterized by the triad of high urine protein losses, hypoalbuminemia, and hypercholesterolemia. Patients often present with periorbital edema, peripheral edema, and/or ascites secondary to decreased plasma protein. This results in decreased plasma oncotic pressure in addition to sodium retention, which is a direct result of the renal disease. The most common cause of nephrotic syndrome in children is minimal change disease.
What is the most likely mechanism of this boy's proteinuria?	The likely mechanism of action is loss of charge barrier at the glomerular membrane due to effacement of foot processes.
What are the most appropriate treatments for this condition?	Prednisone. Although the etiology of minimal change disease is unknown, it is thought to be due to an immune system abnormality. Thus, corticosteroids (prednisone) and immune suppressants are commonly used. Symptomatic treatment should also be initiated for edema, hypercoagulability, infection, decreased intravascular volume, and other clinical manifestations.
What laboratory findings are likely in this condition?	Serum albumin levels would be low, and 24-hour urine protein excretion would be high secondary to the massive loss of albumin at the glomerulus. Patients also often demonstrate severe hyperlipidemia.
After 1 month of steroid treatment, the boy showed no improvement in his renal function, and a renal biopsy was obtained. What is the most likely diagnosis?	The boy likely has **focal segmental glomerular sclerosis,** which is often resistant to steroid treatment. Light microscopy of the biopsy specimen may demonstrate focal areas of glomeruli with segmental sclerosis. Electron microscopy demonstrates foot process derangement.

► Case 9

A 16-year-old previously healthy girl visits her doctor with recent-onset flank pain. She is given ibuprofen and is sent home. Three days later, she develops a fever accompanied by emesis and worsening flank pain. On evaluation, she recalls episodes of urgency as well as decreased urine output. Her physical examination is notable for a temperature of 38.9° C (102.1° F) and costovertebral angle tenderness. Her laboratory findings are as follows:

WBC count: 13,900/mm^3
Neutrophils: 74%
Lymphocytes: 10%
Monocytes: 15%

Platelet count: 181,000/mm^3
Blood urea nitrogen (BUN): 10 μg/dL
Serum creatinine: 1.1 μg/dL
Hematocrit: 33%

Urinalysis: 2+ protein, small leukocyte esterase, many WBCs, 2–5 RBCs/hpf, few bacteria, and WBC casts

- **What is the most likely diagnosis?**

Acute pyelonephritis. This diagnosis is suggested by the presence of flank pain, emesis, high fever, and costovertebral angle tenderness on examination. Pyelonephritis is most common in young children and sexually active women. Men are less likely to develop either pyelonephritis (upper urinary tract infection) or acute cystitis (lower urinary tract infection) in part because of their longer urethras. Other predisposing factors include flow obstruction, catheterization, gynecologic abnormalities, diabetes, and pregnancy.

- **What are the most likely pathogens in urinary tract infections (UTIs)?**

Escherichia coli is by far the most common cause of UTI, causing 50%–80% of cases. *Staphylococcus saprophyticus* is the second most common cause of UTI in young, sexually active women. Other common causative organisms include *Proteus mirabilis, Klebsiella, Serratia, Enterobacter,* and *Pseudomonas.* Group B β-hemolytic streptococcus infection can cause UTI in infants.

- **How can this patient's symptoms be distinguished from those associated with cystitis, urethritis, or vaginitis?**

While pyelonephritis classically manifests as flank pain, costovertebral angle tenderness, nausea, and vomiting with high fever, the classic primary complaint in cystitis is dysuria accompanied by frequency, urgency, suprapubic pain, and hematuria. In contrast, urethritis and vaginitis present with dysuria, discharge, pruritus, dyspareunia, and an absence of frequency or urgency.

- **What are the characteristic laboratory findings in this condition?**

Pyuria is an essential finding for the diagnosis of UTI. Urinalysis typically shows >10 WBCs/mL, whereas significant bacteriuria points toward pyelonephritis rather than cystitis. Hematuria is also common in women with UTI but not in women with urethritis or vaginitis. Additionally, serum tests will show leukocytosis, an elevated erythrocyte sedimentation rate, and an elevated C-reactive protein level.

- **What are the most appropriate treatments for this condition?**

The goal of empiric therapy is to use drugs that achieve high concentrations in the renal medulla. Oral medications include the fluoroquinolones (especially ciprofloxacin) and trimethoprim-sulfamethoxazole. Nitrofurantoin, while useful in cystitis because of its activity in urine, poorly concentrates in tissue and is not particularly useful for pyelonephritis. Intravenous options include ceftriaxone, ciprofloxacin, ampicillin and gentamicin, and piperacillin/tazobactam.

▶ Case 10

A 70-year-old man visits his primary care physician after going to a health fair and discovering that his blood pressure is 170/100 mm Hg. The previous year, his blood pressure was 135/85. The man also has a history of hypercholesterolemia. At the physician's office, he has a blood pressure of 150/100 mm Hg and a heart rate of 80/min, and an abdominal bruit is detected in the epigastric region to the right of midline. Laboratory findings are significant for a serum sodium level of 147 mEq/L and a serum potassium level of 3.3 mEq/L.

What is the most likely diagnosis?	The man most likely suffers from renal artery stenosis, which is often caused by atherosclerotic plaques in older men (secondary to hypercholesterolemia) and fibromuscular dysplasia in young women. This diagnosis is suggested by the relatively sudden onset of hypertension in addition to hypokalemia.
What changes in renin secretion would one expect to see from each kidney?	The kidney ipsilateral to the stenosis will increase renin secretion in response to a perceived decrease in arterial pressure due to decreased blood flow to the juxtaglomerular apparatus. The contralateral kidney will respond to the patient's resulting hypertension by decreasing its renin secretion (see Figure 11-4 below).
How does an elevated plasma renin level lead to hypertension?	In the plasma, renin converts angiotensinogen to angiotensin I, which is converted to angiotensin II by angiotensin-converting enzyme (ACE). **Angiotensin II** acts on vascular smooth muscle to increase blood pressure. Angiotensin II also acts on the adrenal cortex to stimulate the release of aldosterone, which increases renal absorption of sodium to increase blood volume, thus increasing blood pressure.
What electrolyte abnormalities are associated with this condition?	As seen in hyperaldosteronism, hypernatremia is expected as a result of renal sodium retention, and hypokalemia is expected as a consequence of renal potassium losses. (Note that the cause of hypernatremia is actually more complex, as a reset hypothalamic osmostat results in shifting of ADH release and thirst toward higher Na^+ retention.)
What is the diuretic of choice for this condition?	Spironolactone, an aldosterone antagonist, is preferred because of its potassium-sparing properties.
Which classes of antihypertensive drugs directly target the effects of renin?	ACE inhibitors (captopril, enalapril, lisinopril), angiotensin II blockers (losartan), and aldosterone-antagonizing diuretics (spironolactone) achieve this goal.

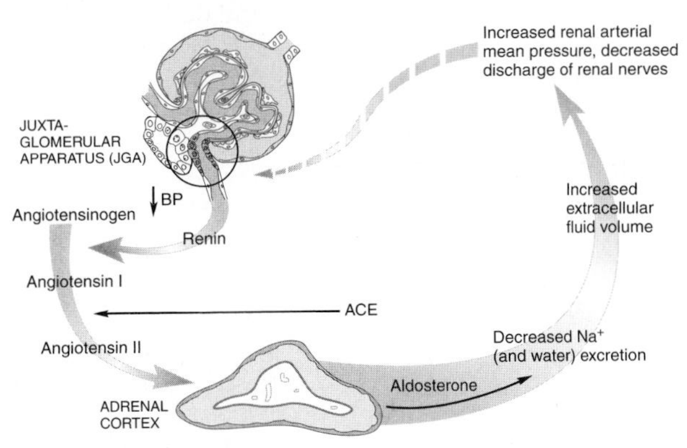

FIGURE 11-4. Renin-angiotensin system. (Adapted, with permission, from Ganong WF. *Review of Medical Physiology*, 20th ed. New York: McGraw-Hill, 2001.)

ORGAN SYSTEMS

RENAL SYSTEM

ORGAN SYSTEMS

RENAL SYSTEM

▶ Case 11

A 64-year-old woman presents to her physician with sudden onset of nausea and severe back pain on her right side. The patient is in acute distress and is unable to find a comfortable position. She has no prior history of back pain. Her temperature is 36.9° C (98.4° F), her heart rate is 90/min, and her blood pressure is 130/80 mm Hg. Relevant laboratory findings are as follows:

Serum

Sodium: 140 mEq/L	Chloride: 100 mEq/L
Potassium: 4 mEq/L	Phosphoric acid: 2.1 mEq/L
Magnesium: 1.8 mEq/L	Glucose: 100 mg/dL
Calcium: 13 mEq/L	Blood urea nitrogen (BUN): 15 mg/dL
Bicarbonate: 25 mEq/L	Creatinine: 1 mg/dL

Urinary pH: 5.85

Urinalysis shows RBCs

What is the most likely diagnosis?	Renal calculi (kidney stones).
How is this condition classified?	Some 85% of kidney stones are **calcium oxalate stones** (see Figure 11-5 on the following page), which are strongly radiopaque. The second most common kidney stones are **struvite** (ammonium magnesium phosphate), which are radiolucent stones associated with *Proteus vulgaris* and *Staphylococcus aureus* infection. Other, less common stones include **uric acid stones** (radiolucent) and **cystine stones** (moderately radiopaque).
What is the pathogenesis of this condition?	Calcium oxalate stones can be caused by hypercalciuria, hyperoxaluria, or hypocitraturia (citrate is a potent inhibitor of stone formation).
What is the pathogenesis of struvite stones?	Struvite stones form in the presence of alkaline urine, created by urease-splitting organisms. Uric acid stones are associated with hyperuricemia, which is seen in gout and in conditions with high cell turnover, such as leukemia or myeloproliferative disease. Cystine stones are observed in congenital cystinuria.
What is the most appropriate treatment for this patient's condition?	Treatment should consist of analgesics, hydration, and thiazide diuretics. Extracorporeal shock wave lithotripsy or surgery may be necessary for stones that do not pass spontaneously.
What hormonal imbalance can cause electrolyte abnormalities?	The high calcium concentration and low phosphate concentration may be a result of excess parathyroid hormone (PTH). A high PTH level increases renal reabsorption of calcium and decreases renal reabsorption of phosphate. It also stimulates renal activation of vitamin D, which increases calcium absorption from the gastrointestinal tract.

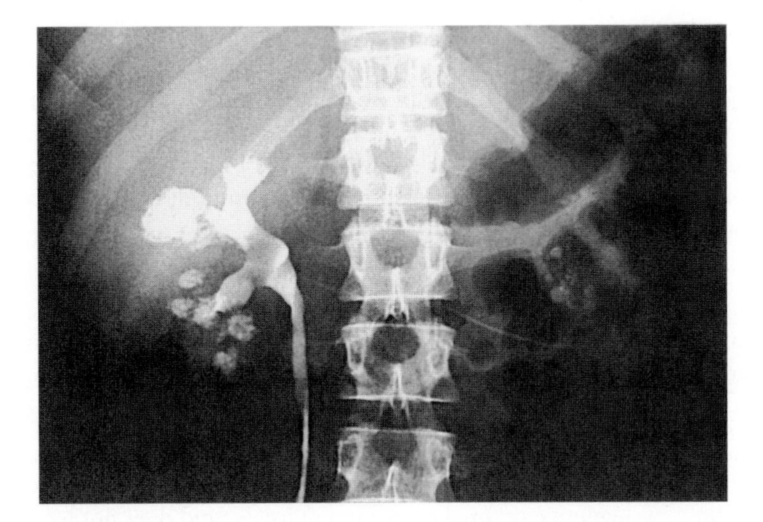

FIGURE 11-5. Kidney stones. (Reproduced, with permission, from Tanagho EA, McAninch JW. *Smith's General Urology*, 16th ed. New York: McGraw-Hill, 2004: 259.)

▶ Case 12

A 60-year-old man with a 30-year smoking history presents to his physician with complaints of cough, fatigue, and a recent 9.1-kg (20-lb) weight loss. An x-ray of the chest reveals a 2-cm hilar mass that is identified on biopsy as small cell lung cancer. On physical examination, the patient has some cachexia but normal skin turgor, no edema or jugular venous distention, and no orthostatic hypotension. Relevant laboratory findings are as follows:

Serum
- Sodium: 130 mEq/L
- Potassium: 4 mEq/L
- Blood urea nitrogen (BUN): 8 mg/dL
- Glucose: 90 mg/dL

Urine
- Sodium: 40 mEq/L
- Osmolality: 610 mOsm/kg H_2O

- **What is the most likely diagnosis?**

This patient is presenting with hyponatremia. The patient has no evidence of renal or extrarenal losses, and does not have evidence of hypervolemia (causing excess water relative to sodium content). The high urine osmolality suggests increased levels of ADH. However, as this patient is euvolemic, the release is inappropriate. Therefore, this patient has syndrome of inappropriate secretion of ADH (SIADH).

- **What are the major causes of this condition?**

- Ectopic ADH production by a tumor, particularly small cell (oat cell) carcinoma of the lung
- Intracranial pathology, such as trauma, stroke, tumors, or infection
- Drugs such as antipsychotic agents, antidepressants, high-dose cyclophosphamide, or thiazide diuretics
- Major surgery
- Human immunodeficiency virus infection

SIADH may also be idiopathic.

- **How is ADH regulated?**

ADH is the main regulator of serum osmolality. ADH causes water channels (eg, aquaporin-2) of the principal cells of the kidney's collecting ducts to open, thereby allowing more water to be reabsorbed. Its release from the posterior pituitary is stimulated by hyperosmolarity and by decreased effective circulating volume.

- **How would one calculate this patient's serum osmolality?**

Serum osmolality = 2 Na^+ + glucose/18 + BUN/2.8 = 268 mOsm/kg

- **What are the most appropriate treatments for this condition?**

Treatment consists of tumor resection. If evidence of SIADH persists or resection is not possible, treatment involves restriction of free water intake or use of hypertonic saline with loop diuretics. An alternative option is demeclocycline, which poisons the collecting tubule, making it unresponsive to ADH.

▶ Case 13

A 5-year-old girl develops a fever of 39° C (102.2° F) 5 days after receiving a renal transplant for focal sclerosing glomerulonephritis. Her kidney was from an unrelated, crossmatched, cadaveric donor. Following the transplant, she was placed on an immunosuppressive regimen consisting of basiliximab, prednisone, azathioprine, and cyclosporine. Blood cultures, including cultures for cytomegalovirus (CMV), are pending.

What is crossmatching, and what is its benefit?

The process of crossmatching determines whether the recipient has antibodies to the donor's WBCs. This measure prevents hyperacute rejection due to preformed antibodies.

If CMV is present, which fraction of a blood sample will have the highest yield for the virus?

Because CMV invades WBCs, these cells will contain the highest titer of the virus. This portion of the blood separates out as the "**buffy coat**" when blood samples are centrifuged. Figure 11-6 below shows a CMV giant cell with multiple hyaline inclusions.

Why is CMV of particular concern in this patient?

The girl is immunosuppressed, and there is a significant probability that she has been exposed to CMV. About 80% of normal adults are infected with CMV yet remain asymptomatic because of their functional immune systems. Thus, there is a high likelihood that the donor may have been CMV positive. As with other members of the herpesvirus family, CMV is more likely to activate in an immunosuppressed host.

What is the mechanism of action of ganciclovir against CMV?

Ganciclovir is a guanosine derivative that inhibits CMV DNA polymerase.

How does infection lead to fever in a normal individual?

Pyrogenic cytokines released by phagocytic cells of the immune system trigger the release of prostaglandins, including tumor necrosis factor-α and interleukin-1, which causes the hypothalamus to increase the set point of core body temperature. A key factor in the ability to mount a fever is the presence of an intact immune system. Infection is often difficult to detect in patients with poor immune function, as such patients' ability to mount a fever is severely blunted.

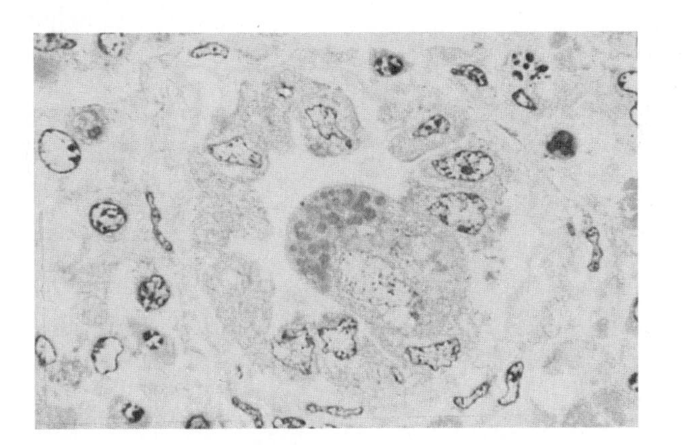

FIGURE 11-6. Photomicrograph of CMV. (Reproduced, with permission, from Bhushan V, Le T, et al. *First Aid for the USMLE Step 1: 2006*. New York: McGraw-Hill, 2006.)

▶ Case 14

An 18-month-old boy is brought to the pediatrician with symptoms of his third urinary tract infection since birth. His mother reports the child has malodorous urine, a low-grade fever, and poor appetite. Urinalysis reveals bacteria on Gram stain.

Describe the anatomy of the kidney.	If one were to slice a kidney in half, the cortex would be most superficial, with the medulla connecting to calyces, which are connected to the renal pelvis.
Explain the anatomical connection between the ureters and the urethra.	There are two ureters that transport urine from each kidney into the bladder. The ureters have three layers of tissue. The most superficial is fibrous tissue, which covers a medial layer of muscle and an inner mucosal layer of epithelial tissue. The urethra exits at the bladder neck at the apex of the trigone. The female urethra is shorter, which predisposes girls and women to urinary tract infections. In male babies frequent urinary tract infections can be a sign of urinary reflux.
Where is the bladder located in males versus females?	The bladder sits behind the pubic symphysis and anterior to the rectum in both males and females. The male bladder lies anterior to the seminal vesicles above the prostate gland, and is anterior to the uterus in females.
What are the two regions of the bladder?	The lower region is the trigone or the base of the bladder. The entry of the ureters marks the base of the trigone. The apex of the trigone is where the urethral orifice is surrounded by the internal urethral sphincter. The upper region of the bladder holds urine that enters the bladder via the ureteral orifices. The bladder can expand vertically and horizontally to hold up to 300–400 cc of urine before voiding.

Describe the innervation of the bladder.	▪ Afferent innervation: via afferent branches of the visceral nervous system: stretch receptors via parasympathetic nerves and pain receptors via sympathetic nerves.
	▪ Efferent innervation:
	  ▪ Parasympathetic innervation: the pelvic splanchnic nerves. The preganglionic axons arise from the lateral horn cells at S2–4 levels; postganglionic cell bodies are in the bladder wall. These efferent nerves cause detrusor contraction and internal sphincter relaxation during micturition.
	  ▪ Sympathetic innervation: the sacral splanchnic nerves. The preganglionic axons arise from lateral horn cell bodies at T10–12 and L1–2 levels. The postganglionic cell bodies are in the inferior mesenteric and hypogastric ganglia. These efferent nerves relax the detrusor and increase the tone of the internal sphincter during bladder filling and prevent reflux of urine into the ureters. In the adult male these efferents also prevent reflux of semen into the bladder at the urethrovesical junction.

Reproductive System

▶ Case 1

A 29-year-old woman in week 28 of her third pregnancy is involved in a minor motor vehicle accident, but does not immediately seek medial attention. Four hours after the accident, she notes lower abdominal pain and vaginal bleeding, and decides to go to the emergency department. Upon presentation, the patient appears quite distressed and says she is experiencing what she believes to be prolonged contractions. Her vital signs are notable for mild hypotension. Relevant laboratory findings are as follows:

Hematocrit: 34%
Platelet count: 8000/mm^3
Plasma fibrinogen: 180 mg/dL

- **What is the most likely diagnosis?**

Abruptio placentae. The presence of painful vaginal bleeding in the late second or third trimester is suggestive of abruption, and the presence of contractions is an additional clinical hint. The laboratory values, particularly the mild thrombocytopenia and decreased plasma fibrinogen (<200 mg/dL), also suggest severe abruption.

- **What is the differential diagnosis of painful vaginal bleeding in the third trimester?**

Abruption often presents as painful vaginal bleeding, while placenta previa is described as painless vaginal bleeding. Other causes of third-trimester painful bleeding include labor and uterine rupture (in which contractions are absent).

- **What is the pathophysiology of this condition?**

Abruptio placentae is the premature separation of a normal placenta occurring after 20 weeks' gestation and before delivery. The rupture of maternal blood vessels at the anchoring villi of the placenta causes a separation from the endometrium in which blood can accumulate. The hemorrhage can be either external or concealed, as shown in Figure 12-1 on the following page (which also shows placenta previa, another common cause of vaginal bleeding in pregnancy). This in turn disrupts the fetal blood supply and, in severe cases, can lead to fetal death.

- **What risk factors are associated with the development of this condition?**

Risk factors typically increase the risk of disruption or weakening of the maternal blood vessels. They include trauma, maternal hypertension, cigarette smoking, cocaine use, thrombophilia, increased parity, and multifetal gestation.

- **What complication is the mother at greatly increased risk for developing?**

Disseminated intravascular coagulation (DIC) occurs in approximately 10%–20% of cases of serious abruption with fetal death. This may be a result of a consumptive coagulopathy. In cases of fetal demise, it is thought that the death of the fetus releases procoagulants into the mother's circulation that provide a trigger for DIC.

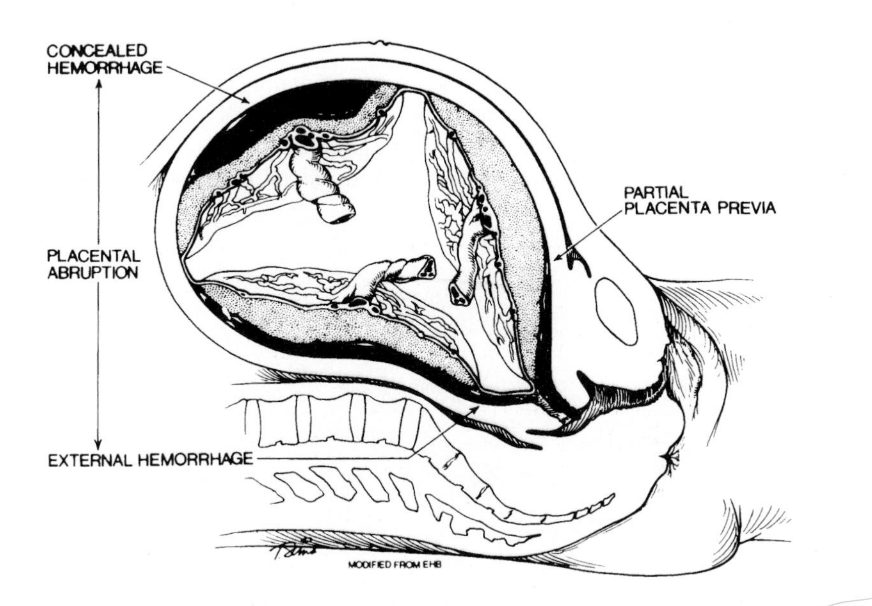

FIGURE 12-1. Layers in abruptio placentae. (Reproduced, with permission, from Cunningham FG, et al. *Williams Obstetrics,* 22nd ed. New York: McGraw-Hill, 2005: 812.)

ORGAN SYSTEMS

REPRODUCTIVE SYSTEM

► **Case 2**

A 22-year-old woman presents to the clinic with complaints of itching; burning on urination; and a green, fishy-smelling vaginal discharge. She has had four different sexual partners in the past year, and says she has "used protection" in each case. Smear of the discharge reveals squamous epithelial cells with smudged borders (see Figure 12-2 below).

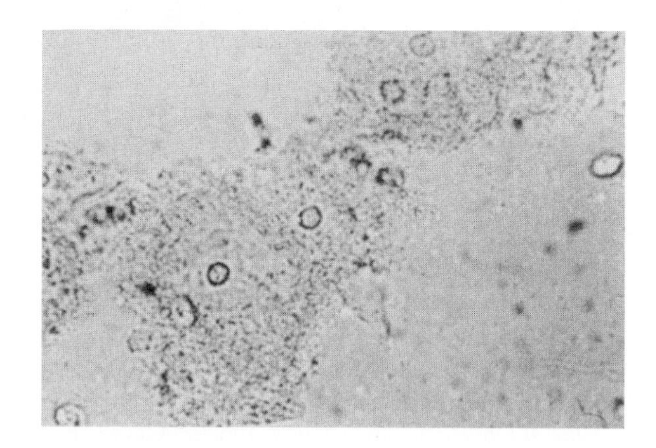

FIGURE 12-2. (Reproduced, with permission, from Kasper DL, et al. *Harrison's Principles of Internal Medicine,* 16th ed. New York: McGraw-Hill, 2005: 767.)

■ **What is the most likely diagnosis?**	Bacterial vaginosis.
■ **What organism causes this condition?**	Bacterial vaginosis is caused by a change in vaginal flora that results in increased numbers of *Gardnerella vaginalis.*
■ **What other conditions should be considered in the differential diagnosis?**	*Candida* and *Trichmonas* are other common causes of vaginitis. The presence of **clue cells,** which are squamous epithelial cells with smudged borders (see Figure 12-2 above), is strong evidence that the infection is bacterial in origin. An elevated pH (>4.5) and a positive **whiff test** (amine release with potassium hydroxide results in a "fishy" smell) may aid in the diagnosis.
■ **What risk factors are associated with the development of this condition?**	Risk factors include multiple/new sexual partners, early age at first intercourse, smoking, and use of an intrauterine device. Diabetics, pregnant women, and women with human immunodeficiency virus infection have an increased risk of developing infection with *Candida.* While bacterial vaginosis is commonly thought of as a sexually transmitted disease, it is also seen in women who have not had intercourse.
■ **What is the most appropriate treatment for this condition?**	Metronidazole treats infections with *Gardnerella* and *Trichomonas. Candida* (yeast) infections are treated with fluconazole.

▶ Case 3

A 17-year-old girl is brought to the emergency department complaining of a 3-day history of nausea and vomiting and intense abdominal pain. Her last menstrual period was 6 weeks ago, but she has a history of irregular cycles. She is not taking oral contraceptives. Her past medical history is significant for an appendectomy at age 13 years. Physical examination reveals a palpable mass in the right lower quadrant. Laboratory tests show her β-human chorionic gonadotropin (β-hCG) level is 1500 IU/L, and the serum progesterone level is <15 ng/mL. Transvaginal ultrasonography, however, reveals no uterine pregnancy.

What is the most likely diagnosis?

Ectopic pregnancy. Ectopic pregnancy occurs with a rate of 17 per 1000 pregnancies. The vast majority (98%) occur in the fallopian tubes, most often (90% of cases) in the ampulla.

What signs and symptoms are commonly associated with this condition?

Nonruptured ectopic pregnancy:
- Abnormal bleeding
- Abdominal/pelvic pain
- Nausea
- Pelvic mass
- Vomiting

Ruptured ectopic pregnancy:
- Local or generalized abdominal tenderness
- Orthostatic hypertension
- Shock
- Shoulder pain
- Tachycardia

What risk factors are associated with this condition?

- Diethylstilbestrol exposure in utero
- In vitro fertilization
- Pelvic inflammatory disease
- Pelvic surgery
- Previous ectopic pregnancy
- Tubal ligation
- Tuboplasty

What are the likely findings of laboratory tests?

The β-hCG level in an ectopic pregnancy is typically <6500 IU/L, which is markedly lower than that in a uterine pregnancy. The serum progesterone level (typically <15 ng/mL) is also much lower than that in a uterine pregnancy.

What are the likely findings on transvaginal ultrasonography?

Transvaginal ultrasonography will show no intrauterine gestational sac, a noncystic adnexal mass, or fluid in the cul-de-sac. A gestational sac is visible with a vaginal probe when the β-hCG level is 1500 IU/L, or with abdominal pelvic ultrasonography when the β-hCG level is 6500 IU/L.

What are the most appropriate treatments for this condition?

The β-hCG levels should be checked every 48 hours. In a normal intrauterine pregnancy, levels of this hormone will double over this time frame; if not, an ectopic pregnancy should be suspected. Methotrexate may be given if the ectopic pregnancy is <3 cm, the β-hCG level is <12,000 IU/L, there is no fetal heart rate, and the mother's liver and renal test results pretreatment are normal. Surgery is indicated if the β-hCG level is higher. Surgery involves removal of part or all of the fallopian tube; the preferred approach for ampullary ectopic pregnancy is salpingostomy (laparoscopic if possible). Segmental resection might be necessary for an ischemic ectopic pregnancy. Salpingectomy is usually reserved for a ruptured ectopic pregnancy.

▶ Case 4

A 26-year-old woman presents to her physician complaining of intense abdominal pain associated with the start of her menstrual periods. She has been trying unsuccessfully to get pregnant for the past 2 years. On questioning, she reports pain with intercourse, especially on deep penetration. Her older sister has a similar history.

What is the most likely diagnosis?	Endometriosis.
What is the pathophysiology of this condition?	In endometriosis, endometrial tissue is found outside the endometrial cavity, usually in the ovary and pelvic peritoneum; see Figure 12-3 on the following page for common sites of endometrial implants. It is theorized that this endometrial tissue is either transported via the lymphatic system such that peritoneal tissue undergoes metaplastic transformation into functional endometrial tissue, or it is transported through the fallopian tubes in retrograde menstruation. Endometrial tissue causes adhesions, fibrosis, and severe inflammation.
What signs and symptoms are commonly associated with this condition?	Cyclic pelvic pain starting 1–2 days prior to the onset of menses and continuing through the first few days of the cycle are characteristic of endometriosis. Dysmenorrhea, dyspareunia, abnormal bleeding, and a history of infertility are also common in these patients. Physical examination typically reveals uterosacral nodularity and a palpable adnexal mass. Laparoscopic evaluation is definitive. Endometrial implants appear as raspberry lesions or **"powder burns"**; these raised, blue or dark brown lesions lead to adhesions. Ovarian cysts can have large collections of old blood called **endometriomas** or **"chocolate cysts."**
What risk factors are associated with this condition?	Endometriosis occurs in 10%–15% of women overall, but is more common (30%–40%) in women with infertility. The risk of endometriosis is 7-fold higher in women who have a first-degree relative with this condition. Endometriosis has also been linked to autoimmune disorders such as lupus. It is less commonly identified in African-American women.
What are the most appropriate treatments for this condition?	Medical treatment includes nonsteroidal anti-inflammatory drugs, oral contraceptive pills, and medroxyprogesterone (to create "pseudopregnancy"). Androgen derivatives or gonadotropin-releasing hormone agonists can be used to induce "pseudomenopause." Surgical treatment may also be necessary in some cases.

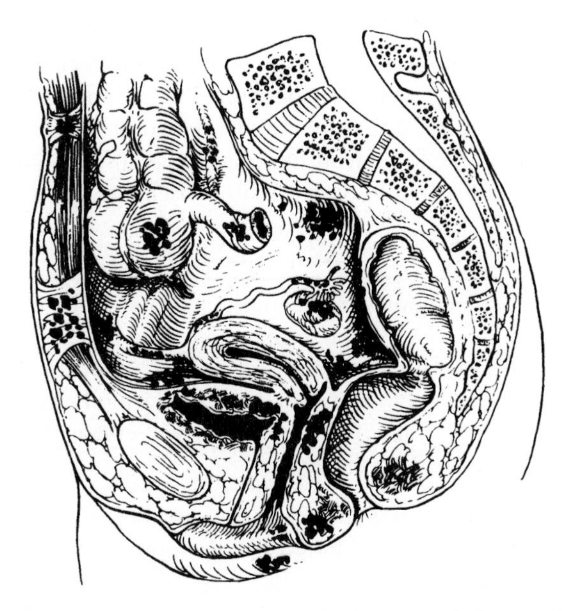

FIGURE 12-3. Frequent sites of endometriosis deposits (dark areas in image). (Reproduced, with permission, from Doherty GM. *Current Surgical Diagnosis & Treatment*, 12th ed. New York: McGraw-Hill, 2006: 1075.)

▶ Case 5

A 24-year-old woman presents to her physician after recently noticing a lump in her left breast that has been associated with some discomfort. The lump moves with touch and she is concerned about cancer, as her mother developed breast cancer at age 62 years. On physical examination, the lump feels firm, has well-defined borders, and is mobile. There are no changes in the skin or nipple and no discharge. No axillary lymph nodes are palpable.

- **What is the most likely diagnosis?**

Fibroadenomas are the most common (benign!) tumor in young women. They often arise quickly, and reabsorb within several weeks to months. Fibroadenomas do not carry an increased risk of breast cancer. Note that the patient's mother's history of breast cancer is not a risk factor for this patient, as the mother was >50 years old when diagnosed.

- **What are Cooper's ligaments?**

The superficial and deep pectoral fascia surrounding the breast are connected by fibrous bands known as **Cooper's suspensory ligaments.**

- **What is the structure of breast tissue?**

Breast tissue is found between the second and sixth ribs and is made of parenchyma and stroma (see Figure 12-4 below). The parenchyma has 15–25 lobes, each of which has 20–40 lobules composed of alveoli. Lactiferous ducts offer drainage to the corresponding lobe. The ducts are dilated immediately before the nipple, which forms the lactiferous sinuses.

- **What are the muscles of the breast tissue, and how are they innervated?**

  - Seratus anterior—long thoracic nerve
  - Latissimus dorsi—thoracodorsal nerve
  - Pectoralis minor—medial pectoral nerve
  - Pectoralis major—pectoral nerve

- **What is the most appropriate treatment for this condition?**

Because these growths are benign, no treatment is necessary. The patient should be followed up in 1–2 months to assess for reabsorption.

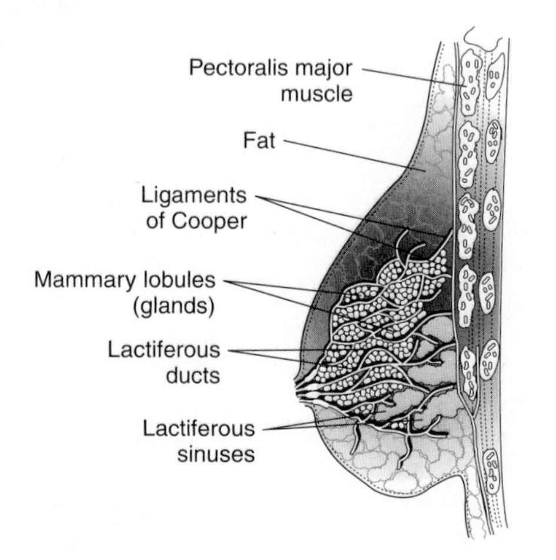

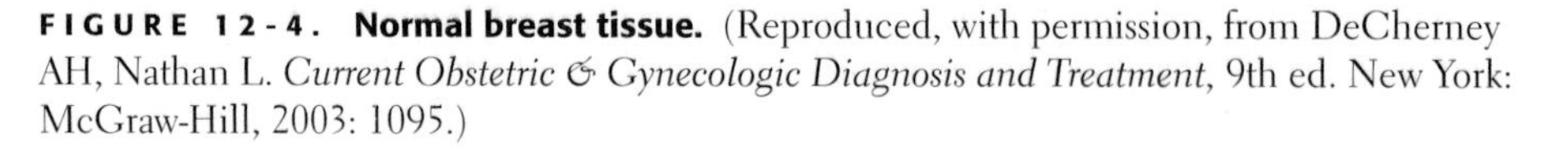

FIGURE 12-4. Normal breast tissue. (Reproduced, with permission, from DeCherney AH, Nathan L. *Current Obstetric & Gynecologic Diagnosis and Treatment*, 9th ed. New York: McGraw-Hill, 2003: 1095.)

▶ Case 6

A 22-year-old woman presents to the emergency department with a 3-day history of fever, abdominal pain, pain on inspiration, and vaginal discharge. Her temperature at presentation is 38° C (100.4° F). The patient admits to being sexually active, but not always using protection. Her last menstrual period ended 5 days ago. She has been with her most recent partner for approximately 1 month. On physical examination, her abdomen is diffusely tender, with more pain in the right upper quadrant, but without rebound. Cervical motion tenderness is present, as is right-sided adnexal tenderness. Relevant laboratory findings are as follow:

WBC count: 11,000/mm^3
Erythrocyte sedimentation rate (ESR): >15 mm/hr
β-Human chorionic gonadotrophin: negative
Alanine aminotransferase: 1.5 × normal

What is the most likely diagnosis?	Fitz-Hugh–Curtis syndrome, a pelvic inflammatory disease (PID) characterized by perihepatitis in association with pleuritic right upper quadrant pain and tubal gonococcal or chlamydia infection.
What is the pathophysiology of this condition?	*Neisseria gonorrhoeae* is responsible for approximately one-third of cases of PID; *Chlamydia trachomatis* causes concurrent infection in another third of cases. Fitz-Hugh–Curtis syndrome is due to a **perihepatitis,** or an inflammation of the underside of the diaphragm and liver capsule. The syndrome is seen in about 5% of patients with PID, and is often mistakenly diagnosed as pneumonia or acute cholecystitis.
What signs and symptoms are commonly associated with this condition?	Patients with Fitz-Hugh–Curtis syndrome present with PID and pleuritic pain in the upper right quadrant that limits chest expansion. Additionally, patients have an elevated WBC count, fever, pelvic pain, cervical motion tenderness, adnexal tenderness, elevated liver enzyme levels, and an ESR >15 mm/hr.
What risk factors are associated with this condition?	▪ Cigarette smoking ▪ High frequency of intercourse ▪ Multiple partners ▪ New sexual partner within 1 month of symptom onset ▪ Recent history of douching ▪ Use of intrauterine device ▪ Young age at first intercourse
What are the likely findings on histology?	Gram staining of the cervical discharge will reveal gram-negative intracellular diplococci. Culture of endocervical samples will reveal N. *gonorrhoeae* and/or C. *trachomatis* infection.
What are the most appropriate treatments for this condition?	Fitz-Hugh–Curtis syndrome is treated with outpatient antibiotics such as cefoxitin, ceftriaxone, or doxycycline. If the patient is pregnant, has a tubo-ovarian abscess, or cannot tolerate oral medications, she must be hospitalized for administering intravenous antibiotics. Surgery is indicated only in cases of tubo-ovarian abscess.

▶ Case 7

A 36-year-old woman at 24 weeks of gestation presents to the clinic for a routine prenatal visit. Her fetus is large for gestational age, and she is scheduled for an oral glucose tolerance test (OGTT). The mother had one previous pregnancy with no complications and is generally healthy, although obese. Results of the OGGT are as follows:

1-hr OGGT: glucose level 144 mg/dL
3-hr OGGT: fasting glucose level 93 mg/dL
glucose level at 1 hour: 172 mg/dL
glucose level at 2 hours: 150 mg/dL
glucose level at 3 hours: 133 mg/dL

■ **What is the most likely diagnosis?**	Gestational diabetes.
■ **What is the pathophysiology of this condition?**	Gestational diabetes occurs in 3%–5% of all pregnancies. Early in a normal pregnancy, there is a normal increase in insulin release. As the pregnancy develops, increases in human placental lactogen, progesterone, cortisol, and prolactin block insulin's action, causing insulin resistance.
■ **What signs and symptoms are commonly associated with this condition?**	This syndrome is most often asymptomatic, and is usually detected between 24 and 28 weeks' gestation by a routine OGTT. Glycosuria, hyperglycemia, and large fetus for gestational age raise the suspicion of gestational diabetes.
■ **What risk factors are associated with this condition?**	■ Age >35 years ■ Family history of diabetes mellitus ■ Fetus large for gestational age ■ Glycosuria ■ Obesity ■ Past history of gestational diabetes ■ Polyuria ■ Recurrent urinary tract infection ■ Several previous still births or abortions
■ **What are the common maternal and fetal complications associated with this condition?**	Maternal: ■ Cesarean section delivery ■ Eclampsia/preeclampsia ■ Glucose intolerance ■ Increased future risk of diabetes mellitus ■ Polyhydramnios ■ Pregnancy-induced hypertension ■ Preterm delivery Fetal: ■ Congenital defects ■ Macrosomia ■ Perinatal mortality (2%–5%) ■ Shoulder dystocia
■ **What are the most appropriate treatments for this condition?**	Affected women should adhere to a sensible diet, such as the American Diabetes Association diet. Fasting blood glucose and 2-hour postprandial glucose levels should be routinely monitored. If levels remain high for 2 weeks, insulin therapy should be started.

▶ Case 8

A 42-year-old African-American woman visits her physician with a complaint of heavy menstrual periods that last for several days. This has been occurring for the past 3 months, and has been associated with pain and fatigue. Physical examination reveals an enlarged uterus with multiple palpable masses. Laboratory tests show her hemoglobin level is 11.3 g/dL and hematocrit is 33.3%.

What is the most likely diagnosis?	Leiomyoma, or uterine fibroids. This diagnosis is suggested by the heavy vaginal bleeding and palpable masses.
What epidemiologic factors are associated with this condition?	The incidence of leiomyoma is greatly increased in African-American women. It is the most common neoplasm in females.
Which cells of the uterus are most commonly affected in this condition?	Smooth muscle cells of the myometrium are most commonly affected, although fibroids can also occur in subendometrial or subperitoneal areas (see Figure 12-5 below). Fibroids within the uterus can be submucosal, subserosal, or intramural. **Submucosal fibroids** are most often associated with abnormal bleeding, while **subserosal fibroids** are most often the cause of "mass-effect" pressure.
How does the size of this neoplasm change with age?	The estrogen sensitivity of leiomyomas correlates with increased size during the first trimester of pregnancy and shrinkage after menopause.
Is this patient at increased risk for uterine malignancy?	Most leiomyosarcomas arise de novo and malignant transformation of leiomyomas into leiomyosarcomas is rare.
What uterine abnormality is associated with an increased risk of endometrial cancer?	**Endometrial hyperplasia,** which is characterized by abnormal glandular proliferation, is considered to be a premalignant lesion. This is caused by increased estrogen stimulation and, like uterine fibroids, often presents with abnormal vaginal bleeding. Its presence, therefore, must be distinguished from abnormal vaginal bleeding secondary to uterine fibroids.

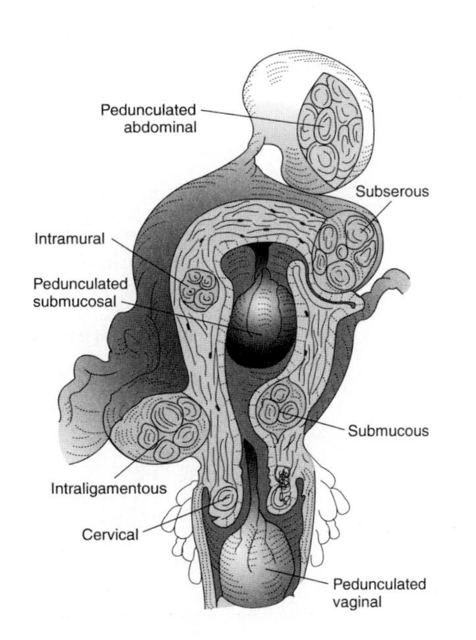

FIGURE 12-5. Myomas of the uterus. (Reproduced, with permission, from DeCherney AH, Nathan L. *Current Obstetric & Gynecologic Diagnosis and Treatment*, 9th ed. New York: McGraw-Hill, 2003: 694.)

▶ Case 9

A 57-year-old woman with a history of eczema presents to her primary care physician with a new rash near the nipple of her right breast. She tells her doctor that the rash first appeared 2 months ago, and she had been treating it with the topical corticosteroid prescribed for her eczema. At first, the rash improved somewhat, but over the past few weeks it has gotten worse and has expanded in size. Physical examination reveals a raw, scaly lesion around the nipple that is beginning to ulcerate. There is also a palpable mass in the affected breast, a few centimeters deep to the skin lesion.

What is the most likely diagnosis?	Paget's disease of the breast, an eczematous skin lesion in the area of the nipple, is associated with underlying invasive or in situ breast carcinoma (see Figure 12-6 below). In about 50% of cases, Paget's disease is associated with a palpable breast mass. Paget's disease is often mistaken for a benign skin lesion, such as eczema.
What is the pathophysiology of this condition?	It is thought that the skin lesion develops from underlying ductal carcinoma cells that migrate through the ducts to the epidermis.
What are the most likely findings on histology?	The classic histologic findings are large cells with a halo of clear cytoplasm surrounding a prominent nucleolus. The cytoplasm stains positive for mucin.
What are the most common sites of metastasis for breast carcinoma?	The most common sites for metastases of breast carcinoma are the lung, the liver, and bone. The ovaries may also be a site of metastatic breast cancer.
What is the lymphatic drainage of the breast?	Knowledge of the lymphatic drainage of the breast is important for understanding the metastasis of breast cancer. Approximately 75% of lymphatic drainage of the breast is to the **axillary lymph nodes,** which include the pectoral (majority of drainage), apical, subscapular, lateral, and central node groups. The nipple drains to the pectoral group. The remaining lymph drains to the infraclavicular, supraclavicular, and parasternal (also known as the internal thoracic) nodes.
Molecular analysis of a biopsy reveals that the cells express c-erbB2 (also known as HER-2/neu) in high levels; what is the significance of this, and how does this affect treatment?	The HER-2/neu protein is a transmembrane growth factor receptor (HER is an abbreviation for **H**uman **E**pithelial growth factor **R**eceptor). Overexpression of this molecule has been associated with a poorer prognosis. A new medication, trastuzumab (herceptin), is a monoclonal antibody directed against this protein. The binding of herceptin to the extracellular portion of the molecule stimulates a cytotoxic immune response, leading to death of the cancer cells.

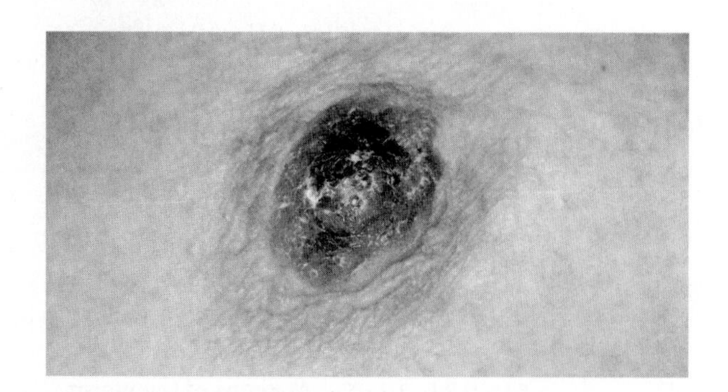

FIGURE 12-6. Paget's disease of the breast. (Reproduced, with permission, from Wolff K, Johnson RA, Suurmond D. *Fitzpatrick's Color Atlas & Synopsis of Clinical Dermatology*, 5th ed. New York: McGraw-Hill, 2005: 495.)

▶ Case 10

A 36-year-old African-American woman in week 34 of gestation presents to the emergency department with a 2-day history of headache, blurry vision, and sudden right upper quadrant pain. She reports her husband has noticed increased swelling of her face since yesterday, and her rings are suddenly too tight. She has been healthy except for pregestational diabetes mellitus. Physical examination is notable for hyperactive reflexes and jugular venous distention. Her blood pressure at presentation is 165/110 mm Hg; 6 hours later the blood pressure is 170/110 mm Hg. Relevant laboratory findings are as follows:

Serum transaminase: 2 × normal
Creatinine: 1.5 mg/dL
Urinalysis: 3+ protein

- **What is the most likely diagnosis?**

Preeclampsia and eclampsia are the two most common causes of pregnancy-induced hypertension (PIH). Preeclampsia can occur at 20+ weeks of gestation.

- **What is the pathophysiology of this condition?**

Systemic endothelial damage is caused by vascular spasm, capillary hyperpermeability, and relatively high levels of thromboxane (vasoconstrictor) relative to prostacyclin (vasodilator).

- **What signs and symptoms are commonly associated with this condition?**

Mild preeclampsia is characterized by 1+ proteinuria and a blood pressure >140/90 mm Hg. Common symptoms include headache, rapid weight gain, edema of the face and hands, jugular venous distention, and hyperactive reflexes. **Severe preeclampsia** is characterized by 3+ proteinuria and a blood pressure >160/110 mm Hg. Common symptoms include visual changes, headache, somnolence, right upper quadrant or epigastric pain, oligohydramnios, elevated liver enzyme levels, thrombocytopenia, pulmonary edema/cyanosis, and intrauterine growth retardation.

- **What risk factors are associated with this condition?**

  - Abnormal placentation
  - African-American ethnicity
  - Age <20 or >35 years
  - Chronic hypertension
  - Chronic renal disease
  - Cohabitation <1 year
  - Collagen vascular disease (eg, systemic lupus erythematosus)
  - Diabetes mellitus before pregnancy
  - Family history of preeclampsia
  - Multiple gestation
  - New paternity
  - Nulliparity
  - Previous preeclampsia

- **What is HELLP syndrome?**

HELLP is a subcategory of preeclampsia that results in a high rate of stillbirth (10%–15%) and neonatal death (~25%). HELLP stands for **H**emolysis, **E**levated **L**iver enzymes, and **L**ow **P**latelets.

- **What treatments are most appropriate for this condition?**

If the baby is term, the fetal lungs are mature, or the case is severe, delivery is the best treatment. Mild preeclampsia is treated with bed rest, close monitoring, and blood pressure control with antihypertensive agents. In severe cases the mother should be hospitalized and magnesium sulfate should be given for seizure prophylaxis (continue 24 hours postpartum) in addition to antihypertensive agents.

► Case 11

A 16-year-old girl is brought to her pediatrician because of an absence of menarche. She has short stature, a webbed neck, and a square chest. Physical examination reveals breast buds and female external genitalia. Her blood pressure is normal in both arms. CT scan reveals a small uterus and atretic, fatty ovaries. There is no known history of this condition in her family.

What is the most likely diagnosis?	Turner's syndrome, characterized by gonadal dysgenesis secondary to the presence of a single X chromosome (XO) (see Figure 12-7 below). This syndrome is the most common cause of primary amenorrhea.
What other conditions can cause primary amenorrhea?	■ Absence of uterus, cervix, and/or vagina (**Mullerian agenesis**) ■ Hypothalamic hypogonadism (secondary to anorexia, exercise, stress, or gonadotropin-releasing hormone deficiency) ■ Ovarian failure (gonadal dysgenesis, polycystic ovary syndrome) ■ Pituitary disease ■ Transverse vaginal septum or imperforate hymen
What diagnostic test are indicated based on the patient's clinical features?	Chromosome analysis. Typically, 20 cells are analyzed to detect whether mosaicism is present. Additionally, no Barr body will be seen.
What other conditions are association with this condition?	Coarctation of the aorta, bicuspid aortic valve, hypothyroidism, sensorineural hearing loss, renal abnormalities, gastrointestinal telangectasias, and osteoporosis have been associated with Turner's syndrome. Mental retardation is not associated with this syndrome.
What are the most appropriate treatments for this condition?	Recombinant human growth hormone and hormone replacement therapy can initiate puberty and complete growth.

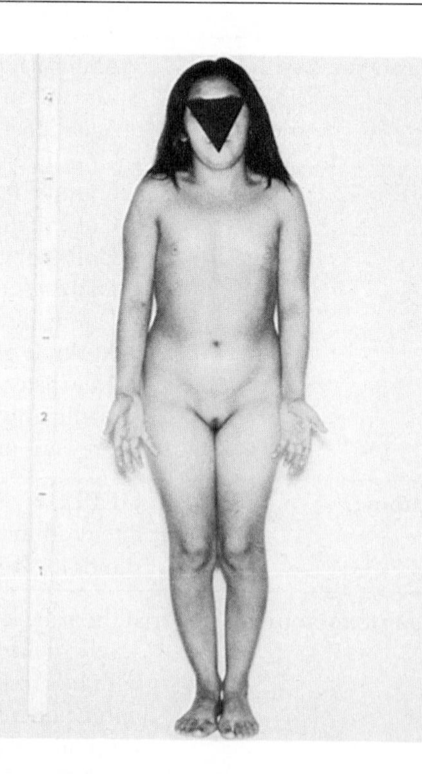

FIGURE 12-7. Turner's syndrome. (Reproduced, with permission, from Bhushan V, Le T, et al. *First Aid for the USMLE Step 1: 2006*. New York: McGraw-Hill, 2006.)

Respiratory System

▶ **Case 1**

A 60-year-old man comes to his primary care physician because of dyspnea on exertion that has been worsening over the past several years. He also reports a nonproductive cough he has had almost daily over the same period. On questioning, the man says he worked for 30 years as a demolition worker in a shipyard, where he stripped and replaced insulating material. On physical examination, chest expansion appears markedly restricted, and there are fine inspiratory crackles that are most pronounced at the lung bases. Also of note are multiple firm, subcutaneous nodules on the man's hands.

What is the most likely diagnosis?	Asbestosis.
What other conditions should be considered in the differential diagnosis?	One should also consider interstitial lung diseases, especially those caused by occupational exposure, such as silicosis, coal worker's pneumoconiosis, and berylliosis. Conditions not related to occupational exposure, including usual interstitial pneumonia and idiopathic pulmonary fibrosis, should also be contemplated.
What is the pathophysiology of this condition?	The pathophysiologic process involves diffuse pulmonary interstitial fibrosis caused by inhaled asbestos fibers. Asbestos fibers penetrate bronchioles and lung tissue, where they are surrounded by macrophages and coated by a protein-iron complex **(asbestos bodies)**; Figure 13-1 shows asbestos bodies with Prussian blue iron stain that are being ingested by macrophages. Diffuse fibrosis around the bronchioles spreads to the alveoli, causing lung tissue to become rigid and airways to become distorted.
What are the most likely findings on x-ray of the chest?	In cases of minor exposure, the only findings may be pleural thickening or calcified pleural plaques. In cases of extensive pulmonary fibrosis, reticular or nodular opacities will be seen throughout the lung fields, most prominently at the bases.
What are the most appropriate treatments for this condition?	There is no definitive therapy for asbestosis. As soon as exposure to asbestos is confirmed, the patient should be removed from the exposure and encouraged not to smoke, as the combination of asbestosis and smoking greatly increases the risk of bronchogenic carcinoma. Corticosteroids may have some benefit, although their use is not well established.

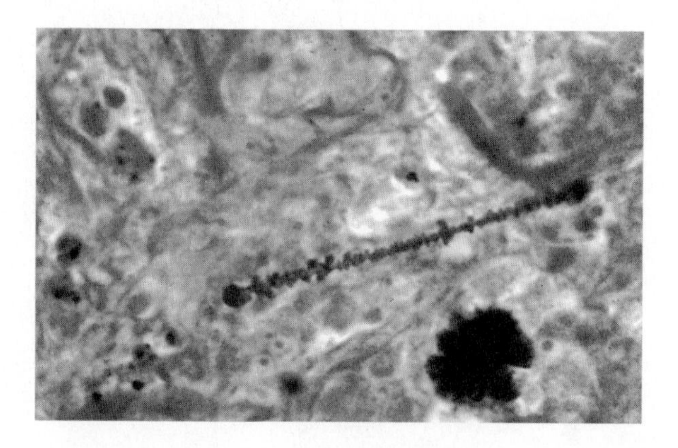

FIGURE 13-1. Asbestos bodies. (Reproduced with permission of the Pathology Education Instructional Resource Digital Library (http://peir.net) at the University of Alabama, Birmingham.)

▶ Case 2

A 7-year-old boy is brought to the emergency department (ED) after awakening in the middle of the night with difficulty breathing. He has a 2-day history of worsening productive cough and wheezing. In the ED, the patient is found to be dyspneic and tachypneic and has a decreased inspiratory-to-expiratory ratio. Lung examination reveals diffuse rhonchi and expiratory wheezes in addition to pulsus paradoxus. He is afebrile and has no recent history of fever. This is the patient's second visit to the ED with this symptomatology; his first visit was 2 years ago.

What is the most likely diagnosis?	Asthma exacerbation. Asthma is a form of obstructive lung disease.
What is the pathophysiology of this condition?	Acutely, tracheobronchial hyperresponsiveness leads to episodic, reversible bronchoconstriction. Specifically, smooth muscle contraction in the airways leads to expiratory airflow obstruction. Chronically, airway inflammation leads to histologic changes in the tracheobronchial tree.
What histologic findings in the lung are associated with this condition?	Histologic examination reveals smooth muscle hypertrophy, goblet cell hyperplasia, thickening of basement membranes, and increased eosinophil recruitment (see Figure 13-2 below; arrow points to plate of cartilage, arrowhead points to infiltrate of inflammatory cells). Dilated bronchi are filled with neutrophils and may have mucous plugs.
What are some common triggers for this condition?	Viral upper respiratory tract infections, various allergens, stress, cold, and exercise are common triggers of asthma exacerbation.
What is the most appropriate treatment for this condition?	Albuterol, a β_2-agonist, helps relax bronchial smooth muscle and decrease airway obstruction.

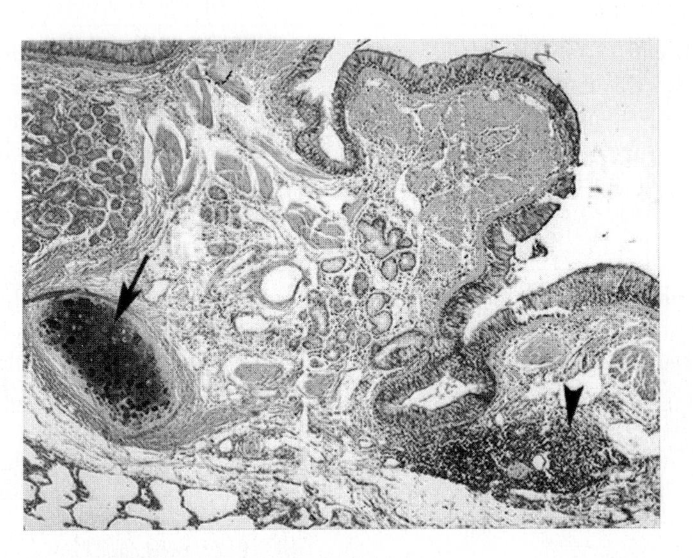

FIGURE 13-2. Histologic findings in asthma. (Reproduced, with permission, from Wilson FJ, et al. *Histology Image Review*. Norwalk, CT: Appleton & Lange, 1997. Copyright © The McGraw-Hill Companies, Inc.)

▶ Case 3

A 50-year-old woman visits a community health clinic because of a 1-month history of cough productive of yellow sputum. On questioning, she says she has had several periods of cough lasting 4–6 consecutive months each year for the past 5 years. She has smoked two packs of cigarettes per day for the past 30 years. On examination, the woman's breathing is shallow, and she is exhaling slowly with pursed lips. Her jugular venous pulse is visible to the jaw line when she is reclined at an angle of 45°. Auscultation of the chest demonstrates wheezing and distant heart sounds. A positive hepatojugular reflux is demonstrated, as is 2+ pitting edema up to her knees. A high-resolution CT scan reveals several hyperlucent areas within the lungs.

- **What is the most likely diagnosis?**

Chronic obstructive pulmonary disease (COPD) with features of chronic bronchitis. The diagnosis is based on clinical findings of a history of productive cough for at least 3 consecutive months over 2 consecutive years accompanied by emphysema (suggested by pursed-lip breathing).

- **What abnormalities would be expected on pulmonary function testing?**

In COPD, the forced expiratory volume in 1 second (FEV_1) is decreased, forced vital capacity (FVC) is normal or decreased, and the FEV_1/FVC ratio is decreased. These findings should be contrasted with restrictive lung diseases, in which decreased vital capacity and total lung capacity result in a FEV_1/FVC ratio of >80%.

- **How would this condition affect the patient's arterial blood gas levels from normal values for pH, $Pa{O_2}$, $Pa{CO_2}$, and $Sa{O_2}$?**

pH will decrease as a result of respiratory acidosis. While pH may be normal in a patient with chronic compensated COPD, it will be low in a patient with an acute exacerbation. Arterial oxygen tension ($Pa{O_2}$) will decrease, arterial carbon dioxide tension ($Pa{CO_2}$) will increase, and oxygen saturation ($Sa{O_2}$) will decrease secondary to impaired gas exchange (from destruction of alveolar septae and pulmonary capillary bed).

- **Why is breathing with pursed lips adaptive in this condition?**

Breathing with pursed lips maintains positive upper airway pressure. Positive upper airway pressure prevents alveolar collapse, which is a common occurrence in emphysema. Respiratory therapy often provides supplemental oxygen therapy via a mask or nasal prongs. Positive airway pressure can be provided by using either continuous positive airway pressure, bilevel positive airway pressure, or intubation and ventilatory support.

- **What complication of this condition do the patient's enlarged neck veins, hepatomegaly, and edema suggest?**

Cor pulmonale. Right heart failure due to chronic pulmonary hypertension leads to systemic venous congestion, which presents with the symptoms mentioned here. This complication occurs only in patients with severe COPD who develop pulmonary hypertension.

► Case 4

A 67-year-old man comes to the emergency department complaining of a 3-day history of cough and fever and a 1-day history of shaking chills. He has smoked about half a pack of cigarettes per day for the past 45 years. For the past 9 months, the man has had an increasingly severe cough that has been productive of clear sputum. His cough is now productive of rusty sputum. On physical examination, he is found to have a respiratory rate of 24/min and his temperature is 37.8° C (100° F). An x-ray of the chest shows lung consolidation (see Figure 13-3 below).

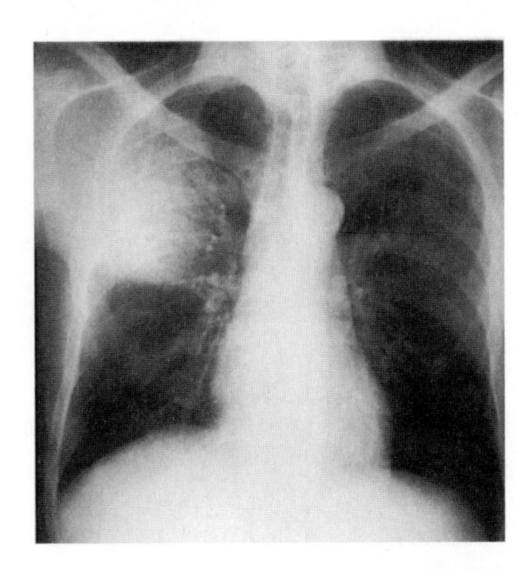

FIGURE 13-3. (Reproduced, with permission, from Bhushan V, Le T, et al. *First Aid for the USMLE Step 1: 2006*. New York: McGraw-Hill, 2006.)

What is the most likely diagnosis?	This patient presents with several of the classic findings of community-acquired pneumonia (CAP): a productive cough, fever, rigors (shaking chills), and tachypnea. He also has risk factors, including advanced age and a significant smoking history, and his 9-month history of mild cough suggests that he has underlying chronic bronchitis.
What are the likely findings on lung examination?	Decreased breath sounds, crackles, dullness to percussion, and increased tactile fremitus are probable findings.
What are the most likely causative organisms?	CAP is most often caused by bacteria, including *Streptococcus pneumoniae* (20%–60%), *Haemophilus influenzae* (3%–10%), *Staphylococcus aureus* (3%–5%), *Legionella* (2%–8%), and *Mycoplasma* (1%–6%), as well as by viruses (2%–15%). Less commonly, they may also be caused by parasites and fungi.
Gram stain of the sputum reveals gram-positive cocci in pairs and short chains. Additional testing reveals that the organism is optochin sensitive, and the Quellung reaction is positive. What is the causative organism?	*Streptococcus pneumoniae. S. pneumoniae* is a gram-positive, encapsulated organism (see Figure 13-4 on page 314); hence the positive Quellung reaction, which is performed by adding anticapsular antisera that cause the capsule to swell. The organism is also catalase negative, α-hemolytic (partial hemolysis; the blood turns greenish), and optochin sensitive (which differentiates it from *S. viridans*, which is also α-hemolytic).

- **What are the most appropriate treatments for this condition?**

Penicillin V or amoxicillin is rarely used in clinical practice because resistance with these drugs is an increasing problem. The typical treatment is either a macrolide in combination with a cephalosporin, or fluoroquinolone monotherapy.

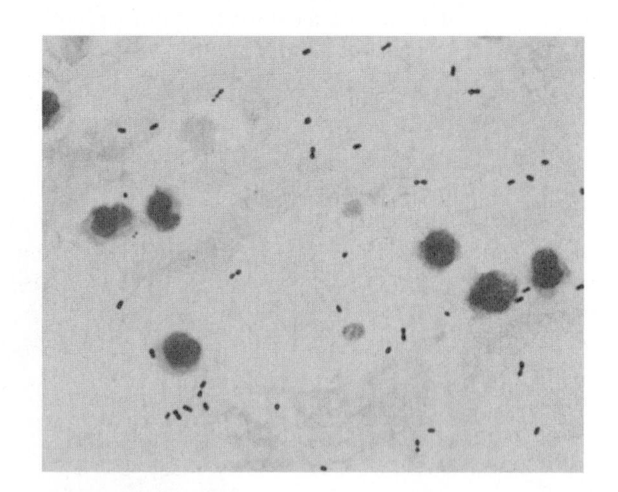

FIGURE 13-4. Histologic findings of *Streptococcus pneumoniae*. (Reproduced, with permission, from Bhushan V, Le T, et al. *First Aid for the USMLE Step 1: 2006*. New York: McGraw-Hill, 2006.)

► Case 5

A newborn boy has been diagnosed by prenatal ultrasound as having a congenital cystic adenomatoid malformation (CCAM) in the right lower lobe of his lung. CCAMs are hamartomas of terminal bronchioles. In view of the risks of CCAM-associated complications, the boy undergoes a right lower lobe resection.

Question	Answer
How many segments of lung will be resected if the entire right lower lobe is removed?	There are five segments in the right lower lobe: superior, medial basal, anterior basal, lateral basal, and posterior basal (see Figure 13-5 below).
Which vessels supply arterial and venous branches to the lungs, and what paths do the branches follow to supply each lung segment?	The lung alveoli are supplied by branches of the pulmonary artery and vein. The bronchial tree also receives its arterial supply from the bronchial arteries (from the aorta) and venous drainage from bronchial veins that feed into the azygos and accessory hemiazygos veins. Pulmonary and bronchial arteries follow the airways into the periphery. Pulmonary veins course in the septa between adjacent lung segments.
When entering the thoracic cavity through an intercostal space, the surgeon preserves the intercostal nerves and vessels, which lie in what anatomic relationship to the ribs?	The intercostal nerves and vessels lie in the costal groove inferior to each rib. They lie between the innermost intercostal and internal intercostal muscles for the length of those muscles.
During development, the pulmonary arteries arise from which aortic arch?	The sixth aortic arch gives rise to the pulmonary arteries as well as to the ductus arteriosus.
During which week of gestation are the bronchial buds formed from the foregut?	Bronchial buds are formed in the fourth week of gestation. Depending on the histology and other associated anomalies, different types of CCAMs are suspected to result from insults at varying stages of development. For example, **type 2 CCAMs** are associated with anomalies such as esophageal fistulas and bilateral renal agenesis. Thus, type 2 CCAMs are thought to arise early in organogenesis, during the fourth week of gestation.

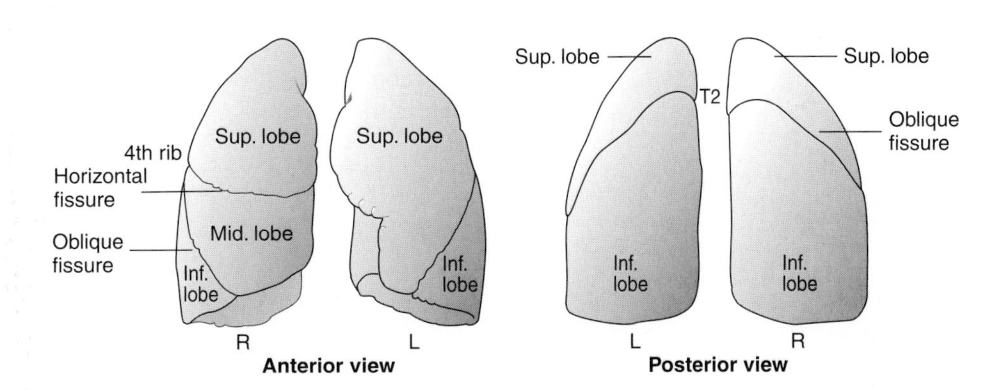

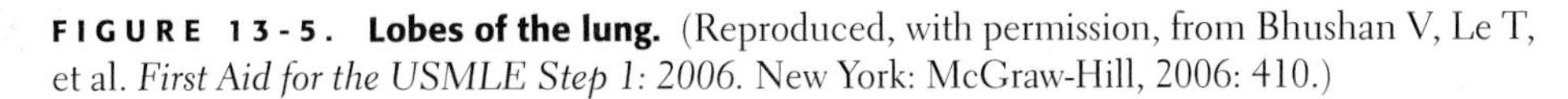

FIGURE 13-5. Lobes of the lung. (Reproduced, with permission, from Bhushan V, Le T, et al. *First Aid for the USMLE Step 1: 2006*. New York: McGraw-Hill, 2006: 410.)

► **Case 6**

A 15-year-old girl who is extremely thin is brought to the emergency department in acute respiratory distress and is stabilized with treatment. On questioning, she reports an increasingly productive cough over the past few days. Her pulse oximetry shows 93% oxygen saturation on 2 L of oxygen, and she often gasps for air midsentence. Examination shows nostril flaring, subcostal retractions, and clubbing of the fingers. A birth history reveals the patient had a meconium ileus.

■ **What genetically transmitted disease does this patient likely have?**	The patient likely has cystic fibrosis (CF), which is caused by loss-of-function mutations in the CFTR (cystic fibrosis transmembrane conductance regulator) protein, a chloride channel found in all exocrine tissues. As a result of these mutations, secretions in the lung, intestine, pancreas, and reproductive tract are extremely viscous. This can result in obstructions in these organs, leading to disease complications.
■ **What test was likely run on this patient in her infancy to confirm the diagnosis?**	A sweat chloride test was most likely conducted. Patients with CF have elevated chloride levels in their sweat.
■ **What is the probable etiology of the patient's current symptoms?**	The lungs in patients with CF are colonized at an early age with various bacteria not normally found in the lung. Therefore, patients suffer from repeated pulmonary bacterial infections, leading to increased production of viscous secretions. Increased secretions, in turn, lead to increased cough and pulmonary obstruction, which can result in acute respiratory distress.
■ **What vitamin supplements do patients with this condition usually require?**	Patients with CF generally require the fat-soluble vitamins A, D, E, and K. The thick secretions block the release of pancreatic enzymes, resulting in pancreatic insufficiency (usually present at birth).
■ **What information would one provide this patient if she asked for genetic counseling?**	CF occurs with a frequency of 1 in 2000 white people; the carrier rate is 1 in 25 white people. CF is an autosomal recessive disease, so all children of a patient with CF will at a minimum become carriers. Some 95% of males with CF are infertile due to defects in the transport of sperm. One or both of the vas deferens are often absent. Infertility affects as many as 20% of women as a result of abnormally thick cervical mucus and amenorrhea from malnutrition.

▶ Case 7

A 70-year-old woman with a 65-pack-year smoking history complains to her physician of worsening dyspnea. The dyspnea has now become so severe she is experiencing shortness of breath at rest. She also admits to an occasional cough productive of small amounts of thin sputum. Examination reveals a thin woman with an increased thoracic anteroposterior diameter. Her lips are pursed as she breathes. She also has an increased expiratory phase and is using the accessory muscles in her neck to breathe.

What is the most likely diagnosis?	Emphysema.
What is the pathophysiology of this condition?	Destruction of alveolar walls results in enlargement of air spaces. As shown in Figure 13-6 below, compared with normal lung (A), the lung in emphysema (B) shows destruction of lung parenchyma and marked dilatation of terminal air spaces. Destruction of lung parenchyma also results in decreased elastic recoil, which increases airway collapsibility, causing expiratory obstruction. As a result, patients with emphysema often find it easier to expire through pursed lips (which maintains a high airway pressure, thereby stenting the airways open)—hence the term "pink puffers."
What findings would be expected on lung and heart examination?	Air trapped in the lungs will cause the chest to be hyperresonant to percussion. These patients will also have decreased breath sounds, wheezing, a prolonged expiratory phase, and diminished heart sounds.
What pattern of lung parenchymal destruction is likely to be found in this patient?	Smoking results in a destruction pattern termed **centrilobular emphysema,** which affects the respiratory bronchioles and central alveolar ducts. **Panacinar emphysema** is associated with α_1-antitrypsin deficiency and results in destruction throughout the acinus.
What pattern would pulmonary function testing likely reveal?	One would expect to see values consistent with obstructive lung disease: dramatically reduced forced expiratory volume in 1 second (FEV_1) and reduced forced vital capacity (FVC), resulting in an FEV_1/FVC ratio of <80%.

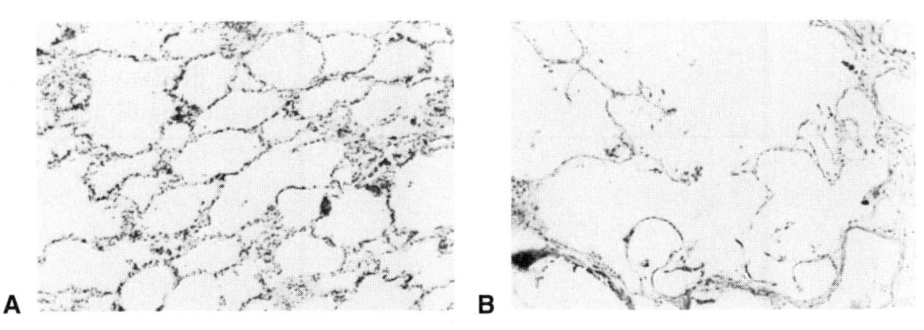

FIGURE 13-6. (A) Normal lung and (B) lung in emphysema. (Reproduced, with permission, from Chandrasoma P, Taylor CR. *Concise Pathology*, 3rd ed. Norwalk, CT: Appleton & Lange, 1998.)

► Case 8

A 4-year-old boy is brought to the emergency department by his mother because he is lethargic and appears to be having difficulty breathing. There is also saliva drooling out of his mouth. Physical examination reveals the patient is febrile, and his lung examination is notable for a high-pitched upper airway wheeze. Further questioning of the patient's mother reveals the child has not received his immunizations.

- **What is the most likely diagnosis?**

This is most likely a case of acute epiglottitis, as suggested by the stridor found on lung examination and the drooling saliva—findings that also suggest obstruction of both the esophagus and the trachea. The obstruction is due to swelling of the epiglottis caused by infection. Given the child's unimmunized status, the most likely cause is *Haemophilus influenzae* infection, specifically the group b subtype.

- **What additional microorganisms can cause this presentation?**

Epiglottitis can also be caused by *Pasturella multocida,* which is often transmitted from dog or cat bites, and herpes simplex virus type 1. However, the child's unimmunized status points to *H. influenzae* as the causative agent.

- **What is the main virulence factor of this organism?**

The polysaccharide capsule is the major virulence factor of *H. influenzae*. The bacterium has both encapsulated and nonencapsulated strains. The nonencapsulated forms are limited to local infections such as otitis media in children and mild respiratory infection in adults (see Table 13-1 on page 319). The encapsulated strains are significantly more virulent and can cause disseminated disease such as meningitis, epiglottitis, and septic arthritis. There are six capsular types, designated a through f. The b-type capsule is the subtype that accounts for roughly 95% of serious *H. influenzae* infections in children.

- **How has the vaccine used to prevent this infection been redesigned to improve its efficacy?**

The **Hib vaccine** consists of a purified b-type capsule conjugated to diphtheria toxin. The diphtheria toxin activates T lymphocytes, which are required for adequate antibody production against the capsular antigen. The original vaccine consisted only of b capsule and was not effective in eliciting an antibody response.

- **What is the likely source of this infection?**

H. influenzae is considered part of the normal flora of the nasopharynx, and the organism may thus be spread by direct contact with respiratory secretions and by airborne droplet contamination. Epiglottitis may also represent a primary infection of the epiglottis rather than invasion from the nasopharynx, as is often the case with meningitis and septic arthritis.

TABLE 13-1. Types of Infection Caused by *Haemophilus*

	H. influenzae		*H. aegyptius*	*H. ducreyi*
	Type B	Nontypable		
Type of infection	Meningitis Epiglottitis Bacteremia Cellulitis Septic arthritis	Otitis media Sinusitis Tracheobronchitis Pneumonia	Conjunctivitis Purpuric fever (Brazilian)	Chancroid (painful ulcers of genitals, lymphadenitis)
Treatment	Ceftazidime Cefotaxime Ceftriaxone Gentamicin	Cephalosporin Fluoroquinolone Azithromycin	Rifampin	Azithromycin Cephalosporin Ciprofloxacin

► Case 9

A 70-year-old man with a history of laryngeal cancer presents to the emergency department with shortness of breath. He complains that for the past 3 days, he has not been able to lie flat to sleep, and last night he woke up suddenly gasping for air. A decubitus chest film shows layering of fluid.

Question	Answer
What is the most likely diagnosis?	A pleural effusion consists of fluid accumulation in the pleural space (between the visceral pleura and the parietal pleura) of the lung. Normally, the pleural space is potential space, with a small amount of fluid.
How is this condition classified?	There are two types of pleural effusion. **Transudative pleural effusions** are caused by increased hydrostatic pressure of the pleural capillaries (as in congestive heart failure), or by a decrease in plasma oncotic pressure, as seen in disorders with decreased plasma albumin levels (such as renal and hepatic failure). **Exudative pleural effusions** are caused by a change in the permeability of the pleural surface (such as secondary to inflammatory or neoplastic changes). These effusions have a high protein content.
What are the common causes of this condition?	Transudative pleural effusion: ▪ Cirrhosis ▪ Congestive heart failure ▪ Constrictive pericarditis ▪ Nephrotic syndrome ▪ Pulmonary embolism Exudative pleural effusion: ▪ Collagen vascular disease ▪ Infection (pneumonia, tuberculosis) ▪ Malignancy (primary or metastatic lung cancer or mesothelioma) ▪ Pulmonary embolism
What are the most likely findings on laboratory testing?	Typically, analysis of pleural effusion fluid includes measuring pH, total protein, lactate dehydrogenase (LDH), albumin, and cholesterol levels. Cytology (Gram stain, culture) will also be performed to identify infectious causes of effusion. Meeting any one of the three **Light's criteria** qualifies the effusion as an exudate: ▪ Protein effusion:serum ratio >0.5 ▪ LDH effusion:serum ratio >0.6 ▪ Pleural LDH level greater than two-thirds the upper limit of serum LDH level
What are the most appropriate treatments for this condition?	**Thoracentesis,** performed by needle insertion into the pleural space, is used for diagnostic and therapeutic purposes. The needle is inserted through an intercostal space superior to the rib, in order to avoid the intercostal nerve and vessels, which lie in the intercostal groove at the inferior border of the ribs. Other treatment options include **pleurodesis,** in which the pleura is made adherent and closed by chemical (such as talc or doxycycline) or physical abrasion, and permanent catheter insertion into the pleural space for periodic fluid drainage.

▶ Case 10

An 18-year-old man comes to the physician complaining of a 3-week history of worsening dry and nonproductive cough. He also has a throbbing headache along with a mild fever and complains of malaise and sore throat. Treatment with penicillin has not relieved his symptoms. Recently, his 16-year-old brother developed similar symptoms.

- **What is the most likely diagnosis?**

Mycoplasma pneumoniae, which causes primary atypical pneumonia (**"walking pneumonia"**), is the most common cause of pneumonia in teenagers (see Table 13-2 below). This organism is the smallest free-living bacterium. It has no cell wall, and its membrane is the only bacterial membrane containing cholesterol.

- **What clinical findings are commonly associated with this condition?**

Infection with *M. pneumoniae* typically results in mild upper respiratory tract disease, including low-grade fever, malaise, headache, and a dry, nonproductive cough. Symptoms gradually worsen over a few days and can last for more than 2 weeks. Fewer than 10% of patients develop more severe disease with lower respiratory tract symptoms.

- **How does this organism cause illness?**

M. pneumoniae is an extracellular organism that attaches to respiratory epithelium. As the superficial layer of respiratory epithelial cells is destroyed, the normal ability of the upper airways to clear themselves is lost. As a result, the lower respiratory tract becomes contaminated by microbes and is mechanically irritated. Close contact allows for spread of the organism.

- **What are the most appropriate treatments for this condition?**

Tetracycline or erythromycin is most commonly prescribed for *M. pneumoniae* infection.

- **What diagnostic tests are useful for confirming the diagnosis?**

A high titer of cold agglutinins (IgM) and growth on Eaton's agar.

TABLE 13-2. Most Common Causes of Pneumonia According to Age

6 Weeks–18 Years	18–40 Years	40–65 Years	>65 Years
Viral (respiratory syncytial virus)	*M. pneumoniae*	*S. pneumoniae*	*S. pneumoniae*
Mycoplasma pneumoniae	*C. pneumoniae*	*Haemophilus influenzae*	Viral
Chlamydia pneumoniae	*S. pneumoniae*	Anaerobes	Anaerobes
Streptococcus pneumoniae		*M. pneumoniae*	*H. influenzae*

► Case 11

A 62-year-old woman presents to the emergency department with acute onset of shortness of breath. She also complains of "stabbing" pleuritic right-sided chest pain. The woman had a stroke 3 months ago but is otherwise healthy. Her temperature is 36.7° C (98.1° F), blood pressure is 90/60 mm Hg, heart rate is 110/min, respiratory rate is 40/min, and oxygen saturation is 77% on room air. Physical examination reveals jugular venous distention, and cardiovascular examination reveals a regular rate and rhythm with no murmurs. The woman's lungs are clear bilaterally with decreased breath sounds in the right middle lobe. She has mild cyanosis in the distal extremities with no clubbing.

What is the most likely diagnosis? Which other etiologies should be included in the differential diagnosis?	This is a case of pulmonary embolism (also known as pulmonary thromboembolism, or PTE). The differential diagnosis includes PTE, myocardial infarction or unstable angina, pneumonia, pneumothorax, exacerbation of chronic obstructive pulmonary disease, pericarditis, and costochondritis or other sources of musculoskeletal pain.
What is Virchow's triad?	One century ago, Rudolf Virchow hypothesized that three factors increased a patient's risk for venous thrombosis: local trauma to the vessel wall, hypercoagulability, and stasis. It is believed that patients with PTE have a predisposition toward developing this condition, which is triggered by a stressor such as pregnancy, obesity, or surgery.
What is the most likely finding on microscopic examination?	Under low-power magnification, characteristic lines of Zahn will be visible in the thrombus.
What test remains the gold standard for diagnosing this condition?	Pulmonary angiography remains the gold standard for diagnosing PTE, as it is the most specific test available for establishing a definitive diagnosis. Lung scanning, however, remains the most frequently used test. A lung scan showing normal perfusion virtually excludes the possibility of a PTE. Patients who have a physical examination and a lung perfusion scan that cannot exclude PTE should undergo pulmonary angiography. **Plasma D-dimer levels** are elevated in >90% of patients with PTE, but this assay is nonspecific and results may also be elevated in conditions such as myocardial infarction or sepsis. The current strategy for diagnosing PTE and deep venous thrombosis is shown in Figure 13-7 on the following page.
What are the most appropriate treatments for this condition?	PTE should be treated with therapeutic levels of heparin for at least 5 days unless there is a contraindication to anticoagulation (eg, recent surgery). In most patients, warfarin and heparin may be started together, with oral anticoagulation continued for at least 3 months. If there is a contraindication to anticoagulation or a high risk of recurrence of PTE, an inferior vena cava filter is recommended.

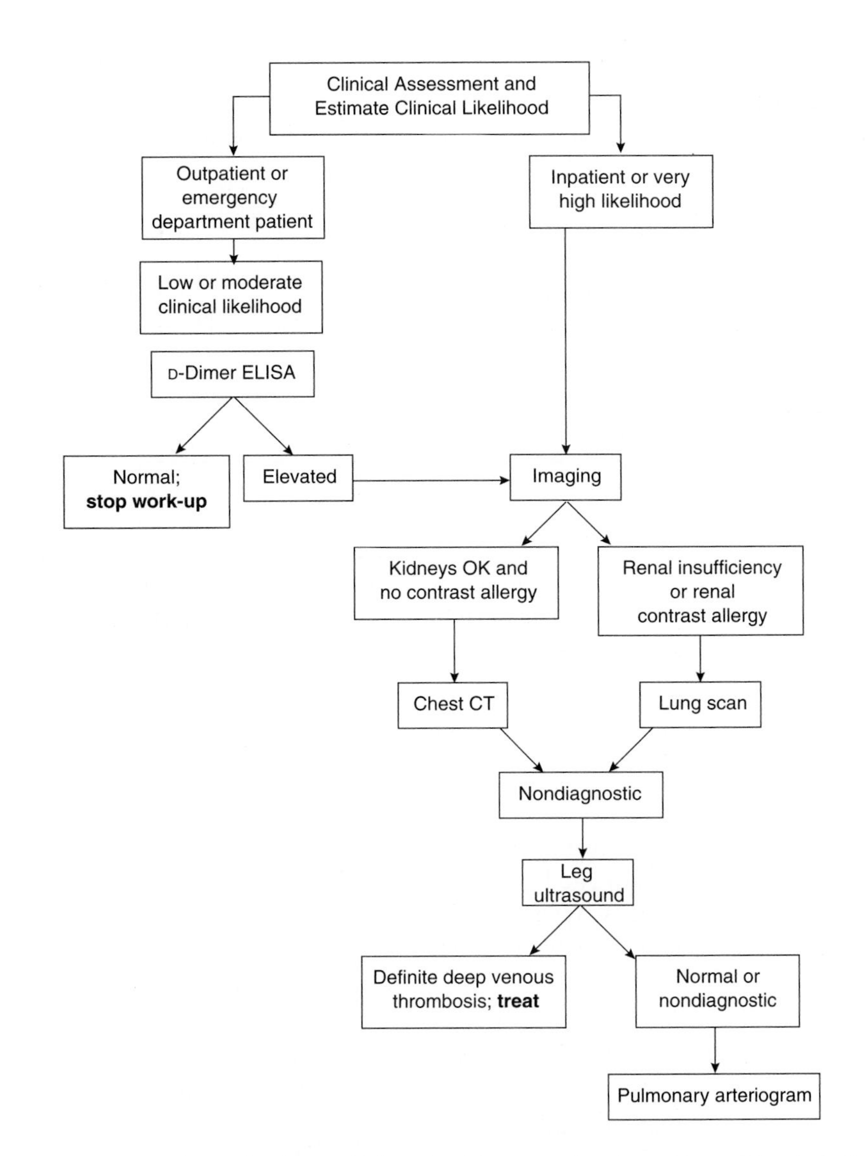

FIGURE 13-7. Diagnosis of PTE. (Adapted, with permission, from Kasper DL, et al. *Harrison's Principles of Internal Medicine,* 16th ed. New York: McGraw-Hill, 2005: 1563.)

▶ Case 12

A 40-year-old woman with a history of interstitial lung disease presents to the local hospital complaining of fatigue and weakness. On admission, she is found to have the following laboratory values:

Serum:
- Sodium: 144 mEq/L
- Chloride: 96 mEq/L
- Bicarbonate: 42 mEq/L
- Potassium: 4.2 mEq/L
- Blood urea nitrogen:creatinine ratio: 18/1.0 mg/dL

Arterial blood gas values:
- pH: 7.32
- Partial pressure of carbon dioxide (P_{CO_2}): 91 mm Hg

What is the most likely cause of these symptoms?	The patient has respiratory acidosis (pH <7.4, P_{CO_2} >40 mm Hg) with a compensatory metabolic alkalosis. Respiratory acidosis can be caused by chronic obstructive pulmonary disease, airway obstruction, and hypoventilation. The likely cause of the patient's acidosis is interstitial lung disease, which can chronically impair gas exchange.
What is the most likely diagnosis?	The patient has a chronic respiratory acidosis, as indicated by the large compensatory increase in bicarbonate, in attempts to correct for an elevated P_{CO_2}. Someone with a more acute process would not be able to compensate this robustly.
In Figure 13-8 on page 325, label the area that corresponds to chronic respiratory acidosis and the area that corresponds to acute respiratory acidosis.	Referring to Figure 13-8, the letter A refers to chronic respiratory acidosis, and the letter B refers to acute respiratory acidosis. Letter C refers to chronic respiratory alkalosis, while letter D refers to acute metabolic alkalosis.
How is this condition distinguished from metabolic acidosis?	In respiratory acidosis, the primary disturbance is an increase in P_{CO_2}, to which the body responds by decreasing renal bicarbonate reabsorption. In metabolic acidosis, the primary disturbance is a decrease in bicarbonate, which is compensated for by hyperventilation, resulting in a decreased P_{CO_2}.
What is the anion gap, and what factors can increase the anion gap in this condition?	**Anion gap** is defined as $[Na^+] - ([HCO_3^-] + [Cl^-])$. Causes of increased anion-gap metabolic acidosis include renal failure, diabetic ketoacidosis, lactic acidosis, and salicylate ingestion. Causes of normal anion-gap metabolic acidosis include diarrhea, renal tubular acidosis, and hyperchloremia.

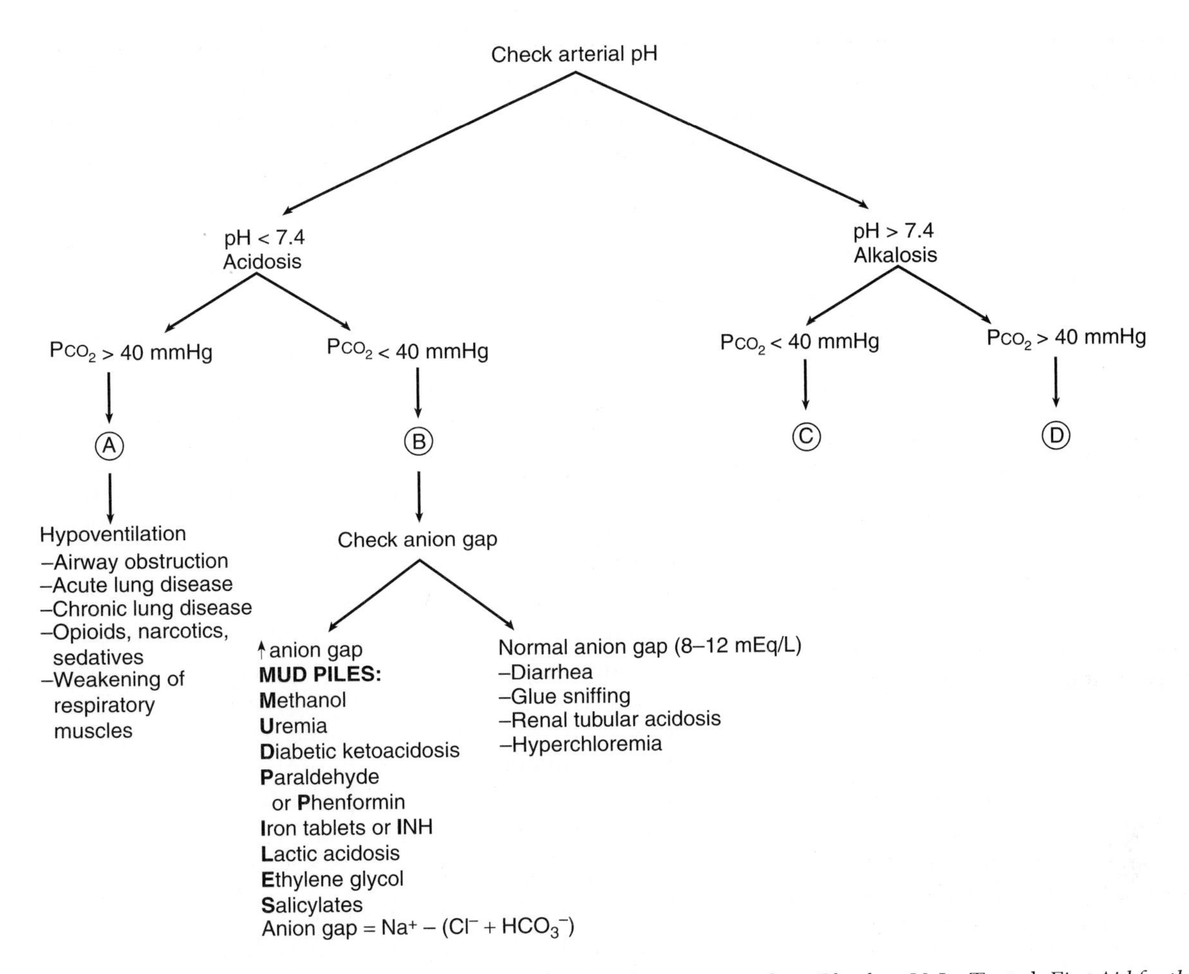

FIGURE 13-8. Acidosis and alkalosis diagram. (Adapted, with permission, from Bhushan V, Le T, et al. *First Aid for the USMLE Step 1: 2006*. New York: McGraw-Hill, 2006: 382.)

▶ Case 13

A 35-year-old black man presents to his primary care physician with progressive dyspnea on exertion. He has no history of congestive heart failure or asthma and has had no known contact with any individuals known to have tuberculosis. His laboratory results reveal normal creatinine kinase (CK), CK-MB fraction, and troponin levels. An x-ray of the chest shows bilateral hilar lymphadenopathy and evidence of interstitial lung disease. A thoracoscopic lung biopsy reveals the presence of several small, noncaseating granulomas in both lungs.

What are noncaseating granulomas, and what diagnosis does their presence suggest?	The granulomas of sarcoid are discrete collections of tissue macrophages, termed *histiocytes,* in the absence of frank necrosis or caseation (as would appear in tuberculosis or histoplasmosis). These granulomas frequently contain multinucleated giant cells and are accompanied by alveolitis. In addition to sarcoidosis, other granulomatous diseases include tuberculosis, histoplasmosis, hypersensitivity pneumonitis, pneumoconioses (eg, beryllioses), and eosinophilic granulomatosis.
What findings would be expected on pulmonary function testing?	In interstitial lung disease, lung compliance is decreased, reflecting increased stiffness from alveolar wall inflammation and fibrosis. Tidal volume and total lung capacity are typically decreased. Diffusion capacity is also decreased as a result of inflammatory destruction of the air-capillary interface. Sarcoidosis is unlike most interstitial lung diseases, in that it has features of both obstruction and restriction.
What are common causes of interstitial lung disease, and what is the most likely cause in this patient?	▪ Antitumor drugs ▪ Connective tissue disease (eg, Wegener's granulomatosis, systemic lupus erythematosus, scleroderma, Sjögren's disease) ▪ Eosinophilic granuloma ▪ Goodpasture's syndrome ▪ Hypersensitivity pneumonitis; "farmer's lung" or "bird-breeder's lung," in which an immune reaction to a microorganism antigen induces a type III or type IV hypersensitivity reaction ▪ Idiopathic pulmonary fibrosis ▪ Prolonged exposure to occupationally inhaled inorganic agents such as silicone, coal, asbestos, talc, mica, aluminum, and beryllium ▪ Radiation-induced disease ▪ Sarcoidosis (which is the most likely cause of interstitial lung disease in this patient)
What are some extrapulmonary manifestations of this patient's interstitial lung disease?	The more common extrapulmonary manifestations of sarcoidosis are in the eye (anterior uveitis) and skin (skin papules and erythema nodosum), but granulomas can also occur in the heart, brain, lung, and peripheral lymph nodes.
What is the most appropriate treatment for this condition?	Corticosteroids.

▶ Case 14

A 55-year-old man comes to the emergency department after he suddenly experienced severe right-sided chest pain followed by profound difficulty breathing. The man informs the physician he has severe emphysema due to an extensive history of tobacco use. On physical examination, the patient is markedly tachypneic and tachycardic. His breath sounds are diminished at the right apex, and his chest wall is hyperresonant to percussion. No tactile fremitus is noted. Arterial blood gas analyses demonstrate a partial pressure of oxygen (PO_2) of 60 mm Hg and a partial pressure of carbon dioxide (PCO_2) of 50 mm Hg.

- **What is the most likely diagnosis?**

Pneumothorax—or, more specifically, secondary spontaneous pneumothorax. Whereas primary spontaneous pneumothorax occurs in the absence of underlying lung disease, secondary spontaneous pneumothorax occurs in the setting of chronic lung parenchymal disruption.

- **What is the pathophysiology of this condition?**

Spontaneous pneumothorax is most likely caused by rupture of a **subpleural bleb,** which allows air to escape into the pleural cavity. A tension pneumothorax ensues when a one-way valve is essentially created, allowing air to gradually accumulate with each inspiration. This air cannot be expelled during exhalation.

- **What diseases most likely underlie this condition?**

The most common underlying condition is chronic obstructive pulmonary disease. Additionally, patients with acquired immunodeficiency syndrome, *Pneumocystis jiroveci* (formerly *carinii*) pneumonia, cystic fibrosis, and tuberculosis are at higher risk for spontaneous pneumothorax.

- **What is the most common clinical presentation of this condition?**

Dyspnea with pleuritic chest pain on the same side of the pneumothorax is a common presentation. Typical physical examination findings include diminished breath sounds, hyperresonance, and absent fremitus over the pneumothorax. Arterial blood gas testing typically shows hypoxia and hypercapnia.

- **What are the most likely findings on radiography?**

Partial collapse of the lung on the side of the pneumothorax with a thin line parallel to the chest wall is occasionally visible. In a **tension pneumothorax,** tracheal and mediastinal deviation can be present away from the pneumothorax. In a **nontension pneumothorax,** however, the trachea and mediastinum will shift toward the side of the collapsed lung.

- **What is the most appropriate treatment for this condition?**

Chest tube (thoracotomy) with parenchymal sclerosing agents.

► Case 15

After a difficult labor, a baby is delivered breech, with her arms above her head. Physical examination reveals the newborn's right hand is slightly contracted, with the fingers curled towards the palm. The infant seems unable to extend the fingers on the right hand.

- **What is the most likely diagnosis?**

Klumpke's palsy. This palsy results from birth injury to the lower trunk of the brachial plexus (C8 and T1 nerve roots). It is a proximal brachial plexus neuropathy.

- **What motor deficits are likely to result from this condition?**

The C8 and T1 nerve roots contribute to the ulnar and median nerves. The muscles affected are the medial part of the flexor digitorum profundus and the flexor carpi ulnaris (these two are the only extrinsic muscles of the forearm supplied by the ulnar nerve), and all intrinsic muscles of the hand, including those innervated by the ulnar nerve (interosseous muscles, the second and third lumbrical muscles, and the adductor pollicis brevis muscles) and those innervated by the median nerve (thenar muscles and the first two lumbrical muscles). Over time, wasting of the thenar and hypothenar eminences occurs. Marked wasting between the metatarsals on both palmar and dorsal surfaces of the hand results from paralysis of the lumbricals and interossei.

- **What sensory deficits are involved in this condition?**

The lower trunk from C8 and T1 contributes to the medial cutaneous nerves of the arm, forearm, and the ulnar and median nerves. Thus, in this case there will be loss of sensation on the medial side of the arm; the forearm; the dorsal and palmar surface of the fifth finger and half of the fourth finger; the palmar surface of the first, second, and third fingers and lateral half of the fourth finger extending onto the nail beds on the dorsal surface as far as the distal interphalangeal joints; and the palmar surface of the hand.

- **What other injuries can cause this condition?**

  - **Thoracic outlet syndrome:** This is a congenital defect in which a cervical rib or a scalenus minimus muscle compresses the lower trunk at C8 and T1.
  - Trauma: Injuries to the inferior brachial plexus are much less common than injuries to the superior brachial plexus; traumatic injury can occur when a person grabs something to break a fall, or a baby's upper limb is pulled too hard during delivery.
  - Tumor infiltration: Tumor infiltration from the apex of the lung **(Pancoast's tumor)** can be associated with compression of the stellate ganglion, resulting in **Horner's syndrome.**

- **What is another nerve lesion that can cause claw hand?**

An ulnar nerve injury will also present with claw hand. However, with ulnar nerve injury only the little finger and the ring finger are clawed because the median nerve is spared (resulting in normal thenar muscles). Also, the sensory deficit involves only the ulnar nerve distribution: the palm and dorsal surfaces of the medial part of the hand and the dorsal and palmar surfaces of the fifth finger and half of the fourth finger.

APPENDIX

CASE INDEX

Index

D

E

I

J

K

L

M

Q

R

S

T

U

V

W

X

Y

Z

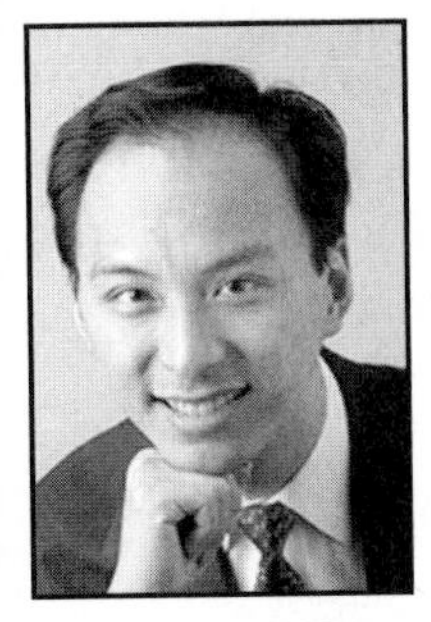
Tao Le, MD

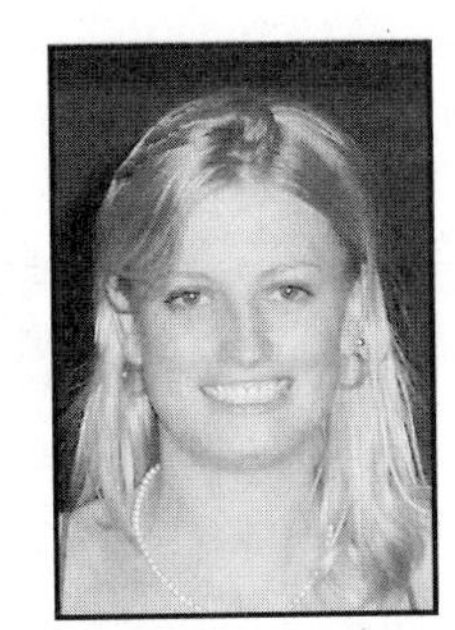
Kendall Krause

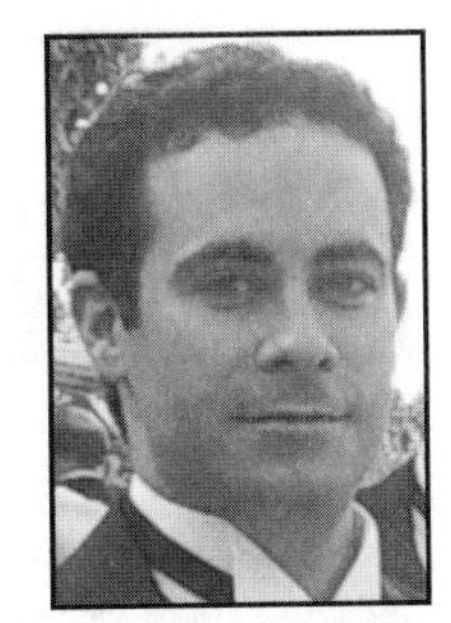
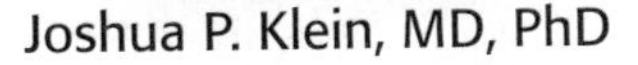
Joshua P. Klein, MD, PhD

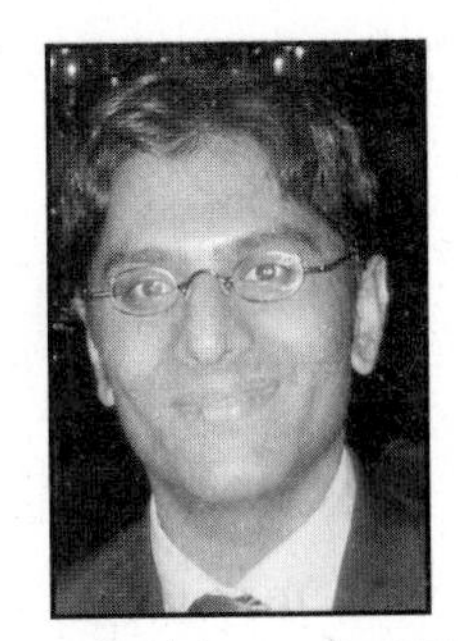
Anil Shivaram, MD

Tao Le, MD, MHS

Dr. Le has been a well-recognized figure in medical education for the past 14 years. As senior editor, he has led the expansion of *First Aid* into a global educational series. In addition, he is the founder of the *USMLERx* online test bank series as well as a cofounder of the *Underground Clinical Vignettes* series. As a medical student, he was editor-in-chief of the University of California, San Francisco *Synapse,* a university newspaper with a weekly circulation of 9000. Dr. Le earned his medical degree from the University of California, San Francisco, in 1996 and completed his residency training in internal medicine at Yale University and fellowship training at Johns Hopkins University. At Yale, he was a regular guest lecturer on the USMLE review courses and an adviser to the Yale University School of Medicine curriculum committee. Dr. Le subsequently went on to cofound Medsn and served as its chief medical officer. He is currently conducting research in asthma education at the University of Louisville.

Kendall Krause

Kendall is currently a fourth-year medical student at Yale School of Medicine. After attending St. Paul's School in Concord, New Hampshire, she completed her undergraduate education at Northwestern University. Before heading off to medical school, she studied public health care delivery in Madagascar, and taught adaptive skiing in her home state of Colorado. During her first two years in medical school, she was an articles editor for the *Yale Journal of Health Policy, Law, and Ethics.* She is currently completing her medical thesis research on high-altitude pulmonary edema at the Colorado Center for Altitude Medicine and Physiology. She hopes to pursue a career in critical care medicine.

Joshua P. Klein, MD, PhD

Dr. Klein is a recent graduate of the MD/PhD medical scientist training program at Yale University School of Medicine. He is originally from Roslyn, New York, and attended the University of Pennsylvania, where he studied biology and music theory. He completed his PhD dissertation in Dr. Stephen Waxman's neurology lab, where he studied activity-dependent modulation of neuronal sodium channel expression. He has authored more than ten journal articles based on his work, and has presented at numerous research conferences. His current research interests are focused on the pathogenesis and neurobiology of epilepsy. He was recently selected as an International Student Delegate of the Academy of Achievement. Following a year of internal medicine at Beth Israel Deaconess Medical Center, he will be a resident in neurology at Massachusetts General Hospital and Brigham and Women's Hospital. Dr. Klein has been an author and editor on multiple *First Aid* projects over the past six years. He can be contacted at joshua.p.klein@aya.yale.edu.

Anil Shivaram, MD

Dr. Shivaram is currently a second-year resident in ophthalmology at Boston Medical Center. He was born and raised in Chicago, Illinois, and attended college at Columbia University, where he majored in Sanskrit. Following his undergraduate studies, he went on to pursue graduate studies at Oxford University and then completed a fellowship in medical ethics at the American Medical Association. During medical school at Yale, his thesis research focused on the migration of retinal microglia in inherited retinal degenerative disorders. When he is not in pursuit of things optical, he spends time pampering his fiancée Lisa, who is finishing her final year of pediatrics residency. This is Dr. Shivaram's sixth year working on the *First Aid* series. He can be reached via e-mail at shivaram@aya.yale.edu.

ABOUT THE AUTHORS